Diabetic Foot Syndrome

Dirk Hochlenert • Gerald Engels
Stephan Morbach • Stefanie Schliwa
Frances L. Game

Diabetic Foot Syndrome

From Entity to Therapy

Springer

Dirk Hochlenert
Amb. Zentrum für Diabetologie
Endoskopie & Wundheilung
Gemeinschaftspraxis
Köln
Germany

Stephan Morbach
Department of Diabetes and Angiology
Marienkrankenhaus GmbH
Soest
Germany

Frances L. Game
Department of Diabetes and Endocrinology
Derby Hospitals NHS Foundation Trust
Derby
United Kingdom

Gerald Engels
Department of Wound Surgery
St. Vinzenz Hospital and MVZ St. Marien
Köln
Germany

Stefanie Schliwa
Institute of Anatomy
Anatomy and Cell Biology
University of Bonn
Bonn
Germany

ISBN 978-3-030-06354-2 ISBN 978-3-319-92055-9 (eBook)
https://doi.org/10.1007/978-3-319-92055-9

Original German edition published by Springer, 2014
Softcover re-print of the Hardcover 1st edition 2018

This Springer imprint is published by Springer Nature, under the registered company Springer International Publishing AG
The registered company address is: Gewerbestrasse 11, 6330 Cham, Switzerland

Preface

The intriguing field of the diabetic foot syndrome (DFS) is evolving rapidly. This book suggests a new classification for the efficient organisation of information. The classification addresses three challenges faced by professionals: (1) Shortening the time to build expertise. (2) Keeping track of the progress made by a wide range of professions. (3) Being specific in discussions and studies dealing with very different clinical pictures of the DFS. All of these issues benefit from a classification system which organises information like leaves on a branch and can be accessed by a simple, visual clue: localisation. The answer to the question 'Why exactly is there an ulcer in this particular location?' or 'Why here?' leads to both, a causal understanding and therapeutic options.

We divided the surface of the foot into areas where ulcers typically arise in a similar way. A manageable number of homogeneous subgroups result in what we named '**Entities of DFS**'. For each entity, we provide reviews in order to merge knowledge from the DFS Register, from the literature and from discussions with members of different specialities and healthcare systems.

To facilitate interdisciplinary understanding, we have also summarised anatomical, physiological and structural aspects of a successful treatment.

We tried to combine the advantages of a typical monograph written by one author and a reference book written by different specialists. Five authors agreed to discuss all the issues and write a common text. It should not be up to the reader to connect the dots and find a way through distinct chapters but for the authors to guide the reader as in a '**travel guide to the diabetic foot**'.

By enhancing clarity, providing a better overview and facilitating exchange and thus progress, it is hoped that the concept of entities will alleviate the burden of the disease and help to keep patients with DFS active and mobile.

This book is aimed at all professionals dealing with people who suffer from a DFS. The manuscript has been corrected by members of various professions in order to ensure a precise use of language and at the same time being easy to understand. We have focused on a visual presentation of the facts and added pictures from many sources including unique anatomic illustrations. However, it was not the aim of this book to present a complete compendium of all aspects of DFS.

In 2014, three of the five authors published a previous version of this book with the same basic concept. In the last 4 years, this German version has been highly successful and many discussions arouse that have led to further insights.

The contribution of deeper anatomical facts, new surgical techniques and the integration of international developments has deepened the understanding and almost doubled the scope of the book. It therefore became more like a new book than a simple translation.

The authors hope you enjoy reading this book and wish you continued success in the treatment of your patients. We are looking forward to sharing your experience and welcome contributions to our online blog.

Köln, Germany — Dirk Hochlenert
Köln, Germany — Gerald Engels
Soest, Germany — Stephan Morbach
Bonn, Germany — Stefanie Schliwa
Derby, UK — Frances L. Game
March 2018

Acknowledgements

To complete a book project of this kind, many people were involved. Their time and commitment were priceless, and we would like to express our gratitude.

In particular, we want to thank our patients who trust in us, were so understanding during our learning curve and allow us to bring a part of their lives to the public eye.

Furthermore, we have to thank all the specialised centres for the documentation of data. A discussion of entities, presented here, would not have been possible without these data.

We have to thank Frank Kamperhoff because without his organisational talent, open-mindedness and farsightedness, the DFS Register and this whole work would be unimaginable.

For their support in the development of this project, we have to thank colleagues who were always willing to discuss and put forward their ideas.

In particular, we would like to mention Prof. Dr. rer. nat. Jürgen Koebke for all his participation and curiosity in answering anatomical and biomechanical questions until his unexpected and sad death.

We took much advice from shoemakers. Our thanks go in particular to the shoemakers Peter Brümmer, Jürgen Stumpf and Herbert Türk, who have allowed us to learn from their particular knowledge of the ancient craft of shoemaking and from their enormous experience.

We have to thank Dr. Alexander Risse for substantial guidance regarding harmonious relationships avoiding the emergence of aggression due to missed or unrealistic goals during interactions with our patients and the concept of 'Leibesinselschwund' as a part of a more general humanistic thinking.

To Dipl.-Psych. Susan Clever we owe advice on the patients' perspective and also on finding individual goals for our therapy, which can include a state of continued ulceration.

We also have to thank Dr. med. Anna Trocha, Dr. med. Johannes Beike, Inge Weß-Baumberger and Ulrike Karabasz for their positive attitude and the many ideas they shared with us.

We like to thank Richard Stow, David Hunt, Carlotta Steinseifer and Rebecca Gollman who helped us in refining the manuscript and Svenja Jansen, Eva Kirchner and Stefan Liedke for their support in processing the anatomical preparations.

Right from the start, we have had great support from Melissa Morton and Wyndham Hacket Pain from Springer for which we enthusiastically thank them.

The reproduction of the complex anatomical phenomena in an understandable graphic representation we owe to the competent work of Dr. med. Katja Dalkowski.

For Fig. 1.1 we thank Dr. med. Dietmar Weber, for Fig. 4.1 Prof. Dr. med. Gerhard Rümenapf, for Fig. 1.3 Dr. med. Thomas Horn, for Fig. 2.8b PD Dr. med Thomas Schaub, for Fig. 21.12 Dr. med. Peter Mauckner and for Fig. 24.2 Dr. Gerry Rayman. We thank for providing the anatomical preparations for the compilation of the Fig. 2.8c, 2.9b, 2.10b, 2.21c, 2.22c, 2.27c, 2.42a and 9.2c which was made possible by Prof. Dr. rer. nat. Jürgen Koebke (†), Centre for Anatomy of the University of Cologne.

Contents

Abbreviations

ABI	Ankle brachial index
ADP	Arteria dorsalis pedis
AF	Arteria fibularis
AHA	American Heart Association
AP	Antibiotic prophylaxis
ATL	Achilles tendon lengthening
ATP	Arteria tibialis posterior
CE-MRI	Contrast-enhanced magnetic resonance imaging
CF	Charcot foot, Charcot arthropathy
CPPPT	Cutaneous pressure pain perception threshold
CRT	Capillary refill time
DFS	Diabetic foot syndrome
DFU	Diabetic foot ulcer
DIP joint	Distal interphalangeal joint
DNOAP	Diabetic neuropathic osteoarthropathy
DSA	Digital subtraction angiography
DWI	Diffusion weighted imaging
ESC	European Society of Cardiology
FDB	Flexor digitorum brevis
FDL	Flexor digitorum longus
FHL	Flexor hallucis longus
GP	General practitioner
HBO	Hyperbaric oxygen (therapy)
ICD	International Classification of Disease
IDSA	Infectious Diseases Society of America
IE	Infective endocarditis
IP joint	Interphalangeal joint
IS	Inpatient Service
i-TCC	Instant TCC
LOPS	Loss of protective sensation
MMPs	Matrix metalloproteinases
MRA	Magnetic resonance angiography
MRT	Magnetic resonance tomography
MTH	Metatarsal head

MTP joint	Metatarsophalangeal joint
NB-TCC	Non-removable bivalved total contact cast
NDS	Neuropathy disability score
NICE	National Institute for Health and Care Excellence
NNT	Number needed to treat
NPWT	Negative pressure wound therapy
NSS	Neuropathy symptom score
OPS	Standardised operation procedure
OS	Outpatient Service
PAD	Peripheral arterial disease
PEDIS	Perfusion, Extent, Depth, Infection, Sensation
PIP joint	Proximal interphalangeal joint
PNP	Polyneuropathy
PTA	Percutaneous transluminal angioplasty
RANKL	Receptor activator of NF-κB ligand
RCW	Removable cam walker
SINBAD score	Site, Ischemia, Neuropathy, Bacterial infection, Area, Depth
TCC	Total contact cast
$TCPO_2$	Transcutaneous oxygen pressure
TIMPs	Tissue inhibitors of metalloproteinases
TMT	Tarso-metatarsal
TMT1 joint	Tarso-metatarsal I-joint, Metatarso-cuneiforme I-joint
UT Classification	University of Texas Classification
VAC®	Vacuum-Assisted Closure Therapy®
WIFi	Wound ischemia foot infection

About the Authors

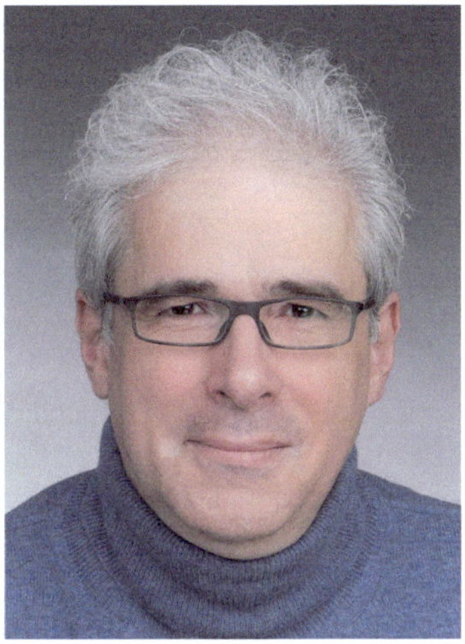

Dirk Hochlenert is specialist in internal medicine and diabetology in an outpatient clinic in Cologne. He organises and conducts postgraduate medical training courses for the treatment of DFS. He manages networks for the treatment of DFS in several regions and organises the DFS Register.

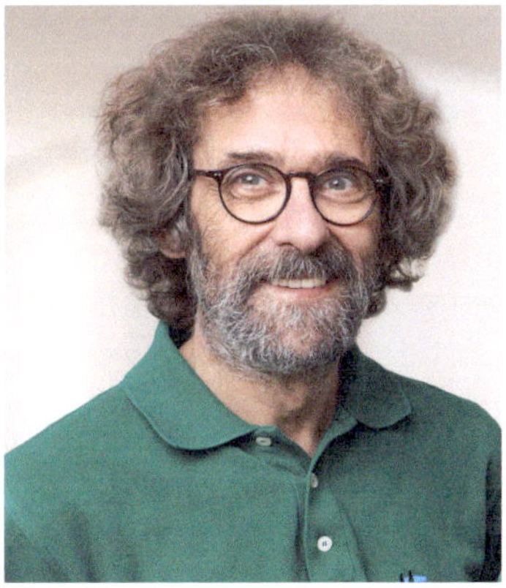

Gerald Engels is Consultant Surgeon in charge of the treatment of DFS in both an outpatient clinic and at the St. Vinzenz-Hospital in Cologne. He is a board member of several associations and together with D. Hochlenert organises postgraduate medical training courses for the treatment of DFS as well as teaching the subject in medical schools.

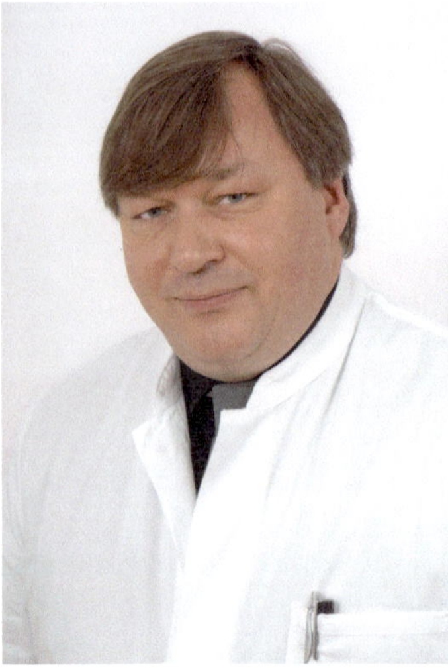

Stephan Morbach is a specialist in internal medicine, diabetology and angiology and Senior Consultant in the Department of Diabetology and Angiology at the Marienkrankenhaus in Soest. He is Corresponding author of several guidelines for the Diabetic Foot and was Chairman of the Diabetic Foot Study Group of the European Association for the Study of Diabetes (EASD) 2004–2008. In the past years, he has served as Vice Chairman of the 'Consultative Section on the Diabetic Foot' of the International Diabetes Federation (IDF) and of D-FOOT International. In the course of the Step-by-Step Programme, he has delivered medical education in several developing countries.

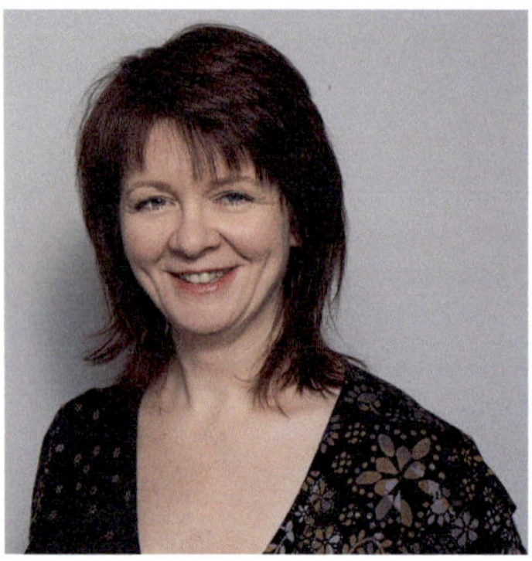

Stefanie Schliwa is certified preparator and anatomist at the Institut of Anatomy at the University of Bonn and specialist in several preparation and dissection techniques. Her work focuses on the visualisation of functional relationships in topographical anatomy, especially that of the foot.

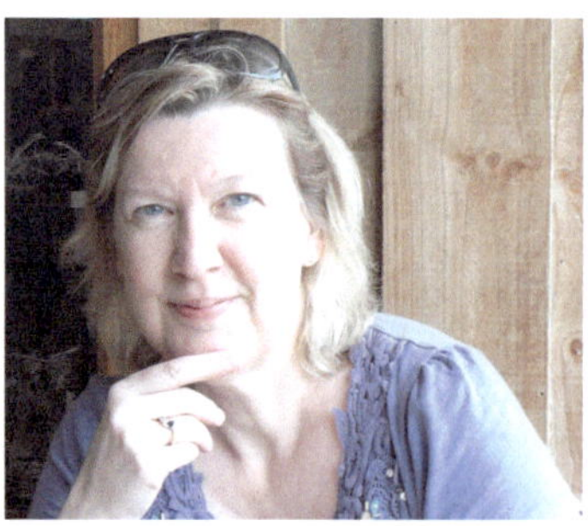

Frances L. Game is Consultant Diabetologist at the Department of Diabetes and Endocrinology and Clinical Director R&D at Derby Teaching Hospitals NHS Foundation Trust. She is also Honorary Professor, University of Nottingham.

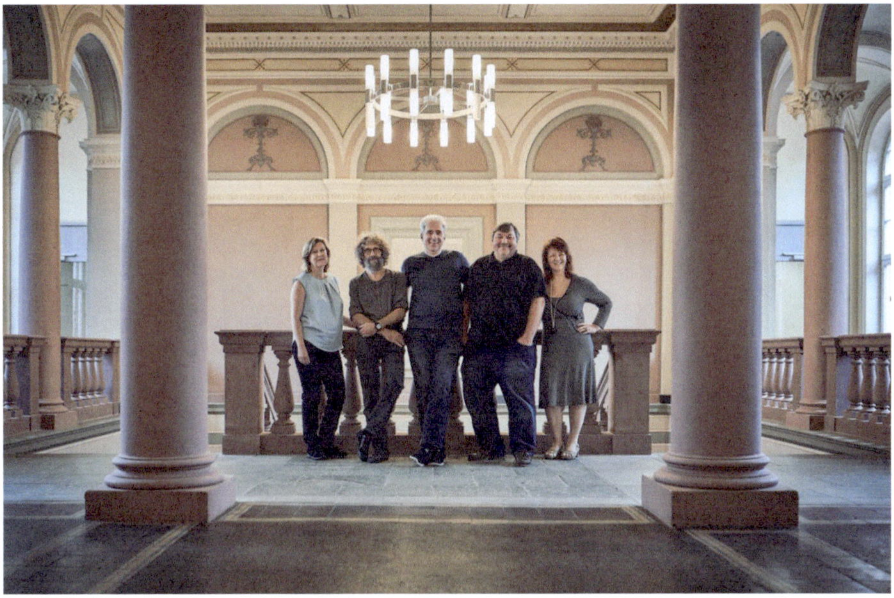

Authors at the Anatomical Institute of the University of Bonn 2017 (Photo by courtesy of Dr. Britta Eiberger)

Introduction 1

This chapter outlines the definition, causes, implications, classifications, epidemiology, economy and perspectives of DFS. The intention is to open up a holistic view of the disease, the people suffering from it and its importance for society.

The defects that allow DFS to develop also permit a view on the marvellous physiological structure the foot represents when everything works as it should. A deeper insight into this aspect is given in the next chapter.

1.1 Overview

Diabetic **F**oot **S**yndrome (DFS) is a consequence of complications of diabetes mellitus and may lead to amputations, restricted mobility, and even death. The term refers to two types of disease: ulcers of the lower extremities including the associated states of risk (Fig. 1.1a) and diabetes-related Charcot foot. The latter is an inflammatory syndrome, characterised by varying degrees of bone and joint disorganisation secondary to underlying neuropathy, trauma, and perturbations of bone metabolism (Fig. 1.1b). The two conditions may occur together. After the first manifestation, DFS will persist for the rest of the patient's life, albeit perhaps in 'remission', as there is currently no possibility of curing the underlying complications of diabetes [1].

One of the most important features of DFS is reduced sensitivity to pain after initial damage. This is also referred to as *'loss of protective sensation'* or *'LOPS'* and is a result of a degeneration of small nerve fibres. The person affected does not show normal pain-preventing behaviour or feel any urgency to call for timely help. This enables the damage to spread. The degree of carelessness is often astonishing for less experienced in dealing with people with reduced sensation of pain. The diabetologist and philosopher A. Risse explains this with the phenomenon of '*Leibesinselschwund*' (vanishing corporal islands) [2]. Put in

D. Hochlenert et al., *Diabetic Foot Syndrome*,
https://doi.org/10.1007/978-3-319-92055-9_1

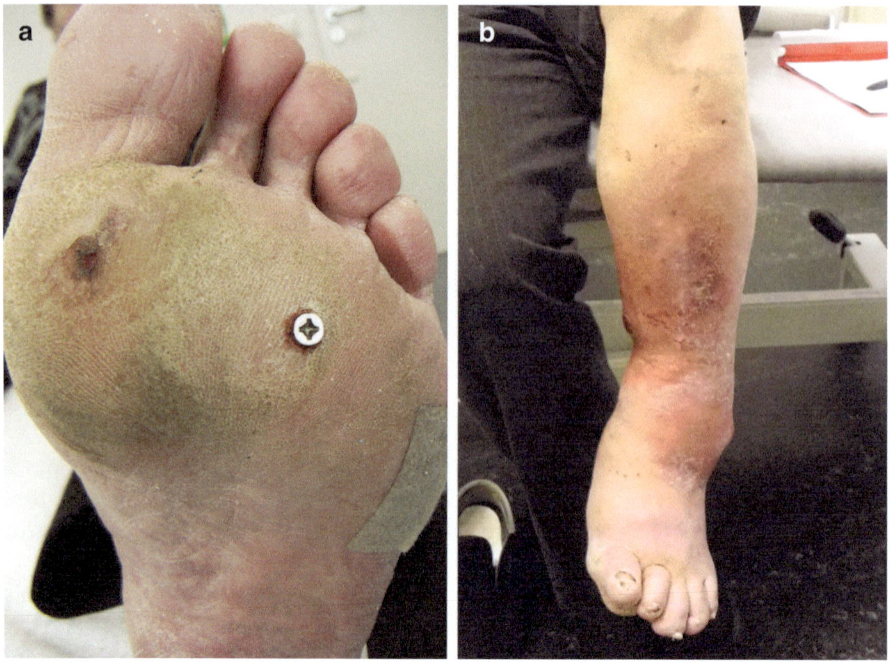

Fig. 1.1 (**a**) Painless injury: This screw remained embedded in the foot for 3 days and was discovered during a routine examination (by kind permission of Dr. Dietmar Weber, Cologne) (**b**) Charcot foot: painless multiple fracture/dislocations of the lower leg and the foot. This injury was presented as 'suspected thrombosis' by a walk-in patient in a major German city after 3 weeks of treatment by a dedicated General Practitioner (GP)

simple terms, this concept describes the loss of affective involvement: the feet seem no longer to belong to the person but are perceived as being parts of the environment.

Damage which affects multiple nerves is referred to as *Polyneuropathy* (PNP). People with diabetes develop symmetrical, predominantly distal and sensory polyneuropathies. As a result, long and small nerve fibres, which transmit information, are affected in equal measure in both legs. Later in the course of the disease, longer fibres and fibres controlling movement also fail. The balance between groups of muscles is deranged because muscles distant from the torso are affected first. This is important for the development of many deformities. The loss of nerves which control autonomic function leads to changes in the skin and its appendages. This results in a failure of the sweat glands that are no longer stimulated by sudomotor nerves (Fig. 1.2).

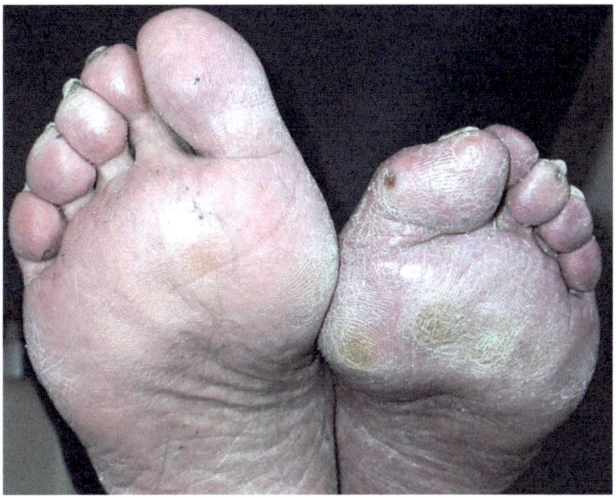

Fig. 1.2 One-sided neuropathy in the left foot as a result of a spinal cord defect with the formation of all alterations typical for polyneuropathy including deformity of the toes and ulcers in the absence of diabetes mellitus (by kind permission of Dr. Thomas Horn)

Other common conditions in people with diabetes might affect tissue repair and thereby enable the damage to extend. The most dramatic consequences arise from peripheral arterial disease (PAD). Deformities, skin problems, oedema, negative effects of completely uncontrolled glucose metabolism and other factors may also prevent repair. For this reason, it is essential not to stop at the verification of the diagnosis of DFS, but to investigate and treat the causes systematically and without delay as soon as DFS is detected.

1.2 Conditions and Triggers

The diabetic foot has numerous causes which may be complementary or secondary to each other. In this book, we split the causes into underlying conditions (prerequisites or requirements) on one hand and triggers on the other, in order to present them in a systematic way.

Feet are continuously damaged, but a healthy foot promptly limits the extent of an injury and repairs the damage. This remarkable resilience may be compromised by underlying *conditions* that provide an answer to the question *'Why does a diabetic foot occur at all?'*. The increased vulnerability is due to a combination of these conditions which characteristically include a reduced and inadequate perception of pain. Other conditions such as poor circulation, swelling, very poor control of diabetes and others limit the repair process.

The risk caused by reduced resilience becomes a reality through a causal precipitant. These *triggers* determine the site of the lesion. Knowing them provides an answer to the question *'Why does a lesion occur at this particular site?'*. Visible signs of the activity of triggers are for example calluses as an initial sign of mechanical stress.

Therapy is targeted at both conditions and triggers. Underlying conditions may be very difficult to improve. In most cases, the treatment aims to prevent the recurrence of triggers in particular.

DFS is caused by conditions and triggers.
Two questions should be answered before starting treatment:
'Why does a diabetic foot ulcer occur at all?' and
'Why does a diabetic foot ulcer occur at this particular site?'

1.3 Progression

Despite a change from resilient to vulnerable, the foot may remain injury-free as long as harmful triggers are kept under control by protective measures. For example, a weakening of protective sensation can be compensated by less physical activity [3] or by better footwear. This balance between triggers and vulnerability on one hand and protection and resilience on the other determines whether the continuous trauma, to which a foot is exposed, will lead to injury or leave the foot unharmed. The phases of changes in this balance are shown in Table 1.1 and Fig. 1.3.

Compensation for an increase in physical stress can be achieved by a thickening of the skin and formation of *calluses*. *Redness* and *blisters* are also superficial results of stress and may be part of a functioning defence mechanism if associated with pain (Fig. 1.3a). In these cases, the affected person is forced to assume a pain-reducing posture, which allows rapid closure of the defect without any further measures being taken.

If, on the other hand, there is temporary *decompensation* and injury to deeper layers of the skin, various defects may arise. Short periods of excessive trauma on areas of skin which have already developed calluses may lead to *haemorrhages within calluses* (Fig. 1.3b). By the time this haemorrhage is discovered, the bleeding has usually stopped and the epithelium has recovered [4].

The phase of inactive diabetic foot is defined by a history of previous uncompensated overload combined with a reduction in resilience.

If this is recognised, preventive measures should be put into place to reinforce the protective mechanisms through patient support, suitable footwear [5] and podiatric care [6–8]. If the overload is intensive or prolonged, the result is more extensive longer lasting damage, requiring a more complex process of repair. The diabetic foot then becomes '***active***'. If this damage affects the skin, it is referred to as *ulceration* (full thickness break of the skin) (Figs. 1.3c and 1.3d). In a

Table 1.1 Phases of the balance between defensive and aggravating factors

	Phase	What happens	Indicators
0	Healthy	Resilient foot, able to withstand normal stress, without external protective measures	**No** signs of diminished resilience
I	Pre-DFS	Increased vulnerability, possibly with signs of compensation	**Reduced resilience** (PNP and possibly further underlying conditions) Possible signs of compensation, e.g. calluses
IIa/ IIb/ IIc	Inactive DFS	Increased vulnerability, with former consequences of decompensation	Reduced resilience Former **decompensated stress**, (a) condition after preulcerative lesions (callosities with **haemorrhaging**) (b) condition after **ulceration** (c) inactive **Charcot foot**
IIIa/ IIIb/ IIIc	Active DFS	Current consequences of decompensation with or without the involvement of deeper hypotrophic regions (bones, joints, corpus adiposum of the heel)	Reduced resilience Current decompensation (a) **superficial ulceration** (b) **deep ulceration** into hypotrophic structures (c) **active Charcot foot**
IV	No foot	Removal of the affected region	**Major amputation**

'*Charcot foot*', the musculoskeletal system is involved, in particular its osseous components.

During the long period of time necessary to restore integrity, repetition of the triggers is likely to occur. In this way, the defects appear as if they were chronic. However, this is not the case, but the lesions are constantly being renewed.

Once the repair is completed, the diabetic foot enters into an inactive state, also referred to as *remission* [1]. In the case of a Charcot Foot, the term 'inactive Charcot foot' is used [9]. The concept of a lifelong disease with active and inactive phases can be applied not only to the Charcot foot but to all aspects of the diabetic foot. Without further protective measures, within 1 year almost 100% of those affected [10] develop at least one reactivation of the diabetic foot. The subsequent terminology is often used: if the new lesions are found at the same site after a short interval, they are referred to as a '*relapse*', if they appear later, they are referred to as a '*recurrence*', if they appear at a different site, they are referred to as a '*new ulcer*'. In this book, the recurrence of an active state is referred to as '*reactivation*'. A lifelong regime of structured measures to prevent reactivation is therefore a core element in the care given to people with a diabetic foot [11]. The progression is shown in Table 1.1. Amputation above the ankle brings the diabetic foot to an end. However, problems with the stump, the prosthesis or the contralateral limb may follow (Fig. 1.3e).

The diabetic foot is a lifelong disease with active and inactive phases.

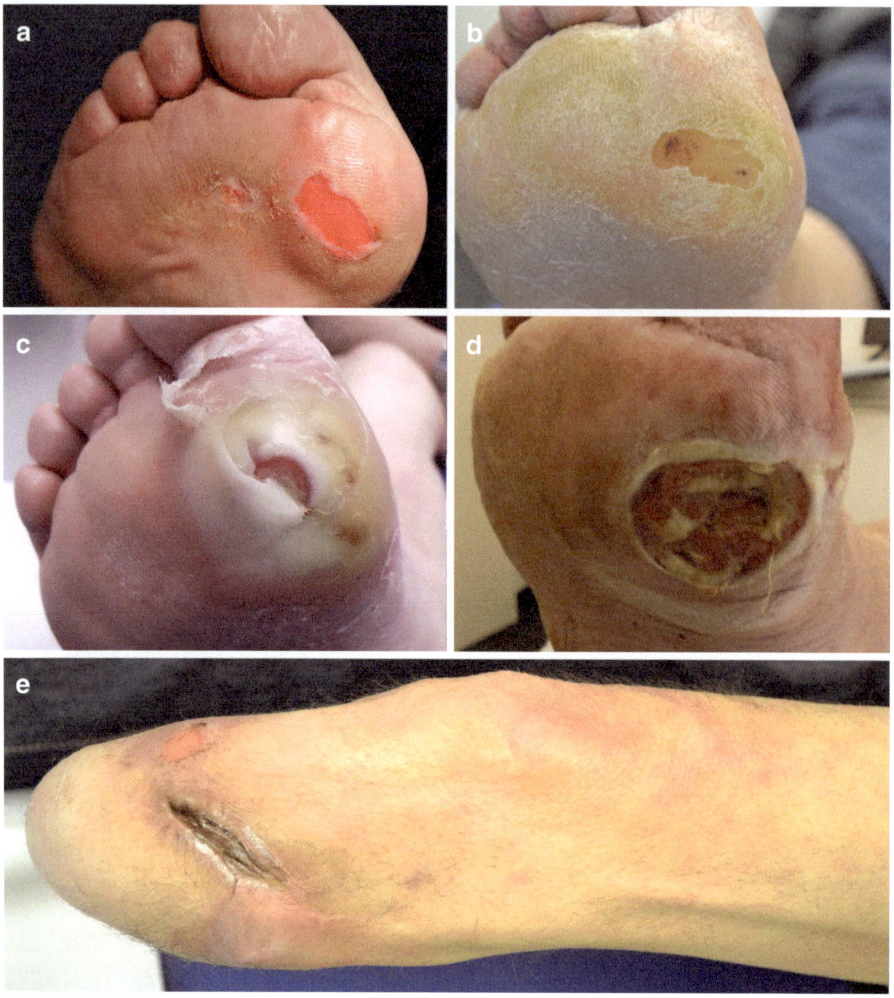

Fig. 1.3 Phases of balance between harmful triggers and protection (Table 1.1): (**a**) Spontaneously burst blister under the medial sesamoid bone, Pre-DFS in Phase I (**b**) Punctuate bleeding in a callus over the medial sesamoid bone as a sign of a previous brief trauma in deeper layers of the skin, inactive diabetic foot, Phase IIa (**c**) Spontaneously erupted blister with ulceration at the base of the blister, active diabetic foot, Phase IIIa (**d**) Deep ulceration with affected bones, active DFS, Phase IIIb (**e**) Stump after amputation of lower leg, ulceration on stump, Phase IV

1.4 Classification

The deep spread of lesions associated with the diabetic foot has traditionally been classified according to Wagner [12, 13] (Table 1.2).

Table 1.2 Classification according to Wagner

Degree	Description
0	Pre- or post-ulcerative lesion completely epithelialised
1	Superficial ulcers
2	Ulcer extends to tendons or articular capsules
3	Ulcer involving bones or open joints or deep abscesses
4	Necrosis of the whole section of parts of the foot
5	Necrosis of the entire foot

Some of the difficulties with this classification are:

- Only ulcers are described, the Charcot foot is not integrated.
- Early stages are not differentiated.
- Stages 1 and 2 are very difficult to differentiate in a clinical setting.
- Stages 3 and 4 are also often difficult to distinguish in a clinical setting. As each ulcer starts with tissue death, the common short description 'partial necrosis' causes misunderstandings.
- Injuries to the heel involving the subcutaneous fat pad are not adequately represented.
- Factors which are important for prognosis such as PAD, infection or concomitant diseases are not represented.
- The use of the classification often deviates from the way it is dealt with in the original text. For example, according to Wagner, a lesion that allows for bone contact using a blunt instrument (probe to bone positive) but without overt osteomyelitis is still Stage 2. However, osteomyelitis may be difficult to determine. On the other hand, the presence of an abscess indicates the advancement to Stage 3 even without osteomyelitis, which is often ignored.

Despite these disadvantages, this classification is still in widespread use. The original text quotation can be found in Appendix A.2.1.

The University of Texas Classification (UT Classification) [14, 15] integrates information on infection and PAD. It uses the numbers 0–3 to describe depth (0 = pre- or post-ulcerative lesion, 1 = not involving tendon, capsule or bone, 2 = reaching tendon or capsule, 3 = reaching bone or joint) and the letters A, B, C and D to describe the absence or presence of the factors infection and ischemia (A = absence of both, B = infection only, C = ischemia only, D = both). A combination which is used in some countries describes the depth of the lesions according to Wagner with information on infection and PAD according to the UT Classification. In deference to the original authors, the combined classification is referred to as 'Classification according to Wagner-Armstrong' (Fig. 1.4). However also UT has some disadvantages as information on neuropathy, ulcer site and area are missing.

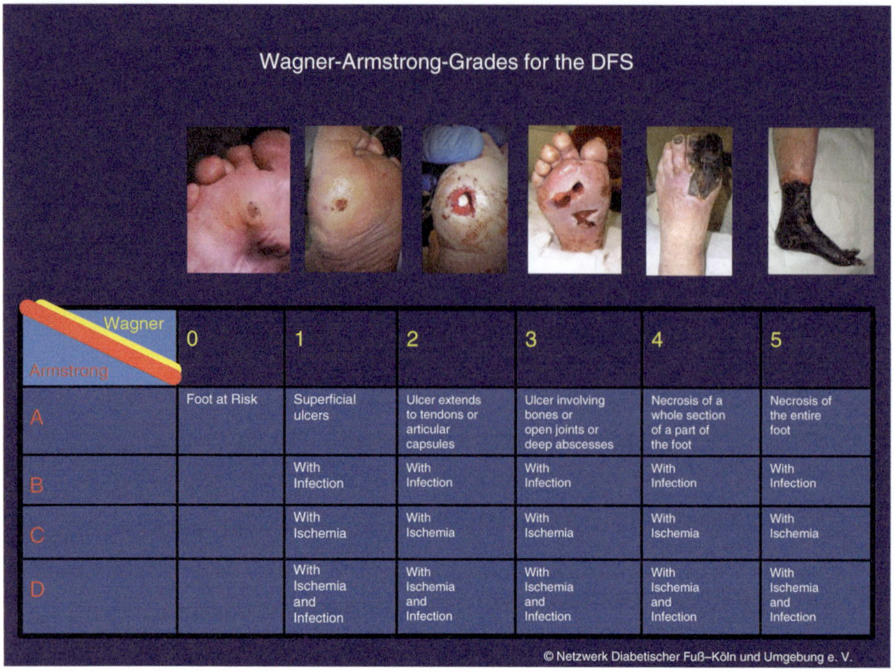

Fig. 1.4 Grading according to Wagner/Armstrong used by the Cologne diabetic foot network

Further classifications are described: The *PEDIS Classification* developed by the IWGDF (International working group on the diabetic foot) is widely used in several countries [16]. It comprises the parameters: (P = Perfusion/ blood flow), (E = Extent/size of ulcer), (D = Depth of spread/tissue loss), (I = Infection) and (S = Sensation/protective sensitivity) The PEDIS Classification is reproduced in Appendix A.2.3. In Germany, the classification according to *Arlt* was common for many years. It differentiates between angiopathic, neuropathic and angioneuropathic diabetic foot [17].

SINBAD [18] is a simple score based on **S**ite (proximal to forefoot = 1), **I**schemia (clinical evidence of reduced pedal blood flow by pulse palpation = 1), **N**europathy (LOPS = 1), **B**acterial Infection (present = 1), **A**rea (>1 cm^2 = 1) and **D**epth (deeper than skin and subcutaneous tissue = 1) and is useful in predicting ulcer outcome and enabling comparison among different centres in different countries.

1.5 Entities

In this book, the authors divide ulcers in the context of DFS into subgroups named '*Entities of DFS*' based on their location. The surface of the foot is divided into areas where ulcers typically arise in a similar way. This classification does not require grades and stages to be memorised. It should allow an intuitive approach using some basic concepts. It organises knowledge similar to leaves at a tree in order to facilitate access and provide overview. If a patient presents with a lesion at a certain location, all background information, tests and therapies may be accessed easily.

The entities of DFS are subgroups of DFS defined by the location. They allow an easy access to causes, prognosis and therapy.

1.6 Epidemiology

The number of people afflicted by DFS is increasing, mainly because the number of people with diabetes is growing at a rate referred to as the 'Diabetes Epidemic' [19]. About 425 million people are affected by diabetes worldwide. In western countries about 10% of all inhabitants suffer from diabetes [20]. Approximately 3% per year experience a new episode of diabetic foot ulcers [21] and 0.1% a new episode of an active Charcot foot [22]. The prevalence of diabetic foot ulcers is 1.6–6.3% and the lifetime risk is 15–25% [23] which means that in a country of 50 million inhabitants, 1 million will suffer from DFS throughout their lifetime.

According to a register of DFS in specialist care [24] about 30% of these episodes of active disease persist for more than 6 months. National UK data have shown that just below two-thirds of patients will be alive and ulcer-free after 6 months of treatment [25].

In specialist care, roughly 1% of the affected patients will experience an amputation above the ankle and about 6–7% an amputation below the ankle. Put in another way, NHS data in the UK (2014–2017) estimates a major amputation rate of 0.81/1000 people with diabetes and a minor amputation rate of 2.1/1000 people with diabetes. Regional variation is however at least eight-fold (2017, publicly accessible at fingertips.phe.org.uk/profile/diabetes-ft).

In the year after the foot has regained ulcer-free status, without specialist care up to 100 new active episodes per 100 people may occur [10], whilst in specialist care the percentage is about 30% [6].

The number of amputations above the ankle is declining in many countries, but the number of amputations below the ankle often increases in the same countries. It is difficult to draw conclusions because of numerous methodological problems [26–29]. However, impressions from daily practice suggest that further improvement in the areas of prevention, amputation, and duration of active episodes should be possible and worthwhile.

1.7 Consequences for the Patient

The diabetic foot imposes limitations on the affected person in many different ways. A few of these are shown in the following overview:

Restrictions for people with a diabetic foot:

- Prolonged duration until remission [30]
- Frequent reactivations [6, 31]
- Demanding therapy in particular offloading, immobilisation and hospitalisation
- Pain
- Amputations
- Loss of mobility and independence
- Loss of employment or the ability to work
- Loss of social contacts [32]
- Costs of other services
- Death

At worst, DFS may end with the death of the patient. DFS might cause death either directly or indirectly. Between 6 and 8% of the patients affected by an active ulcer phase die before DFS becomes inactive [33]. About 70% of people with DFS die within 5 years if they have an amputation [34], 9% don't even leave the hospital alive. Due to methodological problems, it is not easy to determine which of the various possible mechanisms link DFS and death and to which intensity. For premature death, a major role of ischaemic heart disease has been suggested. In a study based on results from death certificates and post-mortem examinations, this was especially pronounced in neuropathic DFU patients [35]. Patients benefit from the introduction of an aggressive cardiovascular risk management programme in DFU clinics. Future implementation of national programmes using such an approach seems recommendable [36].

Among the potential consequences of DFS, amputations above the ankle are a core issue. Less than 50% of patients are able to walk independently after this type of amputation [37]. This is referred to as *major amputation*. In contrast, in a *minor amputation*, parts of the foot are left intact. This wording might be misleading as the term implies that the removal of parts of the foot was of minor importance. Actually, these 'minor' amputations of the foot often alter the stability of the foot and are thought to increase the probability of recurrence. They are very heterogeneous and may reduce mobility or impair the patient's perception of their own integrity. Throughout this book, the authors used the expression '**amputation above the ankle**' or '**amputation below the ankle**' instead.

Health related quality of life (HRQoL), preferably self-reported as a '*patient-reported outcome*' (PRO) is of great importance for healthcare providers when discussing allocation of resources with an institution providing funding for healthcare. More general tools such as the EQ5D or SF-36 are not specific for DFS and not sensitive to slow changes. Hence a lack of difference in the scoring of a patient related outcome of HRQoL, despite clinical improvement [38], may arise if the impact of important clinical outcomes have been overlooked in the tool. More specific tools, easy to apply, sensitive to slow changes, suitable for patients who often have multiple comorbidities and have a poor quality of life, would be welcomed [39].

Over the past decades, the goal of preserving mobility has somehow superseded the aim to close the ulcer bit by bit as the primary target of treatment. Some working groups i.e. in Almelo and Essen (personal report Eric Manning, Almelo, Netherlands and Anna Trocha, Essen, Germany) were early in recognising the conflict between this goal and the common recommendation to limit the number of steps during the month of therapy. They developed cast techniques and physiotherapy to facilitate mobility during the process of ulcer treatment and promoted the slogan '**keep the patient walking**'. When the eradication of ulcers becomes the central focus, more and earlier amputations can be the result.

1.8 Economics and Costs

DFS causes considerable costs accounting for 12–30% of all resources spent for diabetes [21, 26]. In the UK this is approximately £1 billion [40] or £1 of every £140 spent in the NHS per annum. In Germany, the figure is € 2.5 billion [41, 42]. The more complicated the disease has become, the more resources of all types are needed [43]. The treatment of people with DFS has become a significant economic factor for care providers and insurance companies (Healthcare Industry). DFS is a field with a clear and immediate first-hand benefit for patients, insurance companies, and caregivers. For this reason, expertise in this risky and cost-intensive group of diseases should be a core competence for all diabetologists and offers the opportunity to provide great benefits.

1.9 Specialised Treatment

Specialised treatment can lead to a reduction in the frequency of amputations above the ankle, a decrease in reactivations, fewer in-patient hospitalisations, shorter sick leave, and to a reduction in the number of patients needing permanent care [44–46]. It is characterised by rich experience of all members and their intense interaction with all necessary partners [47]. Working groups for the diabetic foot certify facilities which fulfill minimum criteria in Belgium and in Germany [48–50]. In some regions, these facilities have joined forces to set up networks. Networks attempt to guarantee easy access to specialised treatment for every affected person in the region and aim to improve the standard of care [51, 52]. In Germany, a nationwide **'DFS-Register'**, set up in 2003, collects data of treatments in specialised care with extra funding. Data concerning the identification of the entities depicted in this book have been provided by this DFS-Register.

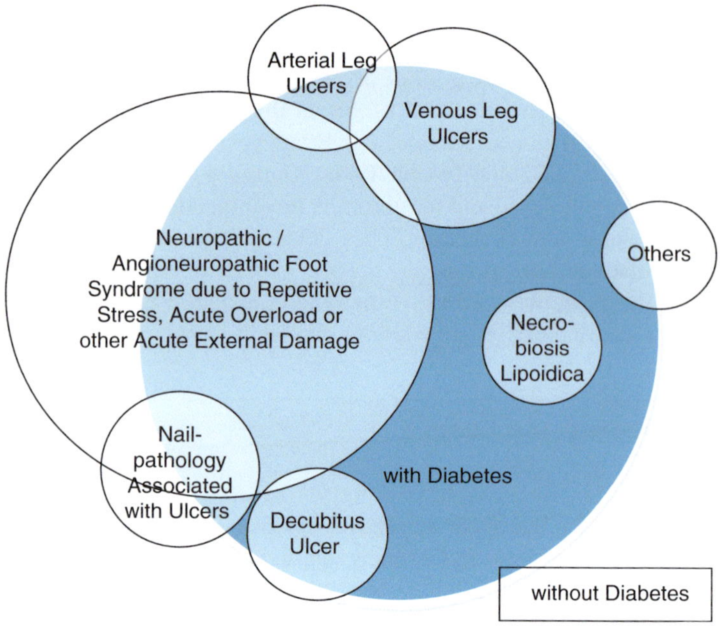

Fig. 1.5 Disorders of patients in a diabetic foot outpatient clinic

1.10 Transitions and Distinctions

The clinical pictures associated with ulcers at the feet overlap in many ways. For example, in the region of the malleoli, diabetic foot ulcers reflect all aspects of the differential diagnosis of crural ulcers. Figure 1.5 shows some of the many overlapping conditions.

The movements of the foot as a structure distal to the malleoli are initiated by muscles situated in the lower leg. The **functional unity of lower leg, ankle joint and foot** is supported by such technical terms as 'foot and ankle surgery'. For this reason, we have attributed lesions in the region of the malleoli to the diabetic foot and lesions on the lower leg to a separate chapter on transitional regions.

On the other hand, many people who are not affected by diabetes have neuropathic and angioneuropathic ulcerations or Charcot feet, that do not differ significantly from those with DFS. Their condition is particularly precarious, as recognition is often delayed, and delivery of care is not tailored to their needs. The provision of footwear, podiatry and other services may be excluded if diabetes is not present, depending on the individual regulations in the healthcare system of the patient's home country.

'Diabetes' and 'foot' are characteristic but not necessary elements of the dysfunctional state we deal with. It is therefore more of a syndrome than a disease. In the literature, 'diabetic foot' and 'diabetic foot syndrome' are used interchangeably. Throughout this book we treat them as equivalent terms.

1.11 Summary

- **From a global perspective, DFS is a challenge where insights in pathogenesis, methods of treatment and effective ways of delivering multiprofessional care are developing at a rapid pace.**
- **For this reason, it is an ideal field of operation for dedicated professionals who are skilled in dexterity and are willing to work in a team.**

1.12 Recommended Lecture

Alberto Piaggesi, Jan Apelqvist: The Diabetic Foot Syndrome

Frontiers in diabetes; v. 26. 0251–5342; Karger, 2017; ISBN 9783318061444

Thoughtful chapters dealing with some core issues of the clinical scenario, the mechanisms in regard to pathology and the organizational tasks of the DFS.

Andrew J. M. Boulton, Peter R. Cavanagh, Gerry Rayman. The Foot in Diabetes

4th edition; Wiley 2006; ISBN 978-0470015049

Complete Textbook dealing with all core aspects of the diabetic foot in distinct chapters written each by dedicated experts in the field. It focuses on practically oriented advice.

Paul Brand, Philip Yancey: The Gift of Pain

Zondervan 1997, **ISBN** 978-0310221449

Brand's perspective explains and integrates the nature of physical pain. It is compelling both from a scientific inquiry and historical point of view, and for its refreshing treatment of the topic of pain. But it is also an explanation of a cornerstone of the diabetic foot by one of the first specialists dealing with it in the western world.

Robert J. Hinchliffe, Nicolaas C. Schaper, Matt M. Thompson), Ramesh K. Tripathi, Carlos H. Timaran: The Diabetic Foot

1 edition (September 8, 2014); Jp Medical Pub; ISBN: 1907816623

Comprehensive coverage of the latest evidence-based investigations, techniques and management of the diabetic foot.

References

1. Armstrong DG, Mills JL. Toward a change in syntax in diabetic foot care: prevention equals remission. J Am Podiatr Med Assoc. 2013;103(2):161–2.
2. Risse A. Phänomenologische und psychopathologische Aspekte in der Diabetologie. Berlin: Walter de Gruyter; 1997.

3. Armstrong DG, Lavery LA, Holtz-Neiderer K, Mohler MJ, Wendel CS, Nixon BP, Boulton AJ. Variability in activity may precede diabetic foot ulceration. Diabetes Care. 2004;27(8):1980–4.
4. Rosen RC, Davids MS, Bohanske LM, Lemont H. Hemorrhage into plantar callus and diabetes mellitus. Cutis. 1985;35(4):339–41.
5. Busch K, Chantelau E. Effectiveness of a new brand of stock 'diabetic' shoes to protect against diabetic foot ulcer relapse. A prospective cohort study. Diabet Med. 2003;20(8):665–9.
6. Armstrong DG, Ingelfinger JR, Boulton AJM, Bus SA. Diabetic foot ulcers and their recurrence. N Engl J Med. 2017;376(24):2367–75. https://doi.org/10.1056/NEJMra1615439.
7. Chantelau E. Alternativen zur Fußamputation bei diabetischer Podopathie. Was ist gesichert? Dtsch Arztebl. 2002;99(30):A2052–6.
8. Plank J, Haas W, Rakovac I, Gorzer E, Sommer R, Siebenhofer A, Pieber TR. Evaluation of the impact of chiropodist care in the secondary prevention of foot ulcerations in diabetic subjects. Diabetes Care. 2003;26(6):1691–5.
9. Rogers LC, Frykberg RG, Armstrong DG, Boulton AJ, Edmonds M, Van GH, Hartemann A, et al. The Charcot foot in diabetes. Diabetes Care. 2011;34(9):2123–9. https://doi.org/10.2337/dc11-0844.
10. Tanudjaja T, Chantelau E. Recurrent diabetic foot lesions—a study of disease activity in high risc patients. In: The diabetic foot, second international symposium Noordwijkerhout 1995; 1995.
11. Waaijman R, de Haart M, Arts ML, Wever D, Verlouw AJ, Nollet F, Bus SA. Risk factors for plantar foot ulcer recurrence in neuropathic diabetic patients. Diabetes Care. 2014. https://doi.org/10.2337/dc13-2470.
12. Wagner FW Jr. The dysvascular foot: a system for diagnosis and treatment. Foot Ankle. 1981;2(2):64–122.
13. Wagner FW Jr. The diabetic foot. Orthopedics. 1987;10(1):163–72.
14. Armstrong DG. The University of Texas diabetic foot classification system. Ostomy Wound Manage. 1996;42(8):60–1.
15. Armstrong DG, Lavery LA, Harkless LB. Validation of a diabetic wound classification system. The contribution of depth, infection, and ischemia to risk of amputation. Diabetes Care. 1998;21(5):855–9.
16. Schaper NC. Diabetic foot ulcer classification system for research purposes: a progress report on criteria for including patients in research studies. Diabetes Metab Res Rev. 2004;20 (Suppl 1):S90–5. https://doi.org/10.1002/dmrr.464.
17. Arlt B, Protze J. [Diabetic foot]. Langenbecks Arch Chir Suppl Kongressbd. 1997;114:528–32.
18. Ince P, Abbas ZG, Lutale JK, Basit A, Ali SM, Chohan F, Morbach S, Mollenberg J, Game FL, Jeffcoate WJ. Use of the SINBAD classification system and score in comparing outcome of foot ulcer management on three continents. Diabetes Care. 2008;31(5):964–7. https://doi.org/10.2337/dc07-2367.
19. Guariguata L, Whiting DR, Hambleton I, Beagley J, Linnenkamp U, Shaw JE. Global estimates of diabetes prevalence for 2013 and projections for 2035. Diabetes Res Clin Pract. 2014;103(2):137–49. https://doi.org/10.1016/j.diabres.2013.11.002.
20. IDF. IDF diabetes Atlas eight edition 2017. 2017. http://www.diabetesatlas.org. Accessed 18 Feb 2018.
21. LeMaster JW, Reiber GE, Rayman A. Epidemiology and economic impact of foot ulcers. In: Boulton AJ, Cavenagh PR, Rayman A, editors. The foot in diabetes. 4th ed. Chichester: Wiley; 2006.
22. Hochlenert D. Qualitätsbericht Netzwerk Diabetischer Fuß Köln und Umgebung 2006; 2007.
23. Reiber GE, Lipsky BA, Gibbons GW. The burden of diabetic foot ulcers. Am J Surg. 1998;176(2A Suppl):5S–10S.
24. Hochlenert D. Qualitätsbericht der Netzwerke Diabetischer Fuß Nordrhein, Hamburg und Berlin. 2017. http://www.fussnetz-koeln.de/Start/Dokus/Qualitaetsbericht_2017.pdf.
25. NHS. National Diabetes Foot Care Audit—2014-2016. 2017. https://www.digital.nhs.uk/catalogue/PUB23525. Accessed 23 Mar 2018.

26. Apelqvist J. The diabetic foot syndrome today: a pandemic uprise. In: Piaggesi A, Apelqvist J, editors. The diabetic foot syndrome (frontiers in diabetes). Basel: S. Karger AG; 2018.
27. Kroger K, Berg C, Santosa F, Malyar N, Reinecke H. Lower limb amputation in Germany. Dtsch Arztebl Int. 2017;114(7):130–6. https://doi.org/10.3238/arztebl.2017.0130.
28. Lombardo FL, Maggini M, De Bellis A, Seghieri G, Anichini R. Lower extremity amputations in persons with and without diabetes in Italy: 2001-2010. PLoS One. 2014;9(1):e86405. https://doi.org/10.1371/journal.pone.0086405.
29. Rumenapf G, Morbach S. Amputation statistics-how to interpret them? Dtsch Arztebl Int. 2017;114(8):128–9. https://doi.org/10.3238/arztebl.2017.0128.
30. Pickwell KM, Siersma VD, Kars M, Holstein PE, Schaper NC, Consortium on behalf of the Eurodiale. Diabetic foot disease: impact of ulcer location on ulcer healing. Diabetes Metab Res Rev. 2013;29(5):377–83. https://doi.org/10.1002/dmrr.2400.
31. Apelqvist J, Larsson J, Agardh CD. Long-term prognosis for diabetic patients with foot ulcers. J Intern Med. 1993;233(6):485–91.
32. Siersma V, Thorsen H, Holstein PE, Kars M, Apelqvist J, Jude EB, Piaggesi A, et al. Importance of factors determining the low health-related quality of life in people presenting with a diabetic foot ulcer: the Eurodiale study. Diabet Med. 2013. https://doi.org/10.1111/dme.12254.
33. Prompers L, Schaper N, Apelqvist J, Edmonds M, Jude E, Mauricio D, Uccioli L, et al. Prediction of outcome in individuals with diabetic foot ulcers: focus on the differences between individuals with and without peripheral arterial disease. The EURODIALE Study. Diabetologia. 2008;51(5):747–55. https://doi.org/10.1007/s00125-008-0940-0.
34. Icks A, Scheer M, Morbach S, Genz J, Haastert B, Giani G, Glaeske G, Hoffmann F. Time-dependent impact of diabetes on mortality in patients after major lower extremity amputation: survival in a population-based 5-year cohort in Germany. Diabetes Care. 2011;34(6):1350–4. https://doi.org/10.2337/dc10-2341.
35. Chammas NK, Hill RL, Edmonds ME. Increased mortality in diabetic foot ulcer patients: the significance of ulcer type. J Diabetes Res. 2016;2016:2879809. https://doi.org/10.1155/2016/2879809.
36. Young MJ, McCardle JE, Randall LE, Barclay JI. Improved survival of diabetic foot ulcer patients 1995-2008: possible impact of aggressive cardiovascular risk management. Diabetes Care. 2008;31(11):2143–7. https://doi.org/10.2337/dc08-1242.
37. Game F. Choosing life or limb. Improving survival in the multi-complex diabetic foot patient. Diabetes Metab Res Rev. 2012;28(Suppl 1):97–100. https://doi.org/10.1002/dmrr.2244.
38. Pickwell K, Siersma V, Kars M, Apelqvist J, Bakker K, Edmonds M, Holstein P, et al. Minor amputation does not negatively affect health-related quality of life as compared with conservative treatment in patients with a diabetic foot ulcer: an observational study. Diabetes Metab Res Rev. 2017;33(3). https://doi.org/10.1002/dmrr.2867.
39. Siersma V, Thorsen H, Holstein PE, Kars M, Apelqvist J, Jude EB, Piaggesi A, et al. Health-related quality of life predicts major amputation and death, but not healing, in people with diabetes presenting with foot ulcers: the Eurodiale study. Diabetes Care. 2014;37(3):694–700. https://doi.org/10.2337/dc13-1212.
40. Kerr M. Improving footcare for people with diabetes and saving money: an economic study in England. Insight Health Economics. 2017. https://diabetes-resources-production.s3-eu-west-1.amazonaws.com/diabetes-storage/migration/pdf/Improving%2520footcare%2520economic%2520study%2520%28January%25202017%29.pdf. Accessed 17 Mar 2018.
41. Hauner H. [Epidemiology and costs of diabetes mellitus in Germany]. Dtsch Med Wochenschr. 2005;130 Suppl 2:S64–65. https://doi.org/10.1055/s-2005-870872.
42. Koster I, Huppertz E, Hauner H, Schubert I. Direct costs of diabetes mellitus in Germany—CoDiM 2000-2007. Exp Clin Endocrinol Diabetes. 2011;119(6):377–85. https://doi.org/10.1055/s-0030-1269847.
43. Prompers L, Huijberts M, Schaper N, Apelqvist J, Bakker K, Edmonds M, Holstein P, et al. Resource utilisation and costs associated with the treatment of diabetic foot ulcers. Prospective data from the Eurodiale Study. Diabetologia. 2008;51(10):1826–34. https://doi.org/10.1007/s00125-008-1089-6.

44. Bakker K, Dooren J. [A specialized outpatient foot clinic for diabetic patients decreases the number of amputations and is cost saving]. Ned Tijdschr Geneeskd. 1994;138(11):565–9.
45. Hochlenert D. Gesundheitspreis NRW 2012: Netzwerk Diabetischer Fuß Nordrhein (ID-Nr.: 236671). 2012. http://www.mgepa.nrw.de/mediapool/pdf/gesundheit/gesundheitspreis_2012/Sonderpreis_Netzwerk_Diabetischer_Fu___Nordrhein.pdf.
46. Schaper NC. Lessons from Eurodiale. Diabetes Metab Res Rev. 2012;28(Suppl 1):21–6. https://doi.org/10.1002/dmrr.2266.
47. Sanders LJ, Robbins JM, Edmonds ME. History of the team approach to amputation prevention: pioneers and milestones. J Vasc Surg. 2010;52(3 Suppl):3S–16S. https://doi.org/10.1016/j.jvs.2010.06.002.
48. Kersken J, Gröne C, Lobmann R, Müller E. Die Fußbehandlungseinrichtung der Deutschen Diabetes-Gesellschaft. Diabetologe. 2009;5(2):111–20. https://doi.org/10.1007/s11428-008-0348-y.
49. Lobmann R, Müller E, Kersken J, Bergmann K, Brunk-Loch S, Gröne C, Lindloh C, Mertens B, Spraul M. The diabetic foot in Germany: analysis of quality in specialised diabetic footcare centres. Diabetic Foot J. 2007;10(2):68–72.
50. Morbach S, Kersken J, Lobmann R, Nobels F, Doggen K, Van Acker K. The German and Belgian accreditation models for diabetic foot services. Diabetes Metab Res Rev. 2016;32(Suppl 1):318–25. https://doi.org/10.1002/dmrr.2752.
51. Hochlenert D, Engels G. Low major amputation rate and low recurrence in networks for treatment of the DFS. In: Abstract Book, X. Diabetic Foot Study Group Meeting Seminaris See Hotel, Berlin-Potsdam, Germany 28–30 Sept 2012; 2012.
52. Risse A, Hochlenert D. Integrierte Versorgung—Neue (?) Versorgungsformen am Beispiel des diabetischen Fußsyndroms. Diabetologe. 2010;2:100–7. https://doi.org/10.1007/s11428-009-0480-3.

The Foot as a Marvel

2

This chapter outlines the structure and function of the foot as well as some commonly seen variations.

The complexity of the foot is evident by features such as its composition of 28 bones. A quarter of the human body's osseous components are found in the feet. Its architecture has to comply with numerous demands as it is designed to support sustained upright walking. For most of the time only one leg carries load. The foot therefore not only features power, endurance and robustness, but it also has to be highly sensitive and be able to balance precisely. On average, 100 million steps are made during a lifetime. This is equivalent to walking more than twice the earth's circumference. The extraordinary resilience of the foot is based on structural and functional characteristics. Knowledge of these characteristics contributes to an understanding of the pathologies and is also needed to find or develop appropriate therapeutic options.

The normal states are described here together with their corresponding deviations in order to concisely show the common features and the differences. For didactical reasons we tried to describe as many anatomical facts as possible using pictures and to keep the text short. When describing different phenomena involving the same anatomical structure, we tried to use one image several times and to give it different colours and descriptive texts to facilitate recognition.

2.1 Evolution

The foot is one of the most characteristic features of mankind [1]. Palaeontological finds, such as the footprints in Laetoli (Tanzania) dating back 3.4 million years, can be classified according to their features (Fig. 2.1). 'Bipedal movement' is a late achievement in human evolution. About 2–4 million years ago human ancestors started out as 'facultative bipeds' and evolved into 'obligate bipeds'. For mankind, this has had the important effect of gradually freeing the hands of load-bearing duties, which in turn has promoted brain development and the advance of human

D. Hochlenert et al., *Diabetic Foot Syndrome*,
https://doi.org/10.1007/978-3-319-92055-9_2

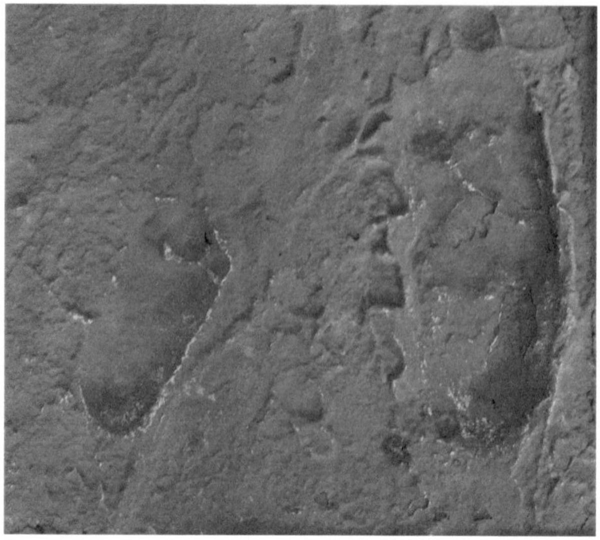

Fig. 2.1 Casting of imprints of two feet at Laetoli

intelligence. The mandatory precondition for a sustained bipedal gait was the positioning of the calcaneus into an upright posture below the talus. This led to the development of the longitudinal arches. The gradual straightening of the calcaneus and therefore the formation of the longitudinal arches can be observed during childhood [2]. Children are born with flat feet. While learning to walk the calcaneus starts to straighten up and therefore the longitudinal arches are formed. The formation of the foot's arches is completed at about the age of ten. The arched foot is unique to humans and represents the last step in human evolution—at least until now.

2.2 Babel

Anatomical language describing the foot is often a bountiful source of confusion. All non-anatomical medical disciplines approach the foot functionally and divide the tarsus into hindfoot (calcaneus and talus) and midfoot (cuneiforms, cuboid and navicular). The metatarsals are classified as part of the forefoot ignoring the literal meaning of their name. For anatomists, by contrast, the forefoot consists only of the toes. The midfoot is formed solely from the 'name-giving' metatarsal bones and the tarsal bones form the hindfoot. While the anatomical classification is merely descriptive, the *functional classification* is closely related to the biomechanics of the bipedal gait. For this reason, only the functional classification will be used in the following chapters.

More confusion arises from the multiple names given to each anatomical structure. A variety of terms are used alongside the official Terminologia Anatomica: traditional Latin terms, national language terms and colloquial terms. The term 'peroneal' for example, still widely used in many countries, was replaced by

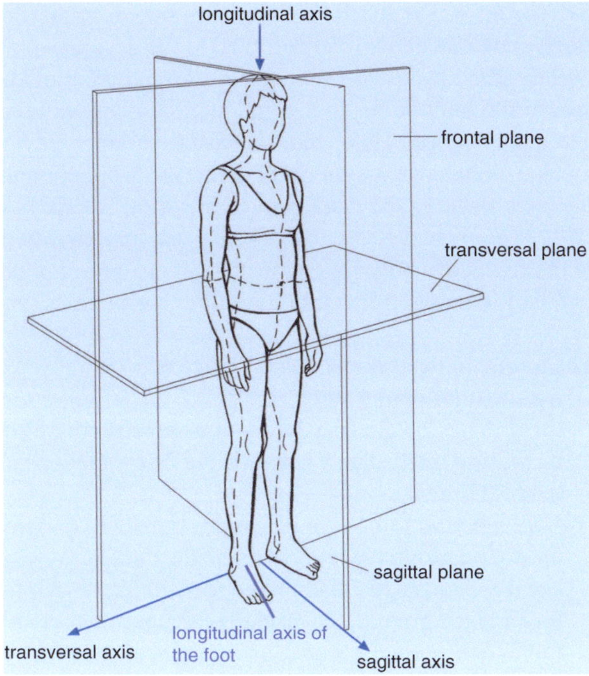

Fig. 2.2 Representation of the planes of the human body

'fibular' in the 1998th Terminologia Anatomica [3]. Traditional expressions will be parenthesised in the course of this book. Synonyms complicate matters further, for example 'plantar fascia' and 'plantar aponeurosis' generally refer to the same structure. In addition, some authors use the term 'aponeurosis' to describe a thicker, central component of the structure and 'fascia' for the thinner, peripheral parts.

Moreover, the description of the *three planes of the body* often differs between sources. In this book, we use the terms sagittal, frontal and transversal for the three planes (Fig. 2.2).

Lowering the foot is referred to as *flexion* (plantarflexion) and lifting movement as *extension* (dorsiflexion). Thereby, the vocabulary describing the foot's movement is the exact opposite of common elocution: a person stretching in the sun flexes the foot in this anatomical context. Additionally, the elevation of the foot narrows the angle between foot and leg. Such a movement is usually not an extension but a flexion. To avoid confusion and to allow a more intuitive language, the terms *dorsiflexion* and *plantarflexion* are often used in English speaking countries to describe this movements of the foot.

Describing the movements of the margins of the foot can also be misleading. With an unloaded foot, the terms *eversion* and *pronation* are often used to describe the lifting of the foot's entire lateral margin. *Inversion* and *supination* refer to a lifting of the entire medial margin. In a clinical setting, the terms *inversion* and *eversion* are typically used when referring to movements of the hindfoot (occasionally also *varus position* and *valgus position*). *Supination* and *pronation* are used for movements of the forefoot. This takes into account the fact that the forefoot is not freely movable under load but fixed to the ground.

The adjective *valgus* refers to a misalignment of the joint in which the convex side of the joint points to the mid-sagittal plane whereas *varus* describes the opposite phenomenon. Here, too, the usual parlance deviates from the rule. The first metatarsophalangeal joint (MTP joint) is not eponymous for its deformity, but rather the bone forming the distal part of the joint: we speak of *metatarsus primus varus*, *hallux valgus* and *hallux valgus interphalangeus* when describing the malposition of the respective bones: first metatarsal, great toe and distal phalanx of the great toe.

The following, frequently used terms sometimes raise questions:

The *torque* indicates how much a force acts on a pivoted body. The farther from the axis of rotation the force is applied, the stronger the torque becomes. The sesamoid bones of the first MTP joint increase the torque of the plantar flexors by increasing the distance between the flexor tendons and the transverse axis of the first MTP joint.

Ground reaction forces are the forces by which the ground supports a body placed on it. The ground reaction forces must act in the same intensity but in the opposite direction as the load on the foot. In the description of the forces between the foot and the ground, the ground reaction forces are often simply equated with the forces acting on the load-bearing parts of the foot.

Stabilisation of joints means the effort to keep the articulating bones in a desired position and to prevent evasive movements. The term 'stabilisation of the hallux in plantar direction' is used when the hallux is pressed onto the ground. 'Stabilisation' also means supporting and maintaining a structure such as the medial longitudinal arch and can be active or passive. A passive stabilisation is achieved by ligaments that cannot vary their own length. Muscles, on the other hand, can contract and the bones bridged by their tendons are actively braced.

2.3 Seven Concepts Explained in Brief

Some basic concepts are outlined here to facilitate an easy access to the detailed descriptions in the following pages. This is to combine deep insight with fluent reading and avoiding repetition (Fig. 2.3).

1. The *gait* is regulated in such a way that most movements are controlled by passive elements and hardly any energy is needed. Two classifications are used equally in this book: the standard and the Rancho Los Amigos nomenclature. The following list compares the respective designations of the gait phases of both nomenclatures for the supporting leg.

    Heel strike = initial contact

   The heel or other part of the foot touches the ground.

    Foot flat = loading response

   The foot reaches plantigrade position.

    Mid stance = mid stance

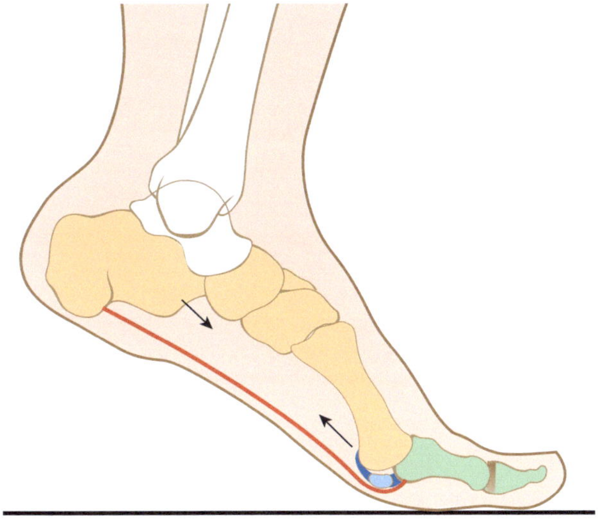

Fig. 2.3 Schematic drawing of a left foot, coloured marking of: plantar aponeurosis (*red*), lamina pedis *(yellow)*, plantar plate of the first MTP joint *(blue) with embedded sesamoid bone (light blue)*, great toe *(green)*

The weight is transferred above the foot.

Heel off = terminal stance

The heel lifts off the ground.

Toe off = pre-swing

Toes rise off the ground.

The first two components are also referred to as *weight acceptance*. The last two components are commonly also referred to as *push off* or *propulsion*. (Details in Sect. 2.6).

2. *Lamina pedis* (*foot plate*) refers to all bones and ligaments from the heel to the MTP joints that are located beneath (distal) the talus. The lamina pedis is twisted and allows the foot to perform two functions: when it is placed on the supporting surface, it is flexible and adapts to the ground; in propulsion, it is a rigid lever. Stiffening is referred to as 'locking', flexibility is referred to as 'unlocking' the lamina pedis. (Details in Sect. 2.4).
3. The parts of the joint capsule situated beneath the MTP joints are thickened to form cushion-like structures called *plantar plates*. Fibres of all structures acting on the MTP joint participate in forming the plantar plates. They position the plantar plate beneath the metatarsal heads (MTHs) and hold the toes in a straight position pressed onto the ground. (Details in Sect. 2.5.4.2).
4. The *plantar aponeurosis* (plantar fascia) connects the heel with the toes and represents a strong supporting component for the longitudinal arch of the foot. When the longitudinal arch flattens, the plantar aponeurosis is tightened, and the toes are pressed to the ground, which is called the *reversed windlass mechanism*. When the heel lifts off the ground, the plantar aponeurosis is stretched around the MTHs and the toes remain pressed to the ground, which is the *windlass mechanism* (Details in Sect. 2.5.4.6).

5. The *toes extend the supporting area of the foot*. This only works if all the bones of a toe are pressed to the ground. For intermediate and end phalanges, this task is accomplished by long toe flexors situated in the calf. For the proximal phalanges this is done by short muscles of the sole of the foot and the windlass mechanism of the plantar aponeurosis (Details in Sects. 2.5.4.2 and 2.5.4.6).
6. The *extensor hoods* wrap around the extensor tendons and the basal phalanges of the toes. The tension of the extensor tendons tightens the extensor hood, which is important for straightening the toes, but also for the pathological development of claw toes. (Details in Sect. 2.5.4.1).
7. *Support and balance*: The metatarsal bones 2, 3 and 4 are very tightly connected to the tarsal bones, while the first and 5th metatarsal bone are more flexible and balance the foot by means of their muscles. (Details in Sects. 2.5.5 and 2.5.6).

2.4 Skeleton

From a functional point of view, the toes and metatarsal bones are referred to as forefoot, the talus and calcaneus are referred to as hindfoot and the remaining tarsal bones as midfoot. In this book, we follow the functional nomenclature (Fig. 2.4). All bones distal (beneath) to the talus up to the MTP joints are combined under the term ‘lamina pedis’ (foot plate).

The *neutral position of the foot* is the *plantigrade position*. In this position, the entire weight-bearing area of the sole, including the heel, is in contact with the ground.

> Upright walking requires two completely opposite functional states of the foot, rigid and flexible, that alternate during the gait cycle.

On one hand, the foot must be able to adapt to any terrain. On the other hand, it must be able to lift the heel off the ground and push the entire body weight forward.

The spatial arrangement of the bones is of fundamental importance for this adaption because, unlike the bones in the hand, they are not arranged in one plane but rather in two. The toes and the metatarsal heads (MTHs) are parallel to the ground (in the transverse plane), while the talus and calcaneus lie on top of each other and perpendicular to the ground (in the sagittal plane). In this way, in the neutral position forefoot and hindfoot are turned 90° to each other (Fig. 2.5).

This is called *twisting of the lamina pedis* and is influenced by the position of the heel (Fig. 2.6). If the heel is turned inwards (inversion), the twisting increases, the medial longitudinal arch becomes higher and the foot becomes more rigid. The lamina pedis is ‘*locked*’. If the heel is turned outwards (eversion), the twisting becomes weaker, the medial longitudinal arch flattens, and the foot becomes softer. The lamina pedis is ‘*unlocked*’.

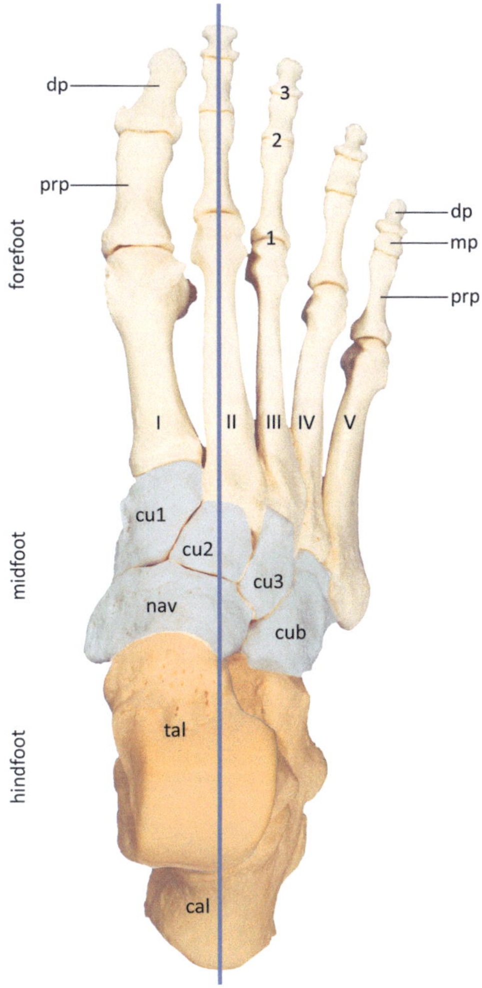

Fig. 2.4 Functional classification of the bones of the foot. Hindfoot *(yellow)* comprised of: talus *(tal)* and calcaneus *(cal)*, midfoot *(blue)* comprised of: navicular *(nav)*, cuboid *(cub)*, medial, intermediate an lateral cuneiform *(cu1, cu2, cu3)*, forefoot *(noncolored)* comprised of: metatarsals 1 to 5 *(I–V)* and toes; distal phalanx *(dp)*, medial phalanx *(mp)*, proximal phalanx *(prp)*; distal interphalangeal joint *(DIP, 3)*, proximal interphalangeal joint *(PIP, 2)*, metatarsophalangeal joint *(MTP joint, 1)*, longitudinal axis of the foot *(blue line)*

Because of this twisting of the lamina pedis, only specific parts of the foot maintain contact with the ground rather than the entire foot. This causes the foot to bulge away from the ground both in the sagittal plane (longitudinal arch) and in the frontal plane (transverse arch). The arches of the foot are stabilised by plantar ligaments and muscles and can yield slightly under the body's weight. This increases the flexibility of the foot skeleton and reduces the risk of fracture.

The *medial longitudinal arch* (also known as the *medial column*) consists of the talus, the navicular, the three cuneiforms and the first to 3rd metatarsal bone (Figs. 2.7a, c). The *lateral longitudinal arch* (*lateral column*) consists of the heel bone (calcaneus), the cuboid and the 4th and 5th metatarsal bone (Fig. 2.7a).

In contrast to the longitudinal arches of the foot, the *transverse arch* runs from the medial to the lateral margin (Fig. 2.7b). It is most pronounced at the height of the

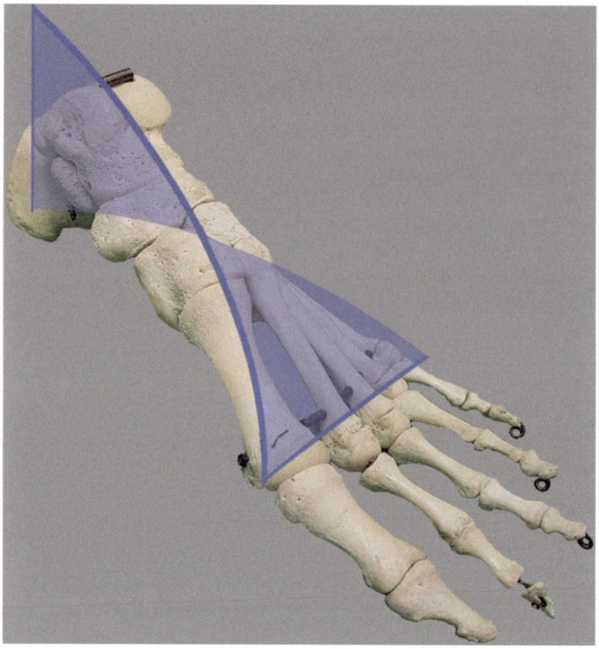

Fig. 2.5 Twisting of the lamina pedis in neutral position of the foot

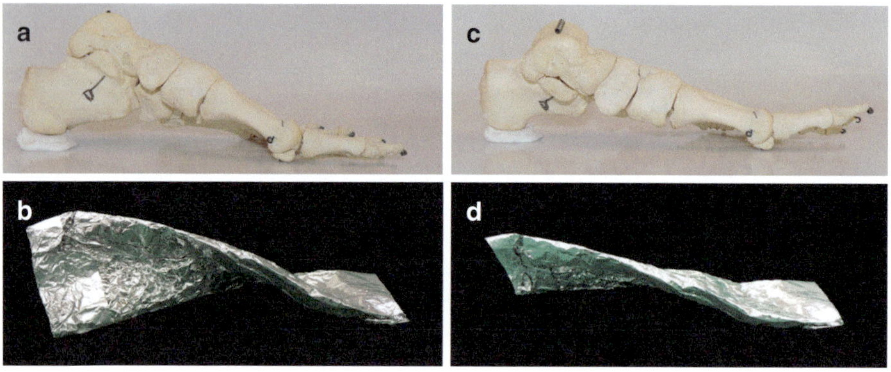

Fig. 2.6 Twisting of the lamina pedis in relation to the position of the heel. (**a**) With an inverted heel, the medial longitudinal arch is raised, and the foot is more rigid. The lamina pedis is 'locked' (**b**) schematic representation of a 'locked lamina pedis' using an aluminium foil model (**c**) With the heel in eversion the medial longitudinal arch is flattened, and the foot is more flexible. The lamina pedis is 'unlocked'. (**d**) Schematic representation of an 'unlocked lamina pedis' using an aluminium foil model

cuneiforms and the cuboid. From here it flattens off towards the toes and ends at the level of the MTHs. With a loaded foot, there is no transverse arch at the level of the MTHs (Fig. 2.8b). All MTHs and the sesamoid bones of the first MTP joint lie on the ground and bear weight. Should a transverse arch at the level of the MTHs be detected under stress, this would indicate a pathological finding.

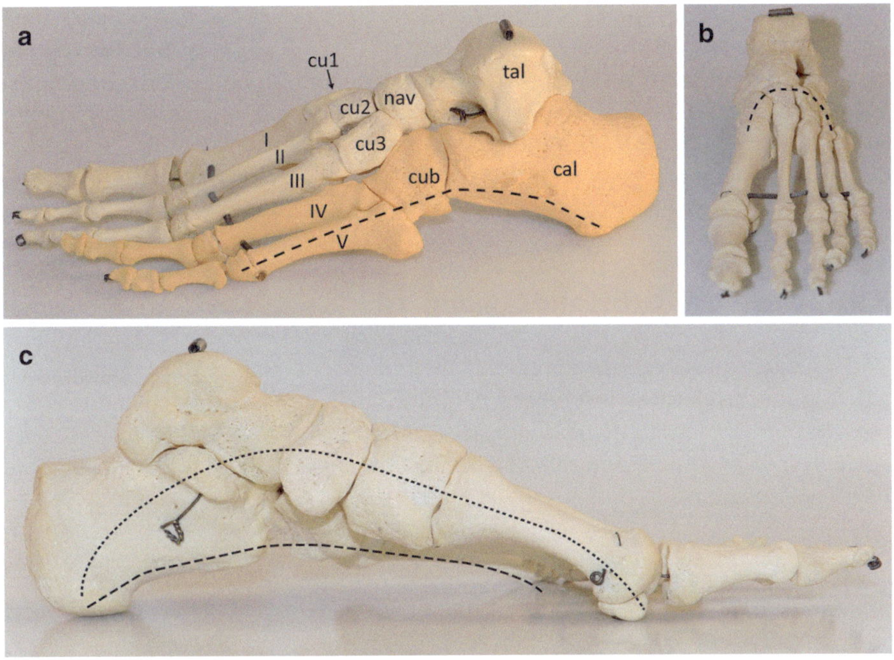

Fig. 2.7 Arches and columns of the foot, (**a**) lateral column *(yellow marked)*: calcaneus *(cal)*, cuboid *(cub)*, metatarsal bones 4 and 5 *(IV and V)*, medial column *(noncolored)*: talus *(tal)*, navicular *(nav)*, medial cuneiform *(cu1)*, intermediate cuneiform *(cu2)*, lateral cuneiform *(cu3)*, metatarsal bones 1 to 3 *(I–III)*, lateral longitudinal arch *(dashed line);* skeleton of a left foot, lateral view, (**b**) transverse arch *(dashed line)*; skeleton of a left foot, ventral view, (**c**) medial longitudinal arch *(dotted line)*, lateral longitudinal arch *(dashed line)*; skeleton of a left foot, medial view

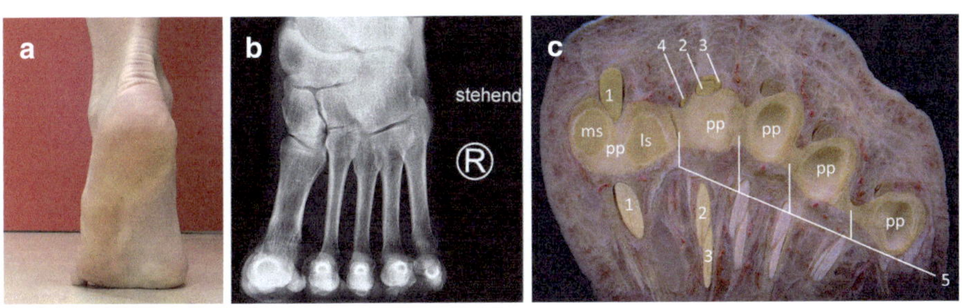

Fig. 2.8 Right foot at propulsion, (**a**) clinical picture (**b**) tangential X-ray of a loaded foot in propulsion. All MTHs and the sesamoids of the first MTP joint are aligned in the transversal plane. There is no transverse arch at the level of the MTHs (X-ray kindly provided by PD Dr. T. Schaub, Institute for Radiology, University of Bonn, Germany) (**c**) Transverse section through the sole of the foot at the level of the plantar plates of the metatarsophalangeal joints (cranial view). The sesamoids of the hallux and the MTHs of the lesser toes are aligned in the transverse plane, plantar plates *(pp)*, lateral sesamoid *(ls)*, medial sesamoid *(ms)*, flexor hallucis longus tendon (*1*), flexor digitorum longus tendon (*2*), flexor digitorum brevis tendon (*3*), first lumbrical (*4*), deep transverse metatarsal ligament (*5*) (specimen kindly provided by Prof. Dr. rer.nat. J. Koebke, Centre for Anatomy, University of Cologne)

Various theoretical *models of the foot* have been created to better understand its complexity through strong simplification. One of these is the 'three-point stand,' which is based on a supposed transverse arch at the level of the MTHs, even under load. According to this concept, a 'splayfoot' is assumed if the 2nd to 4th MTH gets in contact with the ground under load. The use of this model for diagnosis and therapy is an incorrect transfer of a theoretical model into clinical practice.

2.5 Joints, Muscles and Ligaments

This chapter describes the joints and their range of motion. The musculature required for this purpose is arranged into functional groups, extrinsic and intrinsic muscles. Of the multitude of ligaments and smaller articulating structures, only those have been included in this chapter that are necessary for understanding the functional relationships during gait.

2.5.1 Joints of the Ankle

Connecting the foot with the lower leg, the *ankle joint* (*tibiotalar joint*, *tibiocrural joint*) is formed by the upper joint surface of the talus (trochlea tali) and the lower ends of the tibia and fibula. This joint allows movement predominantly in the sagittal plane (plantar flexion up to 50° and dorsal extension (= dorsiflexion) up to 30°) along an axis running through both ankles (Fig. 2.9).

As the foot is movable in all three planes, its range of motion must be increased with additional joints. The talus plays a central role in this process, as it is linked with the lower leg and the lamina pedis. Together with the calcaneus and navicular bone, it forms two joints that are functionally linked, the *subtalar joint* and the *talocalcaneonavicular joint*. In German-language literature, these two joints are grouped together to form the 'lower ankle joint' because they share an oblique axis and are regarded as a functional unit. The entire sole of the unloaded foot can rotate inwards (inversion = lifting of the medial foot margin up to 20°, Fig. 2.10d) and outwards (Eversion = lifting of the lateral foot margin up to 10°, Fig. 2.10c) around this axis (Figs. 2.10a and 2.11).

2.5.2 Extrinsic Muscles

All movements in the above-mentioned joints are controlled by muscle groups that originate at the lower leg and attach to the bones of the foot (Figs. 2.12 and 2.13).

The tendons running in front (ventral) of the transverse axis of the upper ankle joint raise the tip of the foot (dorsiflexion, see also Fig. 2.9d), while those running behind (dorsal) the axis lower the tip of the foot (plantar flexion, see also Fig. 2.9c). Due to the oblique course of the axis of the talocalcaneonavicular joint (lower ankle

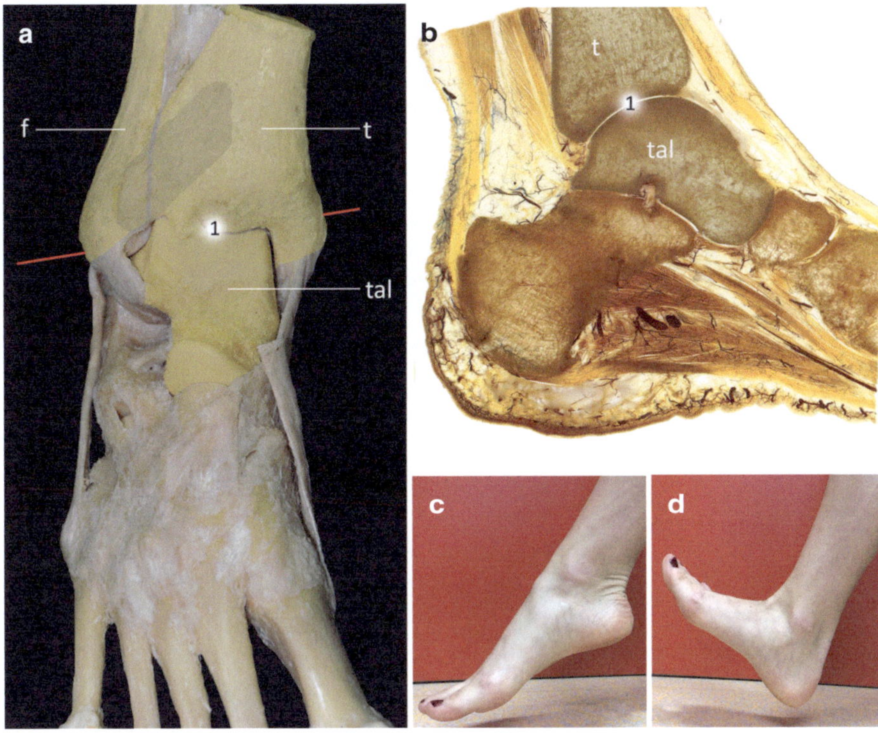

Fig. 2.9 Ankle joint (talocrural joint) (**a**) anatomical preparation of the ankle joint *(1)*, ventral view, associated bones market yellow, tibia *(t)*, fibula *(f)*, talus *(tal)*, transverse axis of the ankle joint *(red line)* (**b**) sagittal plastination slice through the ankle joint *(1)*, tibia *(t)*, talus *(tal)*, (**c**) plantarflexion of the foot (**d**) dorsiflexion of the foot

joint), muscles whose tendons run medially in relation to the axis, rotate the sole of the foot medially (inversion, supination, Fig. 2.14). Muscles whose tendons run laterally to the axis rotate the sole of the foot laterally (eversion, pronation, Fig. 2.14).

2.5.2.1 Extensors

The extensors of the foot (dorsiflexors) are located on the front side (ventral) of the lower leg (Fig. 2.15). If the foot is in the air, the tibialis anterior muscle permits dorsiflexion of the entire foot. This movement is complemented by the long toe extensors (extensor hallucis longus and extensor digitorum longus), which both additionally extend the toes. The tibialis anterior muscle lowers the foot slowly after the heel strike. It holds the medial margin of the forefoot up so that the lateral side of the foot's sole contacts the ground first.

2.5.2.2 Flexors

The flexors of the foot (plantar flexors) are situated in the calf and can be divided into a deep and a superficial component (Fig. 2.16).

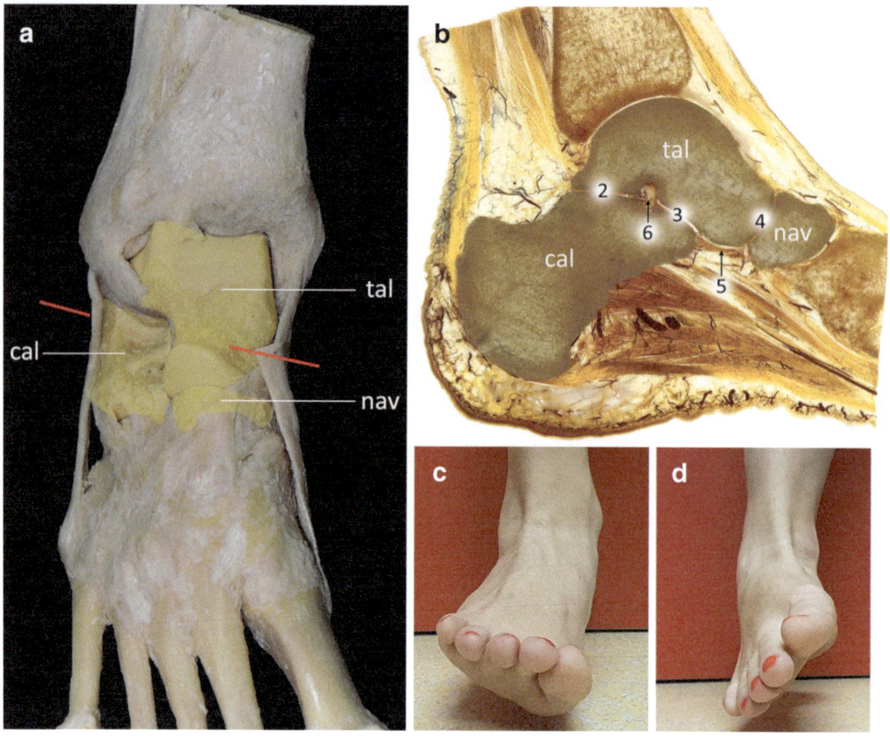

Fig. 2.10 Subtalar and talocalcaneonavicular joint (**a**) anatomical preparation of the talocalcaneonavicular joint *(associated bones marked in yellow)*, talus *(tal)*, calcaneus *(cal)*, *navicular (nav)*, common oblique axis of the subtalar and talocalcaneonavicular joint *(red line)* (**b**) sagittal plastination slice through the subtalar *(2)* and the talocalcaneonavicular joint *(3 and 4)* formed by talus *(tal)*, calcaneus *(cal) and* navicular *(nav)*. Both joints are separated from each other by the interosseous talocalcaneal ligament *(6)*. The articular socket of the talocalcaneonavicular joint is enlarged by the plantar calcaneonavicular ligament *(5)*. (**c**) eversion of the unloaded foot (**d**) inversion of the unloaded foot

The soleus muscle and the gastrocnemius muscle (together called the triceps surae muscle), which form the superficial part, are attached to the calcaneal tuberosity by the Achilles tendon. The deep plantar flexors (tibialis posterior, flexor digitorum longus, flexor hallucis longus) are located between the triceps surae and the bones. Their tendons run behind the medial malleolus to the medial margin of the foot (tibialis posterior) and to the toes (flexor hallucis longus and flexor digitorum longus muscles). Combined, these muscles create plantar flexion and inversion of the foot (see also Figs. 2.9c and 2.10d). For the tibialis posterior muscle, inversion means maintaining the medial longitudinal arch under load. It acts as an antagonist to the fibularis muscles and ensures that the lateral margin of the sole of the foot is pressed onto the ground.

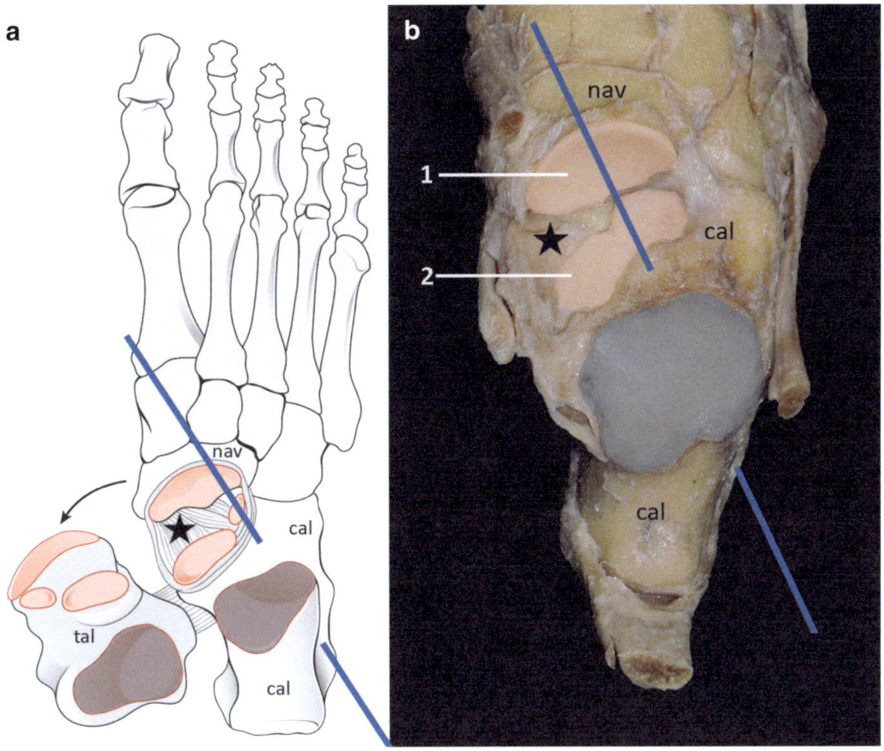

Fig. 2.11 (**a**) Schematic drawing of the lamina pedis and the subtalar and talocalcaneonavicular joint, cranial view. Talus removed and turned upside down so that the talar articular surfaces for calcaneus and navicular are visible. The articular surfaces of the subtalar joint are marked in dark grey, those of the talocalcaneonavicular joint in orange. Talus *(tal)*, calcaneus *(cal)*, navicular *(nav)*, plantar calcaneonavicular or spring ligament *(black star)*, oblique common axis of subtalar and talocalcaneonavicular joint *(blue line)* (**b**) anatomical preparation of the lamina pedis, calcaneal articular surface of subtalar joint *(grey)*, calcaneal articular surfaces *(orange, 2)* and navicular articular surface *(orange, 1)* for talocalcaneonavicular joint, plantar calcaneonavicular ligament *(black star)*, oblique common axis of subtalar and talocalcaneonavicular joint *(blue line)*

2.5.2.3 Fibularis Muscles

The fibularis muscles (fibularis longus and fibularis brevis) are located on the lateral side of the lower leg (Fig. 2.17). They are responsible for lifting the lateral margin of the foot (see also Figs. 2.14d, e). As they run behind the lateral malleolus, they also act as plantar flexors of the foot. The short fibularis tendon extends to the lateral margin of the foot and attaches to the tuberosity of the base of the 5th metatarsal bone (see also Fig. 2.12).

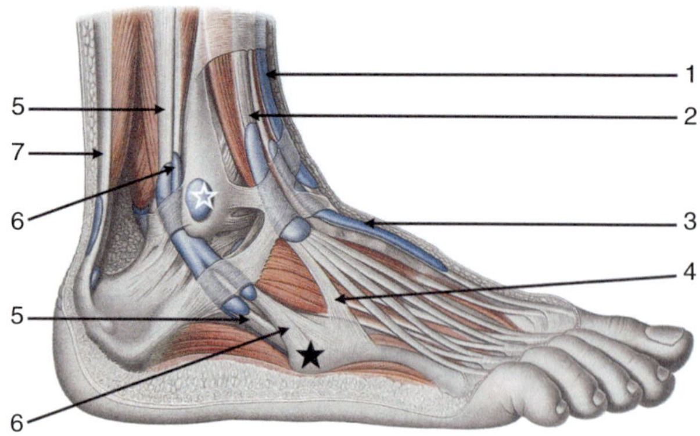

Fig. 2.12 Schematic drawing of extrinsic muscle insertions at the foot (lateral view), tendons of: tibialis anterior *(1)*, extensor digitorum longus *(2)*, extensor hallucis longus *(3)*, fibularis (peroneus) tertius *(4)*, fibularis (peroneus) longus *(5)*, fibularis (peroneus) brevis *(6)*, Achilles tendon *(7)*, lateral malleolus *(white edged star)*, 5th metatarsal base *(black star)*. (source Lanz-Wachsmuth [4])

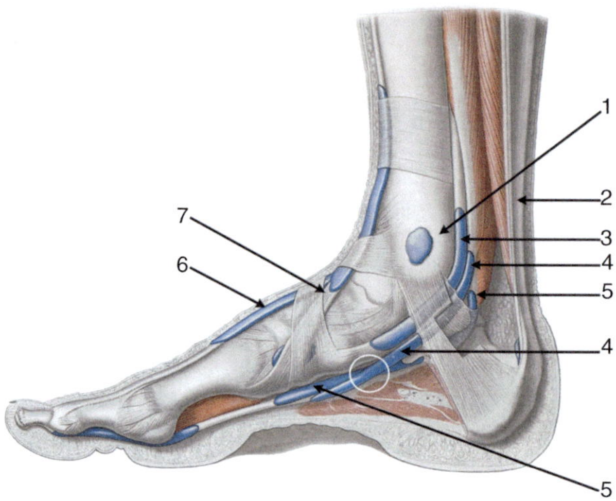

Fig. 2.13 schematic drawing of extrinsic muscle insertions at the foot (medial view), malleolus medialis (1), Achilles tendon (2), tendons of: tibialis posterior (3), flexor digitorum longus *(4)*, flexor hallucis longus *(5)*, extensor hallucis longus *(6)*, tibialis anterior *(7)*, chiasma plantare *(white edged circle, crossover of 4 and 5)*, (source Lanz-Wachsmuth [4])

The fibularis longus tendon also extends to the lateral margin of the foot but does not end here. It crosses the lateral margin of the foot and runs diagonally in the sole of the foot towards its attachment at the base of the first metatarsal bone and the medial cuboid bone (Fig. 2.18). One action thus is that it rotates the medial cuneiform and the first metatarsal with its medial margin to the plantar site (pronation). The double redirection of the tendon at the lateral malleolus and lateral margin of the foot also allows the muscle to attract the first metatarsal and the medial cuneiform towards the 2nd ray. This movements actively stabilises the

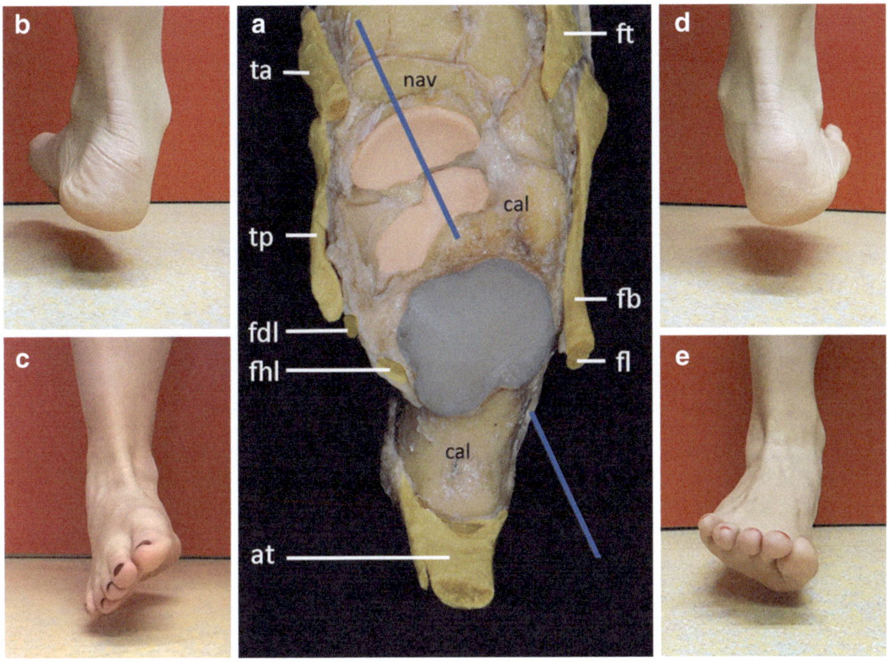

Fig. 2.14 Lamina pedis (**a**) lamina pedis with the combined oblique axis of the subtalar and talo-calcaneonavicular joints *(blue line)*, tendons of inverting muscles extending medially from this axis, tendons of everting muscles laterally, tendons of invertors: tibialis posterior (tp), triceps surae (Achilles tendon, at), flexor digitorum longus (fdl), flexor hallucis longus (fhl), tibialis anterior (ta); tendons of evertors: fibularis longus (fl), fibularis brevis (fb), fibularis tertius (ft) (**b**) inversion of the heel (**c**) supination of the forefoot (**d**) eversion of the heel (**e**) pronation of the forefoot

transverse arch. Therapeutically, this movement could be utilised to counteract a hallux valgus deformity at an early stage. But some argue that this may worsen the rotation [5]. Furthermore, the fibularis longus pulls the first metatarsal bone in plantar direction and therefore presses the first MTH onto the ground during propulsion.

2.5.3 Intrinsic Muscles

In contrast to the long extrinsic foot muscles, which have their origin at the lower leg, the short intrinsic foot muscles originate in the foot and also attach there. All plantar intrinsic muscles stabilise the arches of the foot as well as the first and 5th ray. The most important function of these muscles is the axial alignment and stabilisation of the stretched toes on the ground under load. They are described together with their function during the course of this chapter (Fig. 2.19).

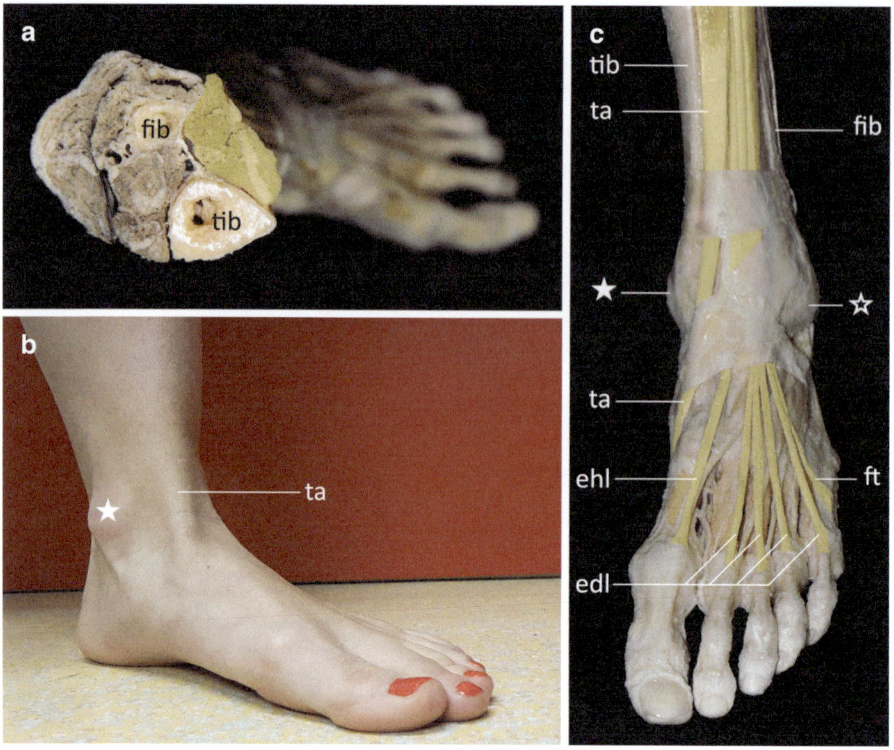

Fig. 2.15 Extensors (**a**) anatomical specimen, cross section through lower leg, fibula (fib), tibia (tib), extensors (*yellow*) (**b**) left foot, tendon of tibialis anterior (ta), medial malleolus (*star*) (**c**) anatomical specimen, ventral view, tibialis anterior (ta), extensor hallucis longus (ehl), extensor digitorum longus (edl), fibularis tertius (ft), tibia (tib), fibula (fib), medial malleolus (*full white star*), lateral malleolus (*white edged star*)

2.5.4 Toes and Toe Joints

The toes increase the contact area of the foot while walking and act as a lever for the foot during propulsion. They can only accomplish these functions if they are pressed onto the ground straight and in a stretched position.

The toes articulate with the distal ends of the metatarsal bones in the metatarsophalangeal joints (MTP joints). These are condyloid joints (= ellipsoid joint), which in principle could allow multidirectional mobility of the toes. Due to massive collateral ligaments, mobility is strongly restricted so that movements are primarily in the sagittal plane. The MTP joints enable plantar flexion of the toes (up to about 40°) and, to a greater extent, dorsiflexion (active about 50°, passive about 90°). In comparison with the metacarpophalangeal joints of the hand, the much greater capacity for dorsiflexion of the toes is an adaptation to the needs of walking during propulsion. The phalanges are connected to each other by interphalangeal joints

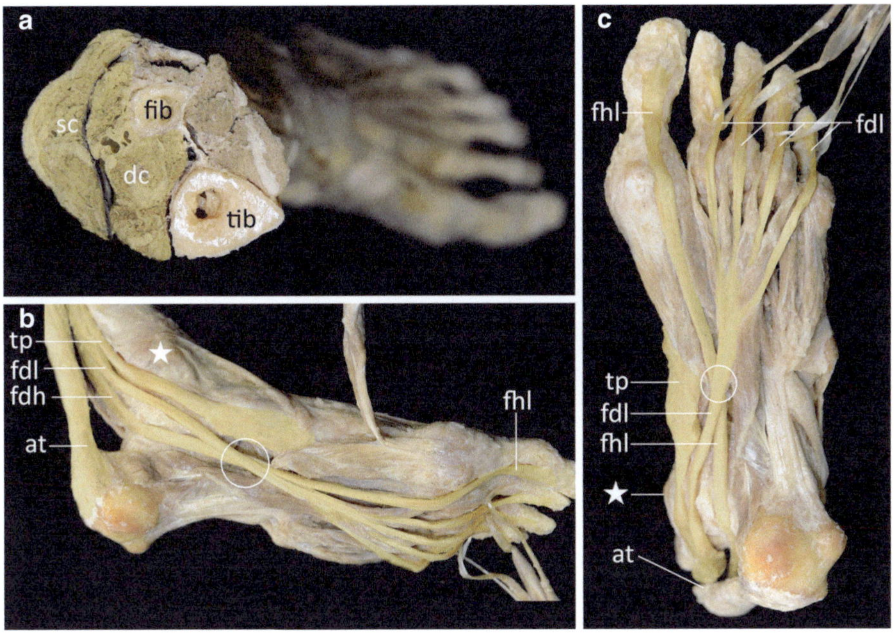

Fig. 2.16 Plantarflexors (**a**) anatomical specimen, cross section through the lower leg, fibula (fib), tibia (tib), flexors (*yellow*), deep compartment (dc), superficial compartment (sc) (**b**) anatomical specimen, medial view, tibialis posterior tendon (tp), flexor digitorum longus tendon (fdl), flexor hallucis longus tendon (fhl), Achilles tendon (at), chiasma plantare (white edged *circle*), medial malleolus (white star) (**c**) anatomical specimen, plantar view, tibialis posterior (tp), flexor hallucis longus (fhl), flexor digitorum longus (fdl), Achilles tendon (at), medial malleolus (full *white star*)

(IP joints), the proximal interphalangeal joints (PIP joints) and the distal interphalangeal joints (DIP joints). In the IP joints, which are hinge joints, the toes can only be plantarflexed and dorsiflexed. Like the thumb, the great toe has two phalanges, the lesser toes have three (Fig. 2.20).

The action of the various tendons on these joints is shown in Fig. 2.20. All tendons that run along the dorsal side of the transverse axes of the toe joints (see Fig. 2.20c) lift the toes from the ground (dorsiflexion of the toes). All the tendons that run on the plantar side (see Fig. 2.20b) press the toes against the ground (plantarflexion of the toes). The effect of the flexor digitorum longus and brevis on the MTP joint is minimal, as they are not directly attached to the proximal phalanx. The plantar flexion in the MTP joint is mainly achieved by the interossei muscles and the plantar aponeurosis (see Fig. 2.20a). A dorsiflexion in the IP joints is only possible starting from a plantarflexed position and ending at the neutral position. 'Overstretching' is prevented passively by the joint capsules and actively by the long tendons of the toe flexors (flexor digitorum longus (FDL) and brevis (FDB) muscle). With a loaded foot, the toes are pressed onto the ground by plantar flexion.

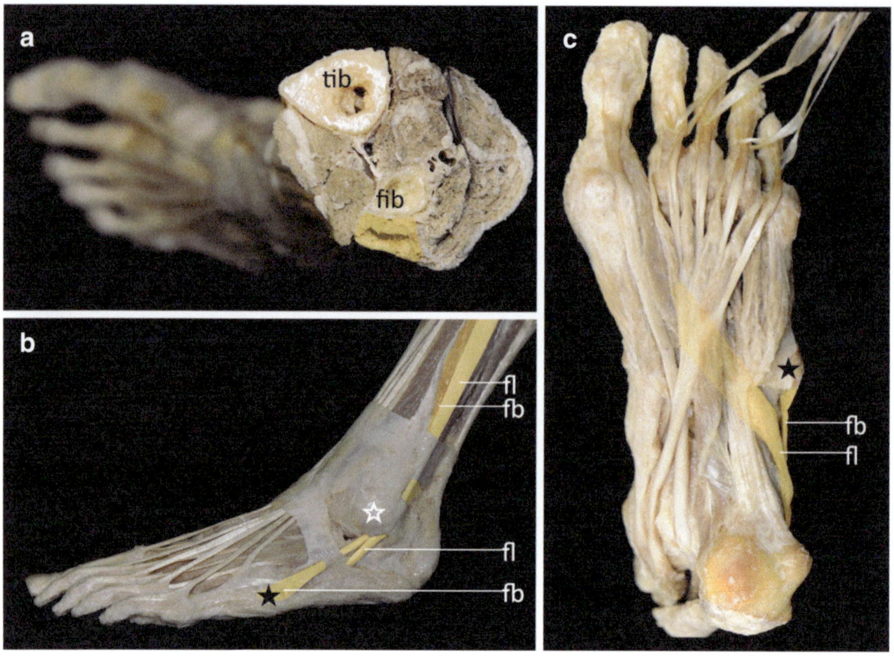

Fig. 2.17 Fibularis muscles (**a**) anatomical specimen, cross section through the lower leg, fibula (fib), tibia (tib), fibularis muscles (*yellow*) (**b**) anatomical specimen, lateral view, fibularis longus tendon (fl), fibularis brevis tendon (fb), lateral malleolus (white edged star), base of 5th metatarsal bone (*black star*) (**c**) anatomical specimen, plantar view, fibularis longus tendon (fl), fibularis brevis tendon (fb), base of 5th metatarsal bone (*black star*)

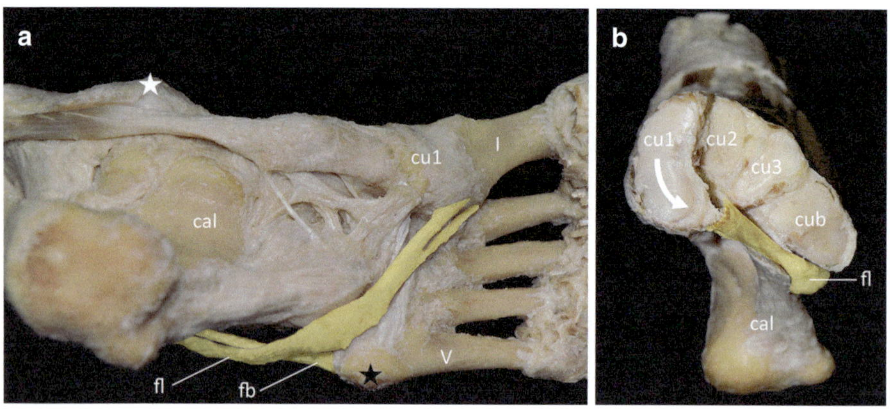

Fig. 2.18 Fibularis longus muscle; active stabilisation of the first ray and the transverse arch by pronating the medial cuneiform and the first metatarsal bone. (**a**) anatomical specimen, plantar view, fibularis longus tendon (fl), fibularis brevis tendon (fb), medial malleolus (*white star*), calcaneus (cal), first metatarsal (I), medial cuneiform (cu1), 5th metatarsal (V), base of 5th metatarsal bone (*black star*) (**b**) anatomical specimen, forefoot exarticulated, ventral view of the transverse arch at the level of the cuneiforms (cu1, cu2, cu3) and cuboid (cub), medial cuneiform (cu1) is pronated (*white arrow*) by fibularis longus tendon (fl), calcaneus (cal)

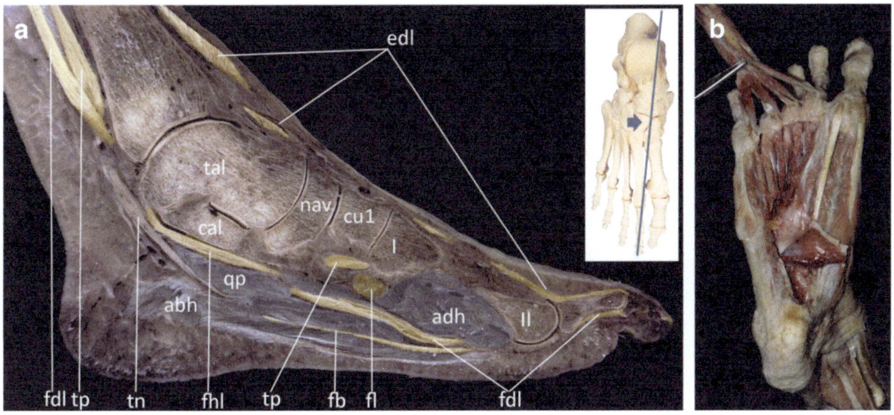

Fig. 2.19 Active stabilisation of the arches of the foot by short intrinsic muscles of the sole (*blue*) and tendons of long extrinsic muscles of the lower leg (*yellow*), (**a**) anatomical specimen, sagittal section, lateral view, tendon of extensor digitorum longus (edl), tendon of flexor digitorum longus (fdl), tibialis nerve (tn), tendon of flexor hallucis longus (fhl), tendon of tibialis posterior (tp), tendon of flexor digitorum brevis (fdb), tendon of fibularis longus (fl), abductor hallucis (abh), quadratus plantae (qp), adductor hallucis (adh), tibia (tib), talus (tal), sustentaculum tali (cal), navicular (nav), medial cuneiform (cu1), base of first metatarsal bone (I), 2nd metatarsal head (II) (**b**) short intrinsic musculature at the sole of the foot, anatomical specimen, plantar view

2.5.4.1 Extensor Hood

The tendons of toe dorsiflexors (extensor digitorum longus and brevis, lumbricals) converge on the dorsum of the toes. They are coated with connective tissue, that also wraps the proximal phalanx similar to a hood (extensor hood) (Fig. 2.21). The extensor hood is firmly anchored on both sides of the toe in the plantar plate of the MTP joint and surrounds the proximal phalanx like a loop. By pulling the extensor tendons, the loop is tightened, and the proximal phalanx is 'pulled up' onto the MTH. This is termed dorsiflexion of the toe in the MTP joint.

2.5.4.2 Plantar Plates and Interossei

The interossei muscles are situated between the metatarsal bones and run towards the toes. Each of the lesser toes (except of the 5th toe) is reached by two interossei muscles. The 5th toe has only one interosseous on its medial side. They pass to the medial and lateral side of the bases of the proximal phalanges and plantarflex the lesser toes at the MTP joints (Fig. 2.22). Together with the plantar aponeurosis, the interossei muscles are also attached to the plantar capsules of the MTP joints, which are thickened by fibrous cartilage to plantar plates. The plantar plates function as pads for the MTHs and are firmly attached to the proximal phalanges. Thus, the traction of the interossei and the plantar aponeurosis will be transmitted to the toes. With a loaded foot this causes the proximal phalanges to be pressed onto the ground with considerable force and the plantar plates to be fixed under the MTHs (see also Fig. 2.20a).

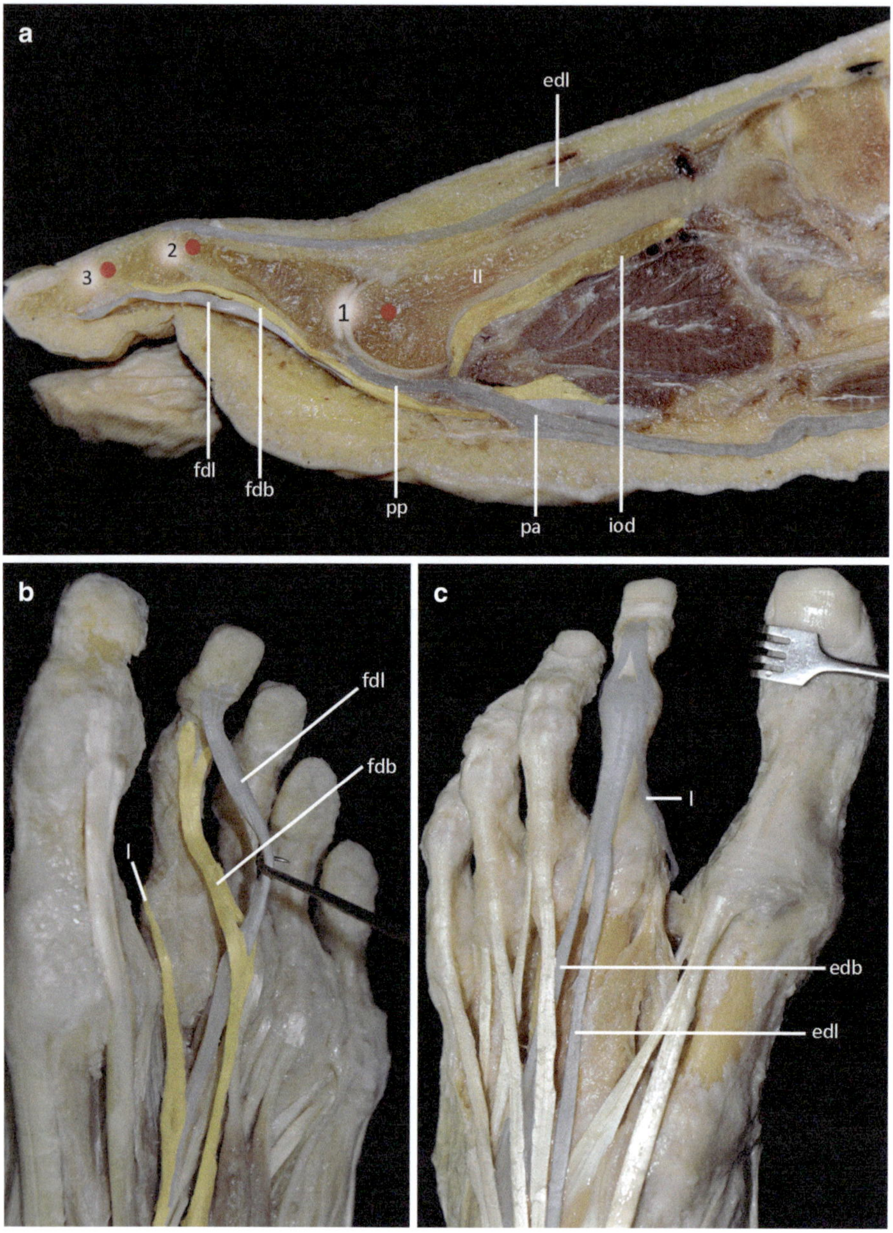

Fig. 2.20 Toe joints and muscles that act on the toes (**a**) anatomical specimen, sagittal section through the 2nd ray, lateral view, MTP joint (1), PIP joint (2), DIP joint (3), transverse axes of the joints (*red dots*), tendons of extensor digitorum longus (edl), flexor digitorum longus (fdl), flexor digitorum brevis (fdb), plantar plate of 2nd MTP joint (pp), plantar aponeurosis (pa), 2nd metatarsal (II), interosseous dorsalis (iod) (**b**) anatomical specimen, plantar view, tendons of flexor digitorum longus (fdl), flexor digitorum brevis (fdb), lumbricalis (l) (**c**) anatomical specimen, dorsal view, tendons of extensor digitorum longus *(edl)* and extensor digitorum brevis *(edb)*, lumbricalis (l)

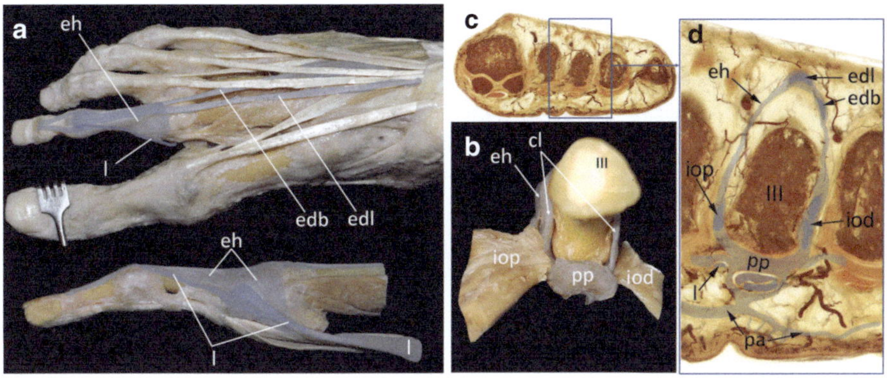

Fig. 2.21 Extensor hood (**a**) anatomical specimen, preparation of the tendons of extensor digitorum longus (edl) and brevis *(edb)*, 1st lumbrical *(l)* and extensor hood *(eh)* (**b**) anatomical specimen, preparation of the 3rd MTP joint, dorsal view, 3rd metatarsal bone (III), extensor hood (eh), collateral ligaments *(cl)*, plantar plate (pp), dorsal interosseous *(iod)*, plantar interosseous *(iop)* (**c**) frontal section at the level of the MTHs, plastination slice (**d**) detail *(blue lined)* of 3rd MTP joint, 3rd metatarsal *(III)*, extensor hood *(eh)*, tendon of extensor digitorum longus *(edl)*, extensor digitorum brevis *(edb)*, plantar interosseous *(iop)*, dorsal interosseous *(iod)*, plantar plate *(pp)*, lumbrical *(l)*, plantar aponeurosis *(pa)*

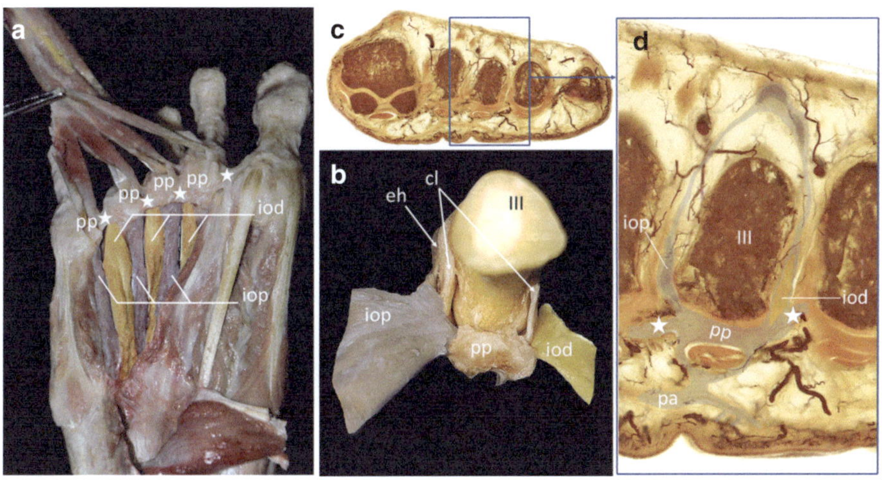

Fig. 2.22 Interossei and plantar plates (**a**) anatomical specimen, plantar view, preparation of the dorsal interossei muscles *(iod in yellow)*, plantar interossei muscles *(iop in blue)*, plantar plates *(pp)* and the deep transverse metatarsal ligament (*white stars*) (**b**) anatomical specimen, preparation of the 3rd MTP joint, dorsal view, 3rd metatarsal bone (III), extensor hood (eh), collateral ligaments *(cl)*, plantar plate (pp), dorsal interosseous *(iod)*, plantar interosseous *(iop)* (**c**) frontal section at the level of the MTHs, plastination slice (**d**) detail *(blue lined)* of 3rd MTP joint, 3rd metatarsal *(III)*, plantar interosseous *(iop)*, dorsal interosseous *(iod)*, plantar plate *(pp)*, deep transverse metatarsal ligament (*white stars*), plantar aponeurosis *(pa)*

The plantar plate can be seen as a kind of nodal point. Here, the structures acting on the MTP joint are interwoven and stabilise the joint. The well-balanced traction of these structures keeps the plantar plates in their position under the MTHs and the toes correctly aligned in the MTP joints. The deep transverse metatarsal ligament connects the plantar plates to each other. Its fibres are interwoven on both sides with the adjacent plantar plates (see also Figs. 2.8c and 2.22a and d).

2.5.4.3 Lumbricals

The lumbricals are important for straight alignment of the 2nd to 5th toe. They originate plantar from the four tendons of the flexor digitorum longus, run along the medial side of the 2nd to 5th toe and attach to their extensor tendons (Fig. 2.23). The extensor digitorum longus is only about a quarter as strong as the flexor digitorum longus and cannot completely stretch the DIP joints without the help of the lumbricals. Due to their position on the medial side of the toe, the lumbricals prevent the lesser toes from deviating laterally and turning with their lateral surface to the ground. This applies especially to the 3rd to 5th toe.

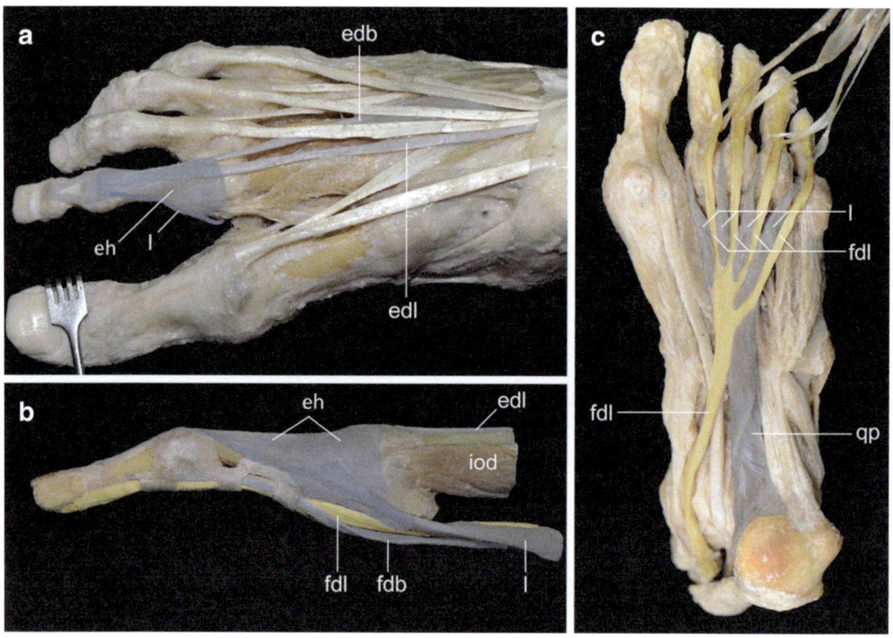

Fig. 2.23 Lumbricals and quadratus plantae (**a**) anatomical specimen, preparation of the extensor hood *(eh)* and the lumbrical *(l)* (**b**) anatomical specimen, preparation of the 2nd toe, medial view, extensor hood (eh), lumbrical *(l)* with its mobile origin at the tendon of the flexor digitorum longus *(fdl in yellow)*, dorsal interosseous *(iod)*, extensor hood *(eh)*, tendon of extensor digitorum longus *(edl)*, extensor digitorum brevis *(edb)* (**c**) anatomical specimen, plantar view, preparation of the four lumbricals *(l)*, quadratus plantae *(qp)* and tendon(s) of the flexor digitorum longus *(fdl in yellow)*

2.5.4.4 Ouadratus Plantae (and Its Insufficiency)

Another intrinsic muscle with an influence on the lesser toes is the quadratus plantae. It also ensures the optimal position of the 2nd to 5th toe in a healthy foot. The quadratus plantae originates with great variability at the calcaneus and attaches laterally to the tendon of the flexor digitorum longus (see also Fig. 2.23c). This enables it to correct the oblique direction of the flexor digitorum longus tendons parallel to the axes of the lesser toes. Without this correction, the flexor digitorum longus would pull the lesser toes medially and turn them with their lateral sides to the ground. Weakness of the quadratus plantae leads to a typical misalignment of the lesser toes (Fig. 2.24).

2.5.4.5 Great Toe, First MTP Joint and Sesamoid Complex

The first ray and to a minor extend also the 5th ray are supported by strong intrinsic musculature. This is a relic from the period in the evolution when the foot was still used for gripping and holding. This musculature now controls the position of the two outer rays (first and 5th) and balances the foot during upright walking under the body's weight. All the intrinsic muscles of the first ray, which are situated in the sole of the foot, press the great toe onto the ground. These are the flexor hallucis brevis, abductor and adductor hallucis (Fig. 2.25a). The two latter also prevent the great toe from deviating medially and laterally. At the level of the TMT-1 joint, the first ray is additionally stabilised by long tendons of extrinsic muscles (Fig. 2.25b).

During the propulsion phase, the toes in the MTP joints are passively dorsiflexed. Consequently, the plantar structures of the first MTP joint carry most of the body's weight at that time (see also Sect. 2.6). For protection of the first MTH, two sesamoid bones are embedded in the plantar plate of the first MTP joint. In addition to their load-bearing properties, they increase the distance between the transverse axis of the first MTP joint and the muscles that plantar flex the great toe (flexor hallucis longus and brevis, abductor hallucis, adductor hallucis). As a result, the torque and therefore the contact pressure of the great toe on the ground are increased. Further protection for the first MTH is provided by a stirrup-configuration built of the proximal phalanx and the sesamoid complex. The ground reaction forces acting on the

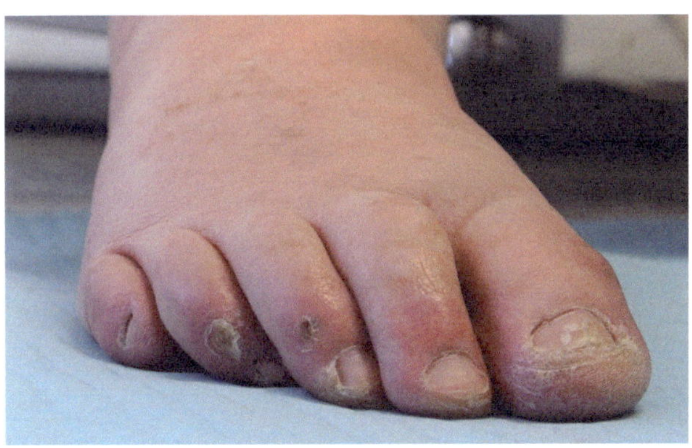

Fig. 2.24 Insufficiency of the quadratus plantae with torsion of D3–D5

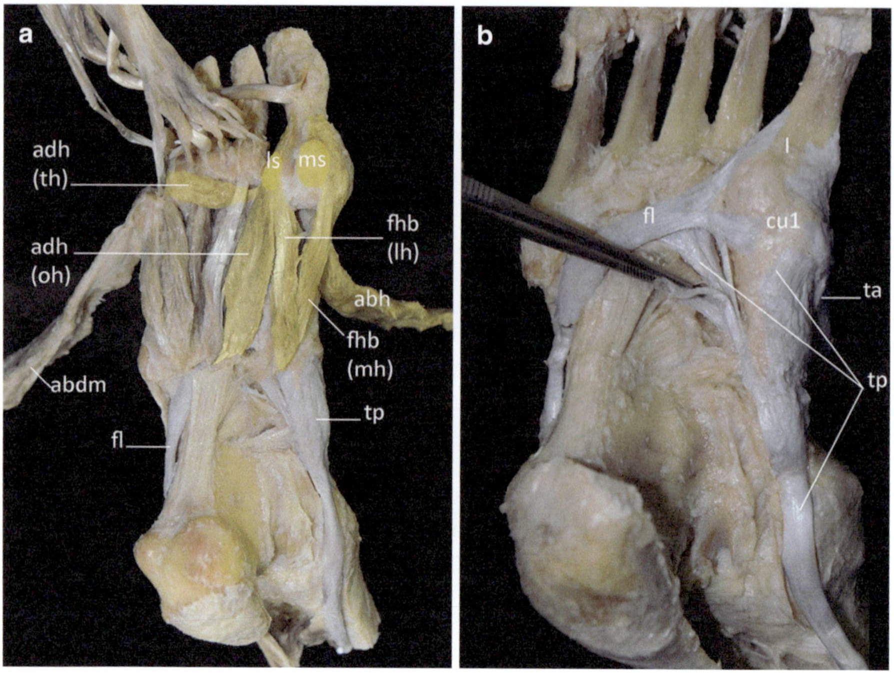

Fig. 2.25 Muscular stabilisation of the first ray (**a**) anatomical specimen, plantar view, intrinsic musculature of the great toe marked in yellow, flexor hallucis brevis *(fhb)* with its medial head *(mh)* and lateral head *(lh)*, abductor hallucis *(abh)*, *ad*ductor hallucis *(adh)* with its oblique head *(oh)* and its transverse head *(th)*, lateral sesamoid *(ls)*, medial sesamoid *(ms)*, extrinsic stabilisers of the first ray *(blue)* tibialis posterior *(tp)*, fibularis longus *(fl)* (**b**) extrinsic stabilisers of the TMT-1 joint and therefore the first ray *(blue)* tendons of: tibialis posterior *(tp)*, fibularis longus *(fl)*, tibialis anterior *(ta)*, first metatarsal *(I)*, medial cuneiform *(cu1)*

first MTP joint are thus shared over a larger area of the first MTH. The long flexor tendon runs in the channel between both sesamoid bones and reaches the base of the distal phalanx. Even under maximum load, the groove between the two sesamoids is preserved. As a result, the flexor hallucis longus tendon stays unaffected during propulsion (Fig. 2.26).

If the long extensor and flexor tendons run anatomically correctly in the longitudinal axis of the first ray and the traction of the abductor and adductor hallucis is well balanced, the flexor hallucis longus will press the distal phalanx against the ground in correctly straightened position. If the interaction of these muscles does not work correctly, the first metatarsal bone deviates medially, while the great toe is pulled laterally and rotates to the ground with its medial side. The sesamoid complex stays where it was (see also Sect. 2.5.5).

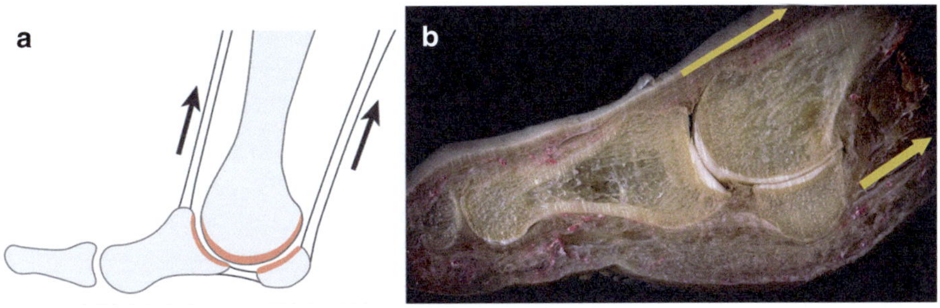

Fig. 2.26 'Stirrup position' of the first MTH (**a**) schematic drawing of the first MTH between the base of the proximal phalanx of the first toe and the sesamoid complex in end position and (**b**) as a sagittal section of an anatomical specimen, as it appears in an unloaded foot (by friendly courtesy of Prof. Dr. J. Koebke, Centre of Anatomy, University of Cologne)

2.5.4.6 Plantar Aponeurosis and Windlass Mechanism

The plantar aponeurosis is a subcutaneous tendinous plate fixed to the heel, which is distally divided into five longitudinal fibre strands, one for each toe. The longitudinal fibre strands are connected to each other by transverse fibre strands and by sagittal septa with the plantar plates of the MTP joints (Fig. 2.27). Due to its connection with the plantar plates, the traction of the plantar aponeurosis is transmitted to the proximal phalanges of the toes.

When the foot is loaded during the gait cycle, the longitudinal arch flattens and so tightens the plantar aponeurosis. Thus, the toes are pressed onto the ground. This passive plantar flexion of the toes in the MTP joints by the plantar aponeurosis is called the *reverse windlass mechanism* (Fig. 2.28).

When the heel is raised, the foot rotates around the transverse axes of the MTP joints. Consequently, the longitudinal strands of the plantar aponeurosis are wound around the MTHs and the toes remain pressed on the ground in their position. The tensed plantar aponeurosis inverts the heel, raises the medial longitudinal arch and shortens the foot, which also stiffens. As the MTHs are used as winches for the plantar aponeurosis, this mechanism is termed as *windlass-mechanism* (Fig. 2.29).

The windlass mechanism is active during propulsion, while the reverse windlass mechanism has its significance during midstance. The reverse windlass mechanism can be seen as a prerequisite for the windlass mechanism.

At the great toe the windlass mechanism is most effective, as the first MTH is the largest in diameter, which is further increased by the sesamoid bones. In this way, the first distal phalanx with its toe pad takes 30% of the weight at the end of terminal stance, 15% is carried by the first MTH and 30% by the head of the 2nd metatarsal bone [6].

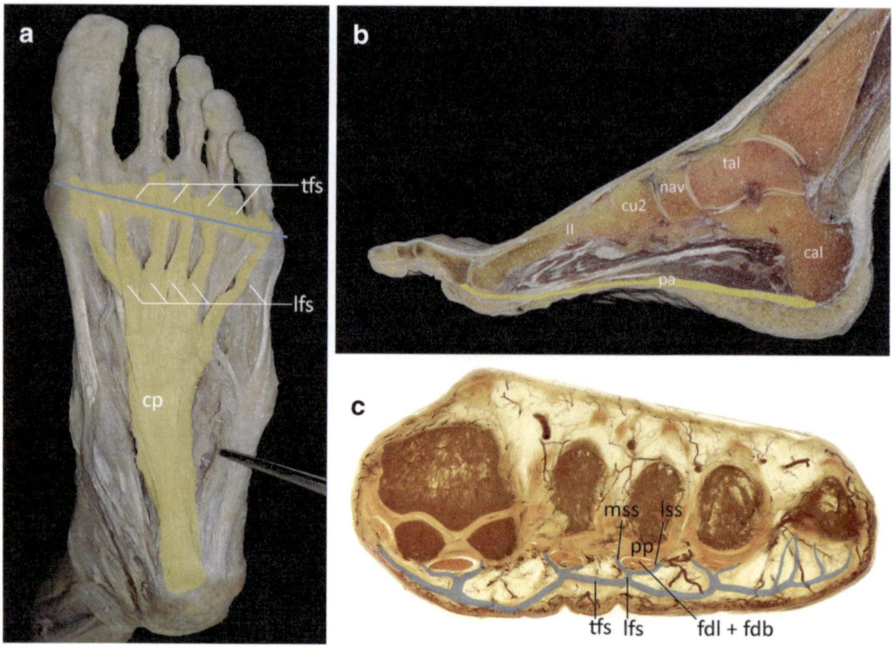

Fig. 2.27 Plantar aponeurosis (**a**) anatomical specimen, plantar view, plantar aponeurosis *(yellow)* with its central part *(cp)*, longitudinal fibre strands *(lfs)* and transverse fibre strand *(tfs)* (**b**) anatomical specimen, sagittal section, medial view, plantar aponeurosis *(pa)*, calcaneus *(cal)*, talus *(tal), navicular (nav)*, intermediate cuneiform *(cu2)*, 2nd metatarsal *(II)* (**c**) frontal section at the level of the MTHs *(blue line in a)*, plastination slice, plantar aponeurosis *(blue)* with its transverse fibre strand *(tfs)*, longitudinal fibre strands *(lfs)* and sagittal septa to the plantar plates of the MTP joints *(medial sagittal septum (mss) and lateral sagittal septum (lss)*, tendon of flexor digitorum longus *(fdl)* and brevis *(fdb))*

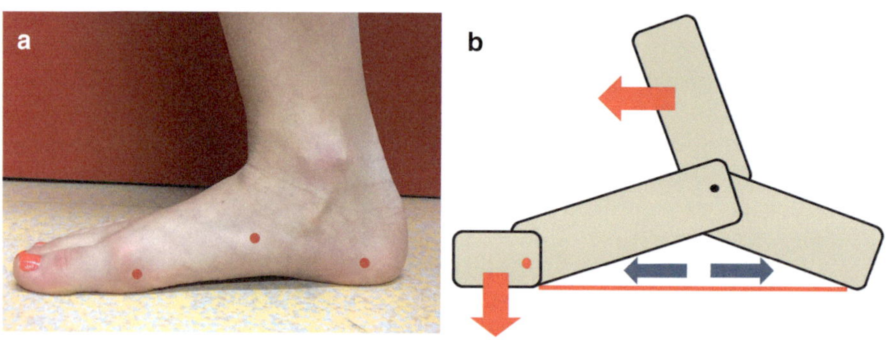

Fig. 2.28 Reverse windlass mechanism (**a**) loaded foot in plantigrade position, *red dots* mark 1st MTH, navicular bone and calcaneal tuber (**b**) schematic drawing: Loading the foot in the plantigrade position activates the reverse windlass mechanism. The longitudinal arch flattens and tightens the plantar aponeurosis. Therefore the toes will pressed to the ground

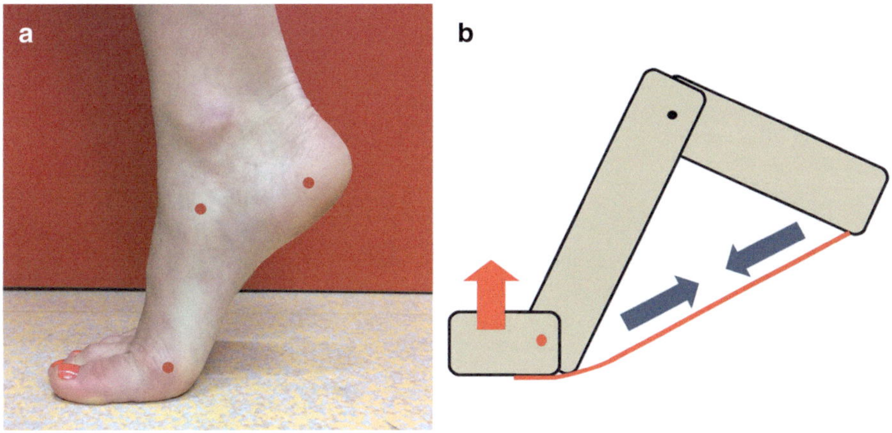

Fig. 2.29 Windlass mechanism (**a**) foot in propulsion, *red dots* mark 1st MTH, navicular, calcaneal tuber, (**b**) schematic drawing: Raising the heel activates the windlass mechanism. The heel inverts and the longitudinal arch rises. The toes are passively dorsiflexed around the axis of the MTP joints (*red dot*) and remain pressed to the ground

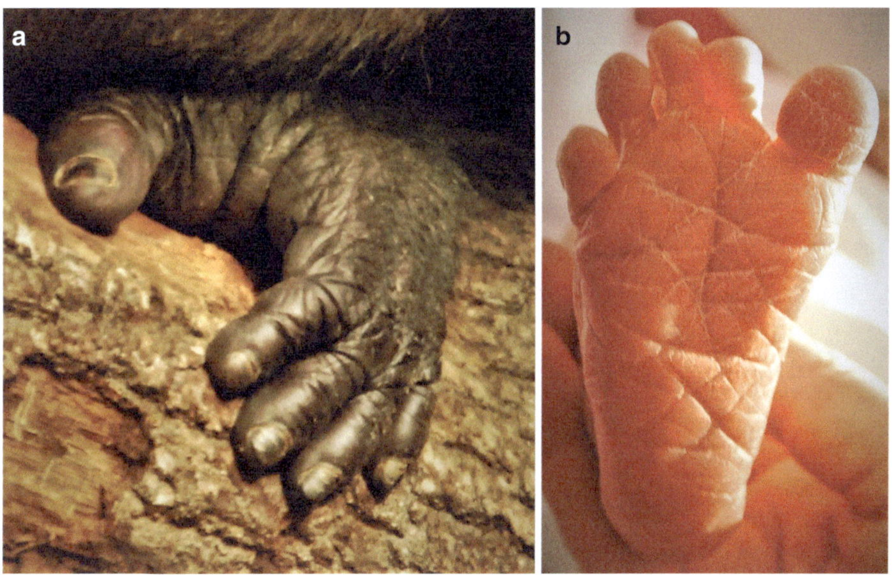

Fig. 2.30 Foot of a (**a**) lowland gorilla (**b**) a newborn baby

2.5.5 Hallux Valgus and Tailor Bunion

The first metatarsal bone can be more or less firmly connected to the medial cuneiform in different individuals. A wide range of motion can be observed in new-borns, in people who have practiced this activity since early childhood and in several primates. Similar to the thumb, in some cases the great toe can even be opposed (Fig. 2.30).

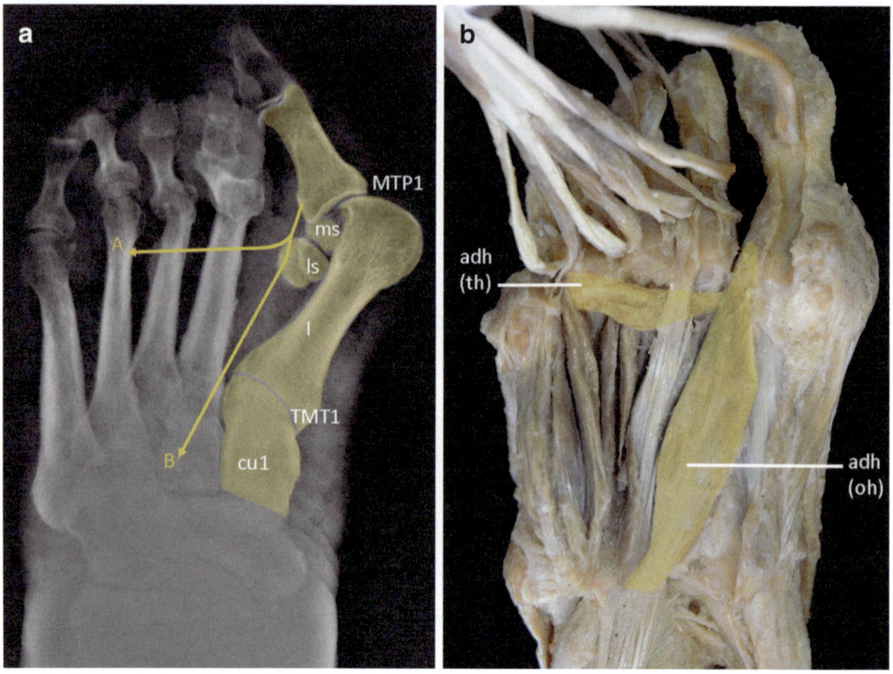

Fig. 2.31 Metatarsus primus varus and Hallux valgus. (**a**) X-ray image, medial cuneiform *(cu1)*, first metatarsal *(I)*, medial *(ms)* and lateral sesamoid *(ls)*, first MTP joint *(MTP1)*, first tarsometatarsal joint *(TMT1)*, direction of the adductor hallucis muscle tension: transverse head *(A)*, oblique head *(B)* (**b**) anatomical specimen, plantar view, adductor hallucis *(yellow)* with its transverse head *(th)* and its oblique head *(oh)*

In a healthy foot, this connection is so firm that lifting or lowering is limited to a maximum of half the shaft's thickness. A range of motion of the first metatarsal bone beyond this is referred to as *hyperlaxity or hypermobility of the first ray* (*Metatarsus primus elevatus*). Hypermobility is a symptomatic, clinically pathological condition, while hyperlaxity remains asymptomatic for a lifetime [7]. The hypermobile first metatarsal deviates more easily into varus position (Fig. 2.31).

Once the bones of the first ray deviate from their axial alignment, the strong muscles of the great toe tend to increase both the medial deviation of the metatarsal bone and the lateral deviation of the great toe. This leads to an irreversible deformity known as Hallux valgus.

A similar deviation but in the opposite direction can be described at the 5th ray as metatarsus quintus valgus. This causes a similar but inverse deformity, which is described as tailor's bunion (bunionette).

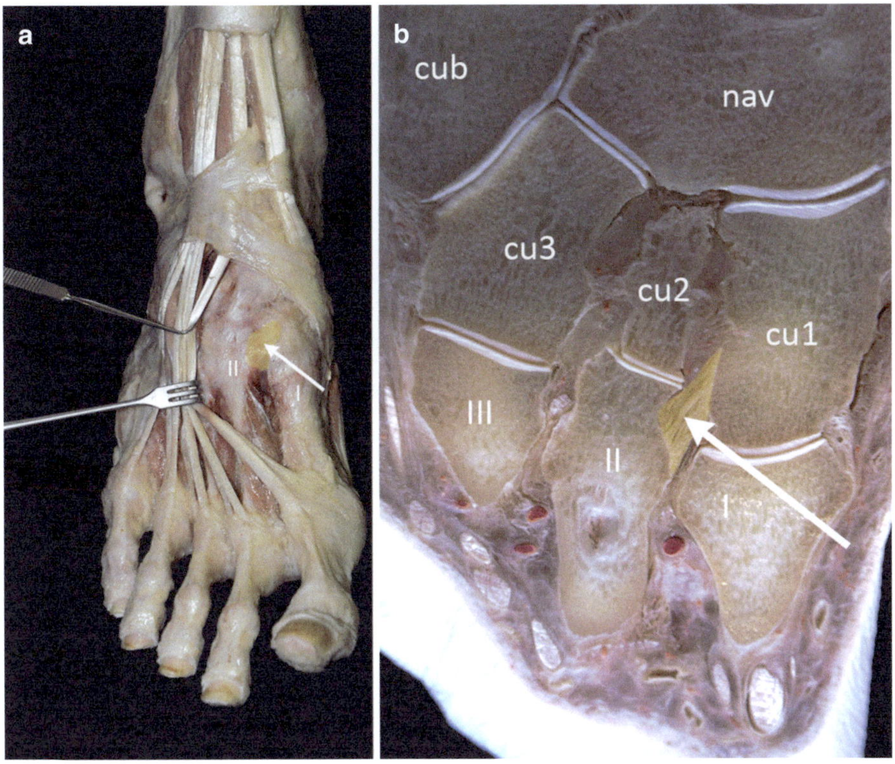

Fig. 2.32 Lisfranc's ligament (**a**) anatomical preparation of Lisfranc's ligament *(arrow)* (**b**) transverse section of the tarsometatarsal region, medial cuneiform *(cu1)*, base of 2nd metatarsal *(II)*, Lisfranc's ligament *(yellow)*, intermediate cuneiform *(cu2)*, lateral cuneiform *(cu3)*, cuboid *(cub)*, navicular *(nav)*, first and 3rd metatarsal *(I, III)* (b: by kind permission of Prof. Dr. rer. nat. J. Koebke, Centre for Anatomy, University of Cologne)

2.5.6 Overload of the 2nd Metatarsal

In order to compensate for the greater mobility of the first metatarsal bone, the first ray is provided with stronger muscles for stabilisation. When these muscles weaken, the first MTH and the great toe can no longer be pressed firmly enough to the ground when walking. As a result, the 2nd metatarsal bone is put under more strain. Because its base is pivoted between the three cuneiforms, it cannot move and is overloaded easily. This leads to pain, ligament fatigue and tears as well as bone fractures. Additionally, the base of the 2nd metatarsal bone is connected to the medial cuneiform by a strong ligament. This ligament is termed the Lisfranc's ligament and can tear when overloaded (Figs. 2.32, 2.33 and 2.34).

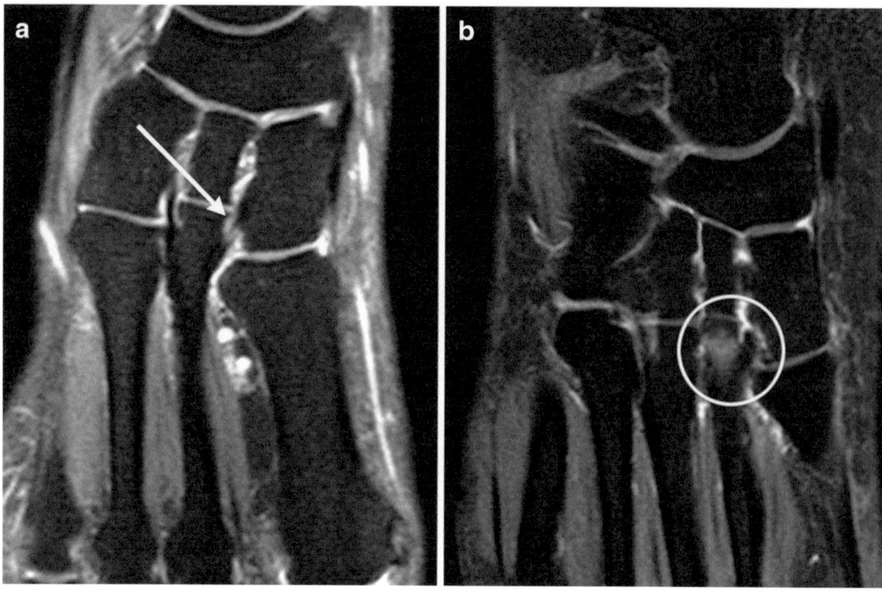

Fig. 2.33 (**a**) MRI with normal Lisfranc's ligament (**b**) rupture of the Lisfranc's ligament and bone marrow oedema of the basis of 2nd metatarsal (*white circle*) as shown by MRI

Other functional limitations may exacerbate the overload. The ability of the toes to bear weight is limited in a claw toe formation. The foot ends at the MTHs from a functional point of view, which significantly increases the load there. In addition, shortening the calf muscles leads to increased strain on the forefoot and thus also on the 2nd metatarsal. To compensate, the shaft (diaphysis) thickens, which can be recognised by seasoned radiologists in X-ray images (Fig. 2.35).

In some cases, the 2nd MTH protrudes significantly further in distal direction than all other MTHs (overly long second ray). This is not pathologic, but due to the greater leverage and increased pressure on the head, it may lead to overloading of the bone and soft tissue beneath the 2nd MTH (Figs. 2.36 and 2.37).

2.6 Gait Cycle

The bipedal gait is a rhythmic pattern of fine, coordinated movements in which the body is balanced over the supporting leg. The forward movement of the body is primarily governed by the forward movement of its centre of gravity and maintaining balance is achieved through alterations in the position and orientation of the legs. When standing upright, the centre of gravity is located centrally in the pelvis at the height of the 2nd sacral vertebra.

A gait cycle (100%) consists of two phases. During 'stance' (60%), the foot of the supporting leg is on the ground. It can be further divided into '*single limb support*' (only one foot has contact to the ground) and '*double limb support*' (both feet have contact to the ground). In the swing phase (40%), the foot is lifted off the

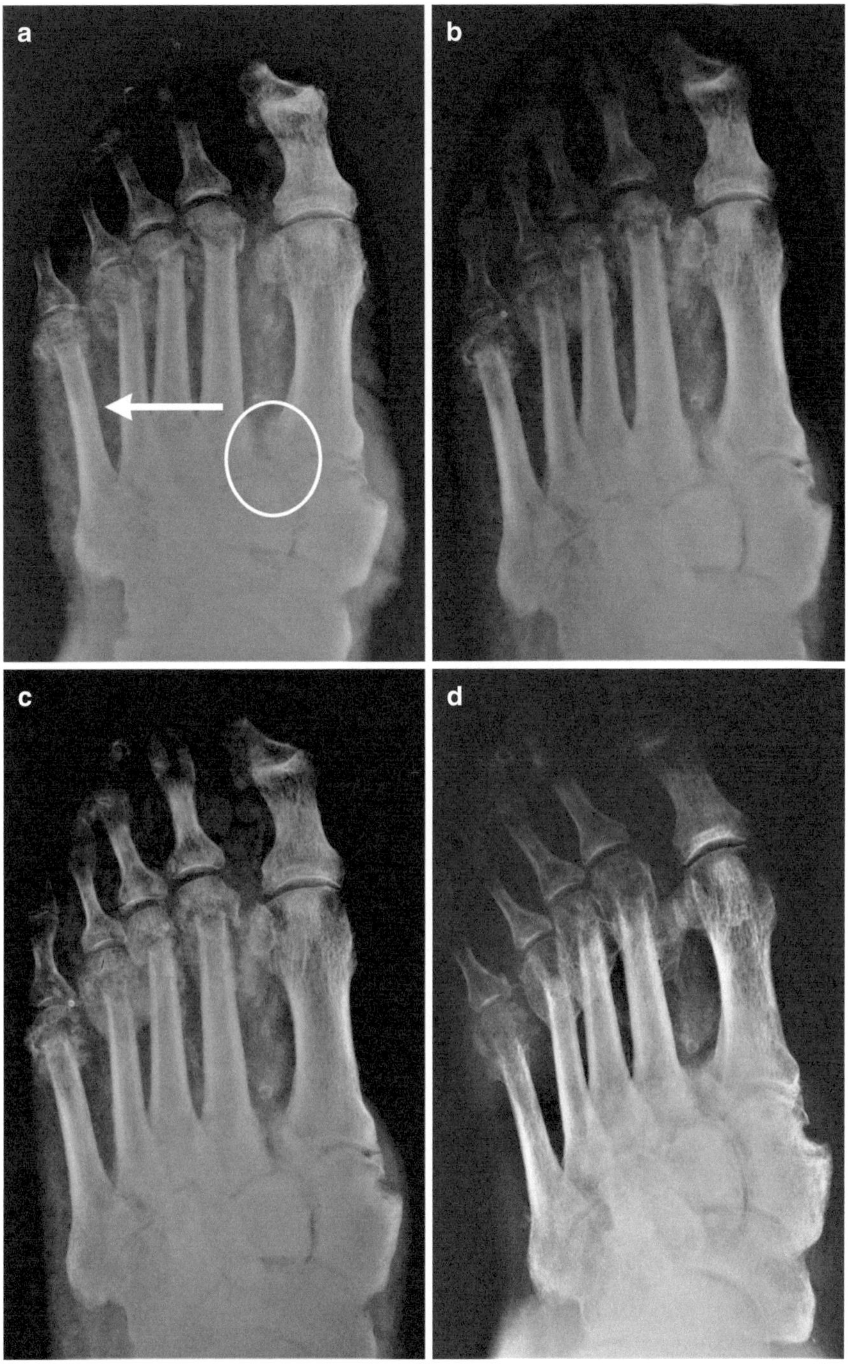

Fig. 2.34 Overload resulting in fractures of the 2nd to 5th metatarsal, rupture of Lisfranc's ligament (*white circle*) and homolateral dislocation (*white arrow*) of the 2nd to 5th metatarsal (progression in conventional X-ray (**a**) month 0, (**b**) month 2, (**c**) month 5 and (**d**) month 12)

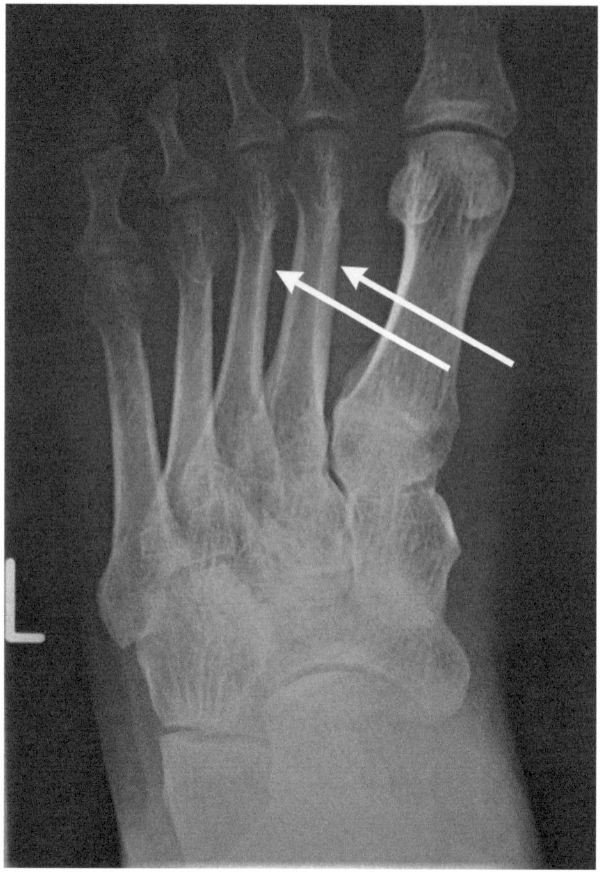

Fig. 2.35 Overload of the 2nd metatarsal. Thickening of the medial corticalis (*arrows*) as a sign of biomechanical overload in the metaphysis of the 2nd and 3rd metatarsal bone

ground and is guided past the supporting leg (Fig. 2.38). These phases can be further subdivided in different ways. Running differs from walking in that it has an additional flight phase during which neither foot has contact to the ground.

The body's centre of gravity moves with approximately constant height, speed and direction. Requirements concerning stability, forward locomotion and energy conservation limit the diversity of possible movements. The anatomical structures are designed to perform according to these needs. In this way, muscles must only provide about 30% of the energy required for locomotion [8].

2.6.1 Heel Strike (=Initial Contact)

In the phase of initial contact, the heel strikes the ground. The calcaneus is slightly everted (turned laterally) and the talus is held firmly in the 'bone fork' of the lower leg, which includes the malleoli (ankles). The spool-shaped upper joint surface of the talus, the trochlea tali, is wider at the front than at the back. During weight transfer, this wider part is fixed firmly in the ankle fork. This means that the upper ankle

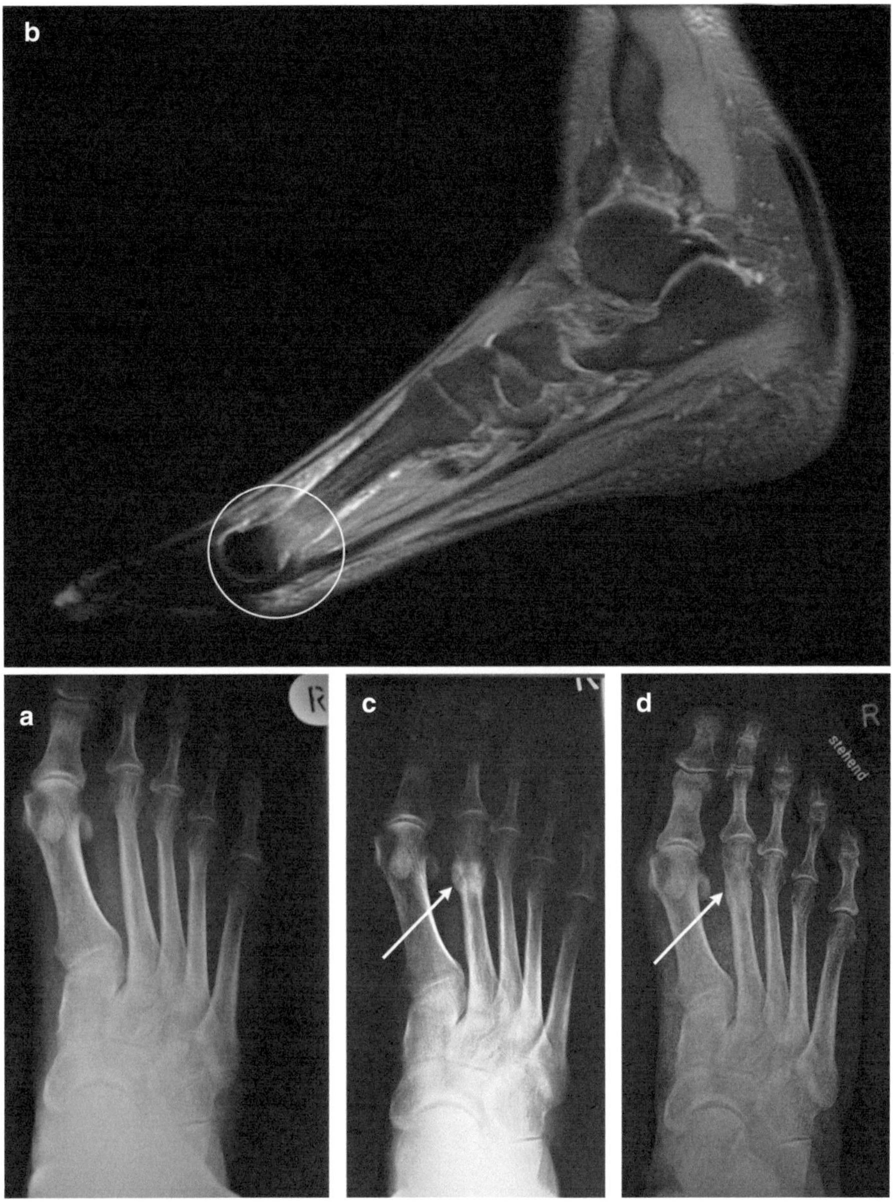

Fig. 2.36 (**a**) A 57-year-old patient (without neuropathy) with severe pain after a long hike, radiologically inconspicuous 2nd metatarsal, (**b**) MRI, performed due to the clinical complaints and inconspicuous X-ray with evidence of osteo-oedema of the distal 2nd metatarsal (*white circle*) (**c**) month 3 and (**d**) month 7 in conventional X-ray

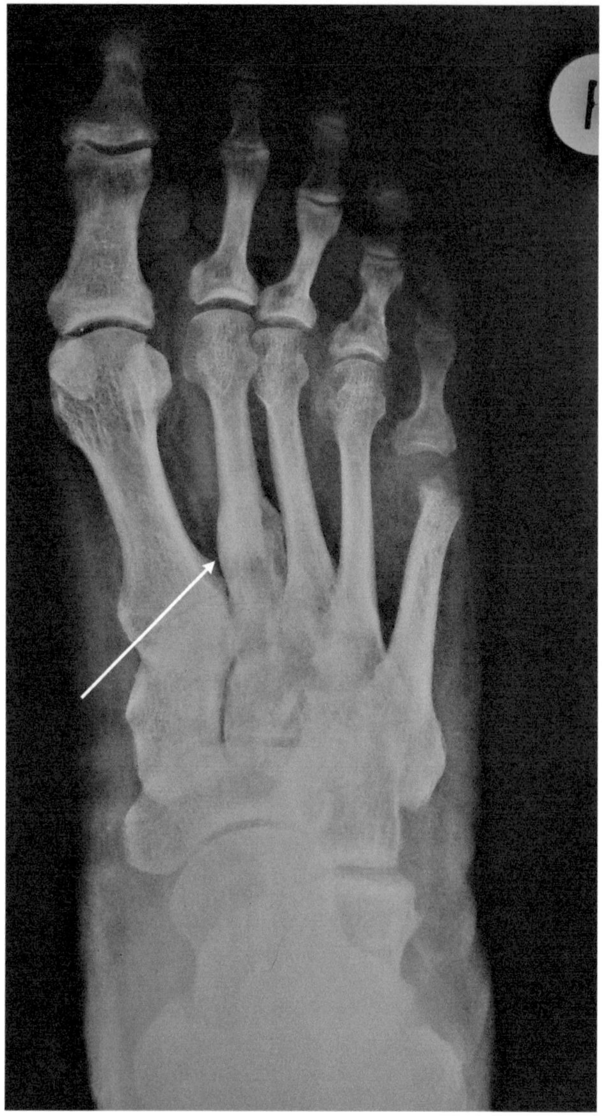

Fig. 2.37 Consolidated, occult fracture of the 2nd metatarsal (*white arrow*) as a result of biomechanical overload (concomitant finding in a patient with DFS and a plantar lesion with fistula and osteomyelitis of the 5th metatarsal head)

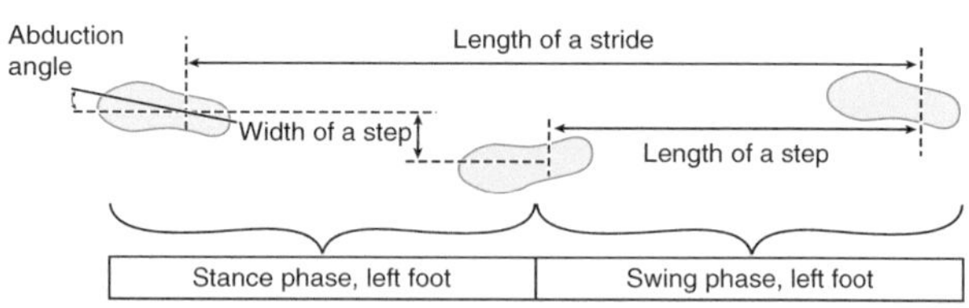

Fig. 2.38 Step sequence

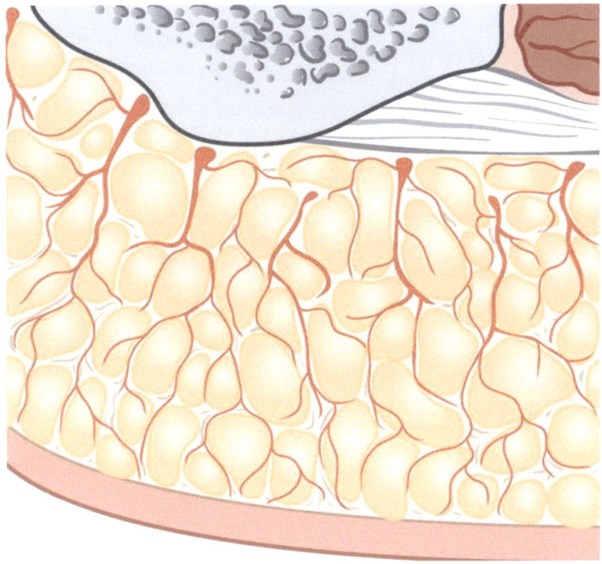

Fig. 2.39 Schematic illustration of the heel pad

joint is stable when the heel has only a limited contact surface with the ground and does not allow lateral movements of the foot.

The two-centimetre-thick *fat padding of the heel* is used to cushion the heel (Figs. 2.39 and 2.40a). Adipose tissue under the foot is divided into compartments by connective tissue septa. In this way, it acts similar to a tautly elastic gel cushion. Such cushions are available in a thinner design for use under the entire weight-bearing surface of the sole. In contrast to the tissue between them, the septa are well vascularised. The vessels in the septa represent the micro-circulatory bed of the lower leg arteries. A deep ulcer is therefore often a manifestation of a relevant arterial occlusive disease (Fig. 2.40b and c).

2.6.2 Loading Response (=Foot Flat)

In the loading response phase, the foot reaches the plantigrade position. While the centre of gravity moves forward, the sole of the foot makes first contact with the ground along its lateral margin. The controlled lowering of the foot is permitted by the tibialis anterior muscle. Compared to humans, water birds walk on their toes and have no equivalent to the human heel. They cannot control the impact of the forefoot and therefore 'waddle' (Fig. 2.41). With paralysis of the tibialis anterior muscle, the foot loses its ability to be lowered slowly and therefore crashes onto the ground, similar to a water bird waddle.

During the first part of this phase, the lateral part of the sole of the foot contributes to support the foot and the medial part does not. The predominance of lateral versus medial ground reaction forces leads to a pronation of the forefoot. The medial

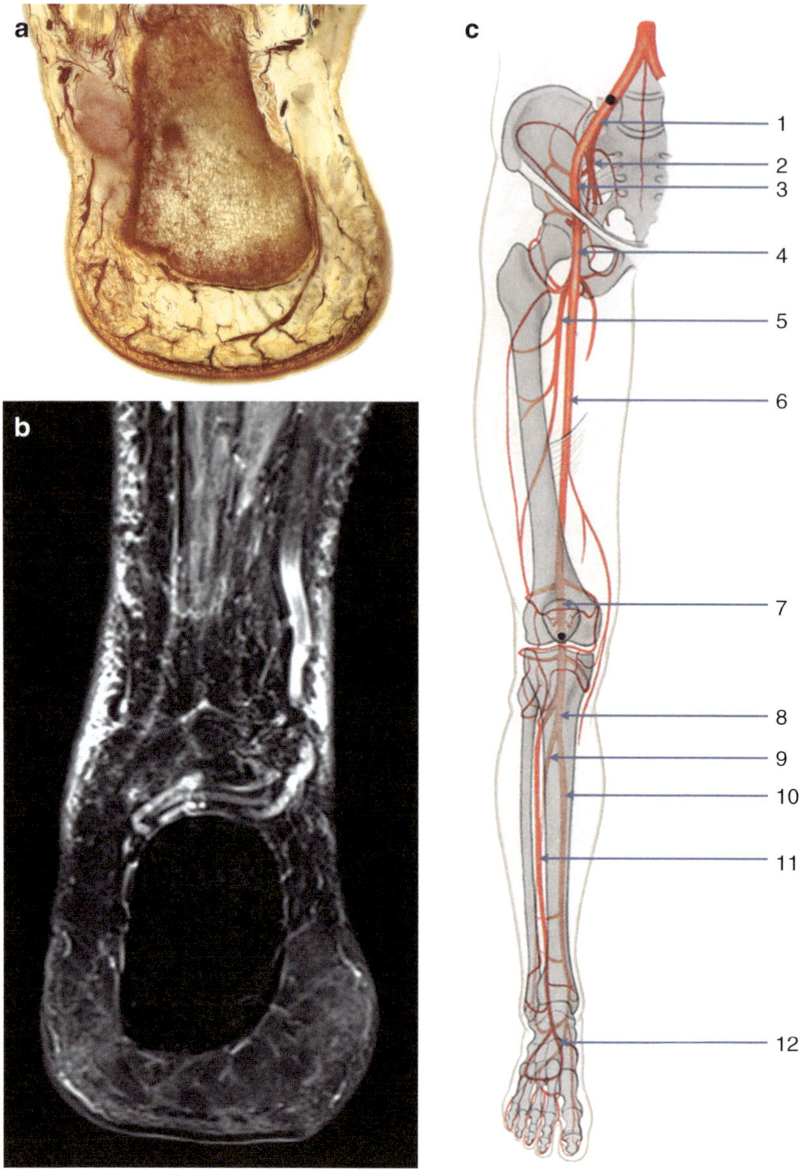

Fig. 2.40 Heel pad and its arterial supply (**a**) frontal plane plastination slice with vessel injection (**b**) CT after contrast agent injection (**c**) arterial supply of the leg: A. iliaca communis (*1*), A. iliaca interna (*2*), A. iliaca externa (*3*), A. femoralis communis (anatom. A. femoralis, (*4*)), A. profunda femoris (*5*), A. femoralis superficialis (anatom. A. femoralis (*6*)), A. poplitea, p-I-segment (*7*), Truncus tibiofibularis (anatom. A. tibialis posterior (*8*, *10*)), A. fibularis (*9*), A. tibialis posterior (*10*), A. tibialis anterior (*11*), A. dorsalis pedis (*12*) (source Lanz-Wachsmuth [4], ((**a**) by friendly permission of Prof. Dr. rer. nat. J. Koebke, Anatomisches Zentrum der Universität zu Köln)

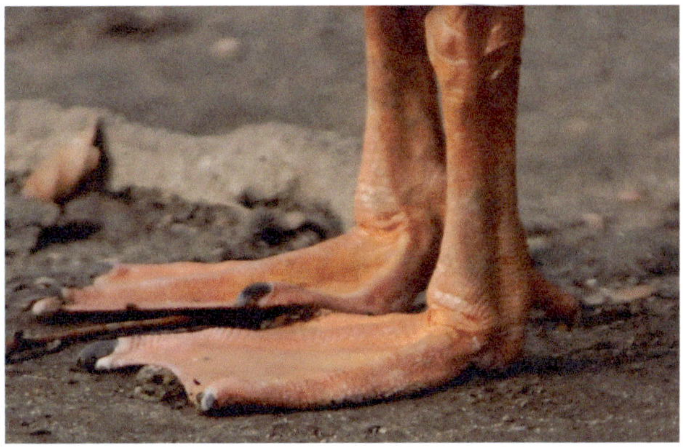

Fig. 2.41 Feet of a greylag goose

foot margin is lowered and the MTHs successively touch down from lateral towards medial. This movement is driven by gravity and guided by the fibularis longus and brevis muscles.

2.6.3 Midstance

The foot is in plantigrade (level) position with the centre of gravity above it. The opposite leg does not have contact with the ground and is in the swing phase. Due to the body's weight and the forward shift of its centre of gravity, the medial longitudinal arch flattens. The plantar aponeurosis is taut and presses the toes against the ground. In this phase of the one-legged stance, the foot is balanced by the fibular muscles (pronators) and the tibialis posterior (supinator). Further flattening of the longitudinal arch and thus pronation of the forefoot is limited by the tibialis posterior muscle and its tendon. Without the effect of this muscle, a part of the medial foot margin would touch the ground, as is the case with a flat foot.

2.6.4 First Part of Propulsion: Terminal Stance

As the centre of gravity continues its shift forward, the tension of the Achilles tendon increases. The heel lifts off the ground and terminal stance starts. Terminal stance is the first part of the phase called propulsion. The foot rotates around the transverse axis of the MTP joints, whereby the toes are passively dorsiflexed. Using the windlass mechanism, the heel is inverted and the lamina pedis is locked.

The following mechanisms contribute to inversion of the heel:

- Windlass mechanism of plantar aponeurosis
- Course of the tibialis posterior tendon around the medial ankle
- Spiral course of the Achilles tendon

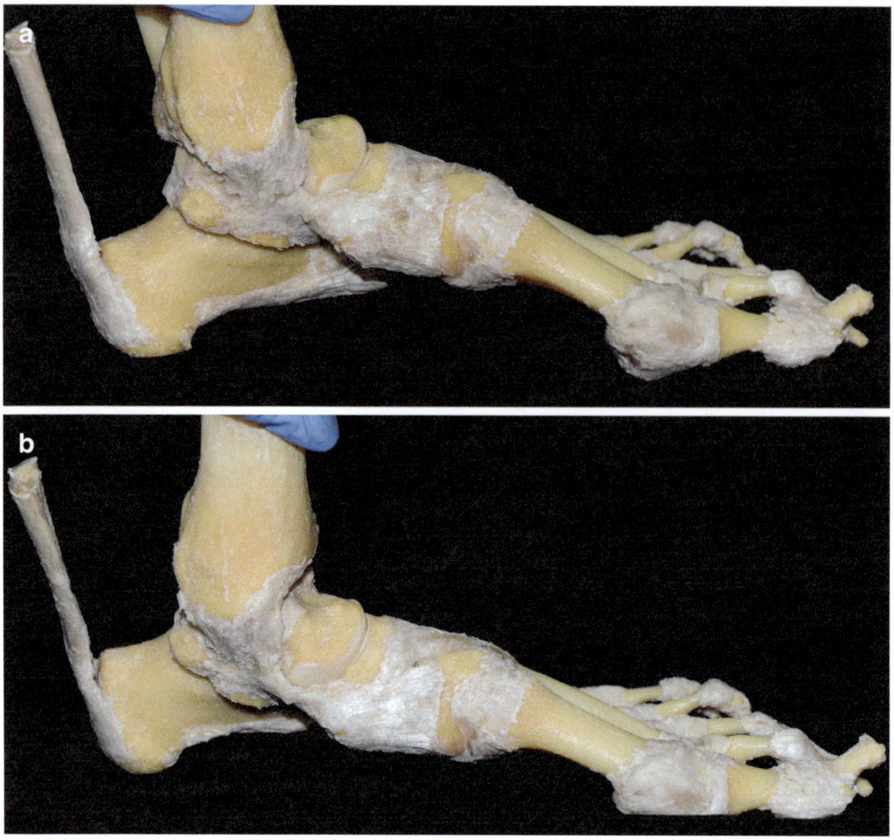

Fig. 2.42 'Locking' and 'unlocking' of the lamina pedis (**a**) 'locked' lamina pedis, outward rotation of the lower leg and abduction of the talus with calcaneus in inverted position (**b**) 'unlocked' lamina pedis, inward rotation of the lower leg and adduction of the talus with calcaneus in inverted position

The movements of the calcaneus and talus are interconnected and cannot be separated from each other. With the inversion of the calcaneus, the talus is rotated laterally around its vertical axis to its 'final position'. As a result, the distal tarsal bones also reach the end of their range of movement and are maximally tilted in the tarsal joints. This leads to a rigid grouping of all bones below the talus also known as 'the locking of the lamina pedis'. The foot is stiffened and can be used as a lever in the following phases (details in the Sect. 2.7.1) (Fig. 2.42).

If the locking mechanism is incomplete or starts too late, the foot remains flexible and cannot function as a lever. This type of foot is often abduced to allow forward movement but powerful propulsion is not restored. If the locking mechanism starts too early in the gait cycle, the foot is supinated and rigid with a propensity to overload the 5th MTH.

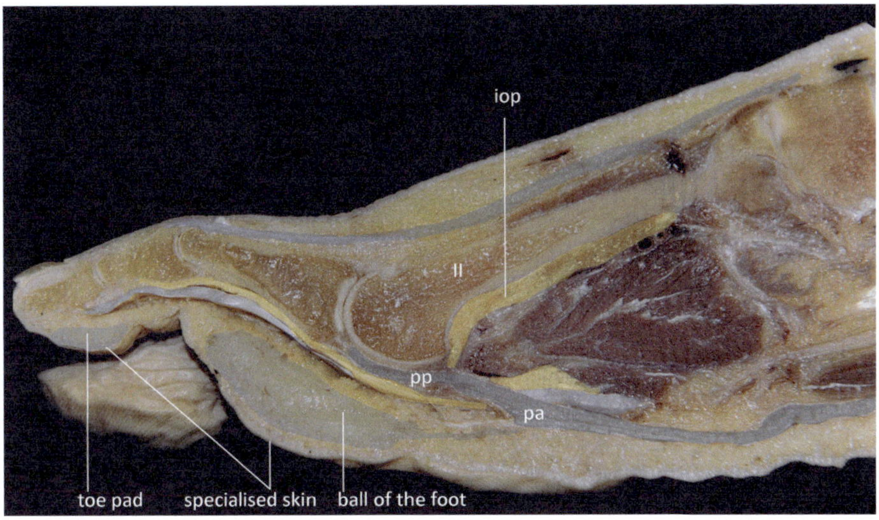

Fig. 2.43 Cushion complex of the toe, sagittal section of the 2nd ray, lateral view, plantar plate *(pp)*, plantar interosseous muscle *(iop)*, plantar aponeurosis *(pa)*, 2nd metatarsal *bone (II)*

While the lamina pedis is locked, the ankle joint is mobile, and the body can be better balanced over the fixed foot. At this point in the gait cycle, the ankle joint is particularly vulnerable to sports injuries.

When the heel is lifted off the ground, the centre of gravity is above the forefoot. The MTHs and toes support the entire body weight. This phase is crucial in preventing the development of pressure ulcers under the MTHs. The windlass mechanism of the plantar aponeurosis transfers pressure from the MTHs to the toe pads and thus protects the MTHs from overloading. Additionally, the MTHs are protected during propulsion by a cushioning complex consisting of plantar plates, fat pads ('balls of foot') and the special pressure-resistant skin of the sole of the foot. This cushioning complex is held in place under the MTHs by the interossei and the plantar aponeurosis (Fig. 2.43).

2.6.5 Second Part of Propulsion: Pre-swing

The centre of gravity advances continuously until the MTHs are finally lifted from the ground. At this moment, only the toes, especially the great toe, carry weight. At a walking pace, the opposite leg is already in contact with the ground. This marks the beginning of the 'pre-swing phase.' The knee is bent, which immediately relieves the foot. With faster walking and larger steps, this rapid reduction of pressure occurs later. By contrast, with slower and shorter steps it occurs earlier. Therefore, the MTHs are stressed less during strolling than at a faster walking pace. The pre-swing phase ends when the toes are lifted off the ground (Fig. 2.44).

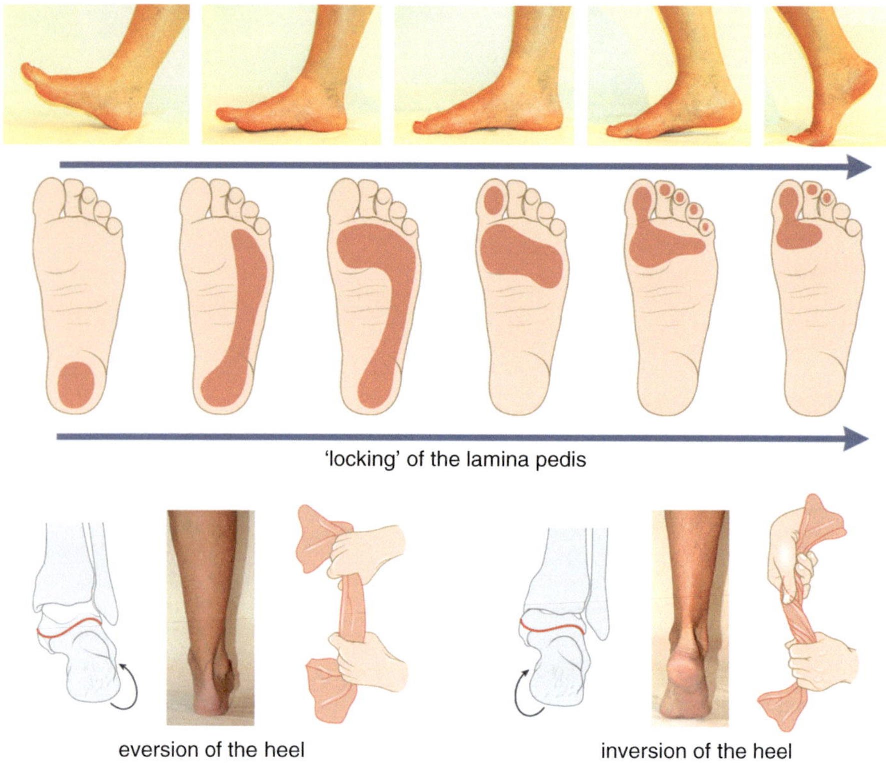

Fig. 2.44 Schematic representation of the individual periods of a step (*gait cycle*)

2.7 Deformities

Proximal deformities of the foot generally determine the conditions under which the distal parts of the foot accomplish their work. For this reason, this text starts with the hindfoot deformities.

2.7.1 Hindfoot Deformities

The two most significant deformities of the foot are pes planovalgus and pes cavus. These complex deformities involve the whole foot and have their cause often in the proximal part of the foot. They are therefore traditionally categorised as hindfoot deformities. With a weight-bearing foot, the heel is incorrectly aligned in valgus position in the first case and in varus position in the latter. Both may be induced by adult-onset muscle disorders that are often caused by diabetes and neuropathy. These deformities and their consequences might be modified by supporting aids, training and operations.

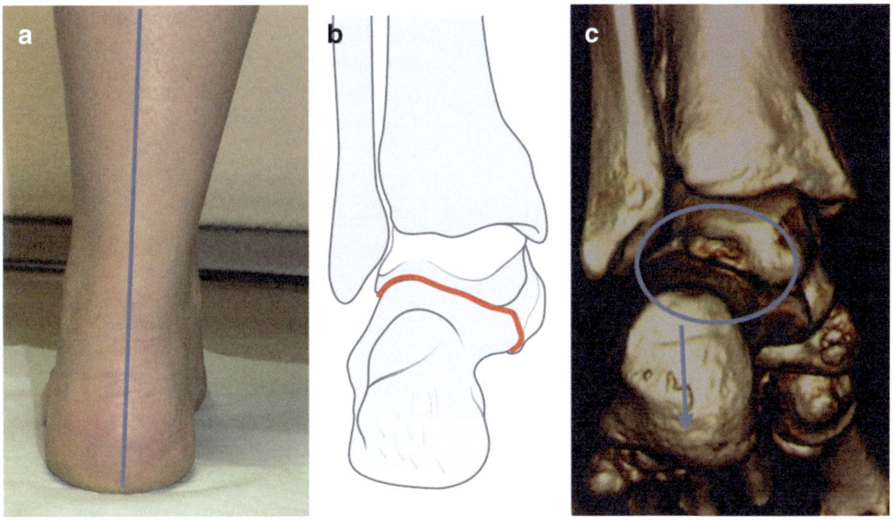

Fig. 2.45 Normal position of the hindfoot and the talocalcaneonavicular joint under load (**a**) clinical picture, (**b**) schematic drawing, the subtalar joint line is marked in red (**c**) three-dimensional CT reconstruction, the subtalar joint is marked by a circle

First, the deformity of the foot, as well as its consequences, are discussed in this subsection. A closer look at the influence of concomitant muscular disorders on the respective deformity follows in the next subsection.

To diagnose deformities of the hindfoot, the heel of the standing patient is examined. The focus is on whether the heel is straight, inverted or everted in relation to the lower leg. The patient is also asked to stand on tiptoe. If the suspected misalignment returns to normal, it is probably clinically insignificant (Fig. 2.45).

2.7.1.1 Pes Planovalgus (Flat Foot)

With a pes planovalgus, loading of the foot leads to an extreme stress on the talocalcaneonavicular joint and opens it medially. This joint is essential for the stability of the medial column. If it yields, the medial longitudinal arch collapses and parts of it touch the ground. The collapsed medial column forces the calcaneus into eversion (valgus position). Thus, the lamina pedis unlocks and the foot remains flexible during propulsion (Fig. 2.46). During childhood, flat feet are a physiological finding. In the first 10 years of life, the calcaneus gradually straightens up. As a result, the longitudinal arch is formed and the lamina pedis is twisted.

2.7.1.2 Pes Cavus (High Instep, High Arched Foot)

With a pes cavus, the heel inverts earlier and to a greater extent than normal. This locks the lamina pedis prematurely in course of the gait cycle. The foot stiffens when it should still be flexible and adaptable. The inversion of the heel also supinates the midfoot and shifts the load laterally (Fig. 2.47). As a result, the calcaneocuboid joint and the lateral margin of the forefoot are overloaded. Pressure ulcers

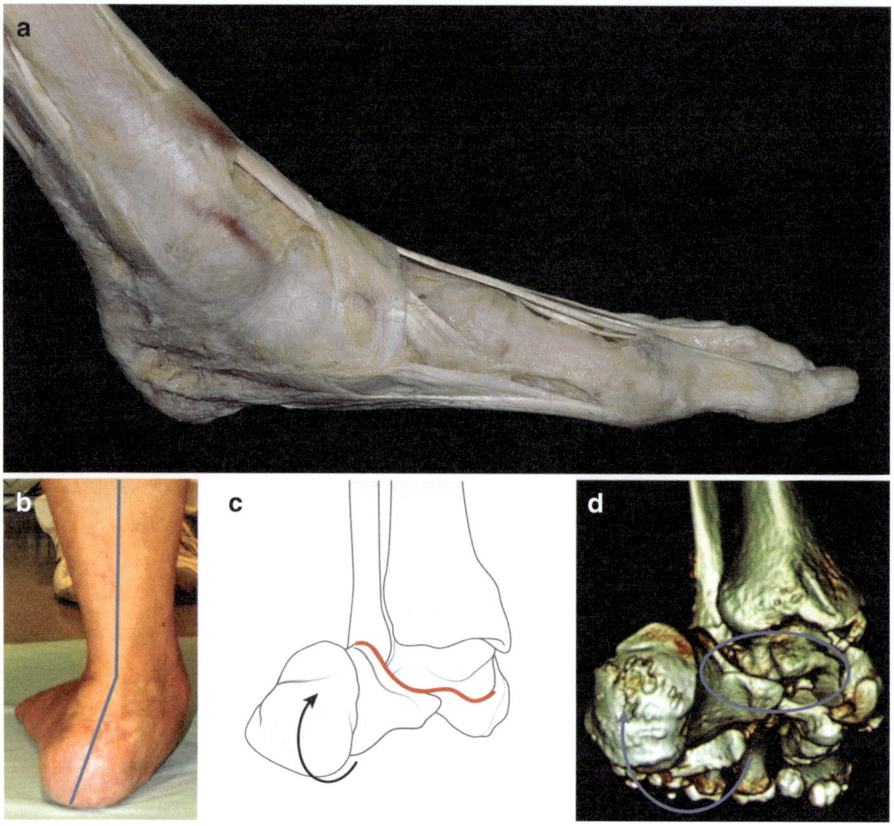

Fig. 2.46 Pes planovalgus (flat feet) with a collapsed medial column and calcaneus shifted in everted position under load (**a**) anatomical specimen (**b**) clinical picture (**c**) schematic drawing (the subtalar joint line is marked in *red*) (**d**) three-dimensional CT reconstruction (subtalar joint is marked by a *circle*)

are therefore typically located somewhat more laterally at the 5th MTH when compared to patients with plantigrade-oriented feet (see also Chap. 3; Sect. 3.4.1).

2.7.2 Muscular Causes of Hindfoot Deformities

Two frequently occurring and biomechanically significant muscle disorders are the shortening of the muscles forming the triceps surae (gastrocnemius and soleus) and the weakness of the tibialis posterior muscle.

2.7.2.1 Shortening of the Gastrocnemius and Soleus Muscle

There are many different causes of the development of a pes equinus deformity. A common cause is the shortening of the gastrocnemius or soleus muscle in people with DFS, often confused with a shortening of the Achilles tendon. Depending on the importance of these muscles as strong plantarflexors, the entire forefoot may be

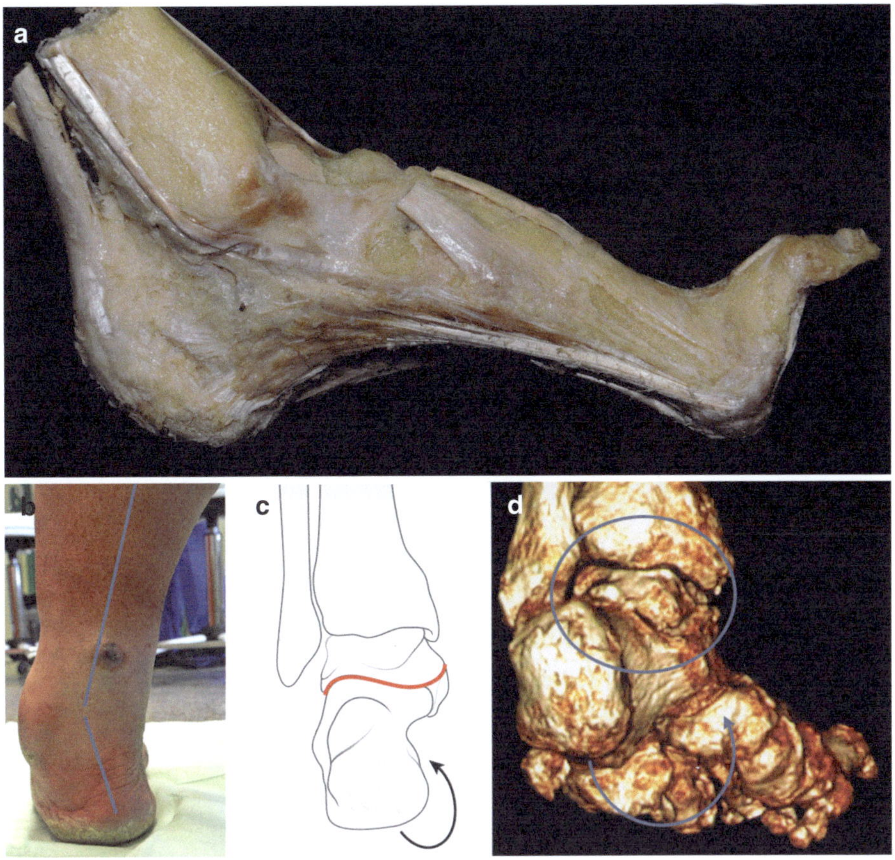

Fig. 2.47 Pes cavus (high arched foot) with reinforcement of the medial longitudinal arch, inversion of the hindfoot (varus position) and metatarsal stiffness (**a**) anatomical specimen (**b**) clinical picture (**c**) schematic drawing, (subtalar joint line is marked in *red*) (**d**) three-dimensional CT reconstruction (subtalar joint is marked by a *circle*)

overloaded. The shortening and the cause of it can be identified by the Silfverskjöld test (see Chap. 3, Sect. 3.4.1.3). In some cases, the shortening of the above-mentioned muscles is combined with a pes cavovarus deformity. In this combination, the heel is inverted permanently when the foot is loaded. As a result, the Achilles tendon is displaced more medially and this, in turn, inverts the heel even further. In a kind of a vicious circle, both deformities are reinforcing each other. As a consequence, the calcaneocuboid joint can be overloaded in such a way that the joint capsule tears and the joint becomes instable. The effects of the muscle shortening in combination with a planovalgus deformity are represented below.

2.7.2.2 Tibialis Posterior Dysfunction

Tibialis posterior dysfunction describes a relative weakness of the eponymous muscle (see Sect. 2.5.2.2) and is one of several reasons for a flat foot deformity in adulthood. When the foot is loaded, the medial longitudinal arch collapses and exerts

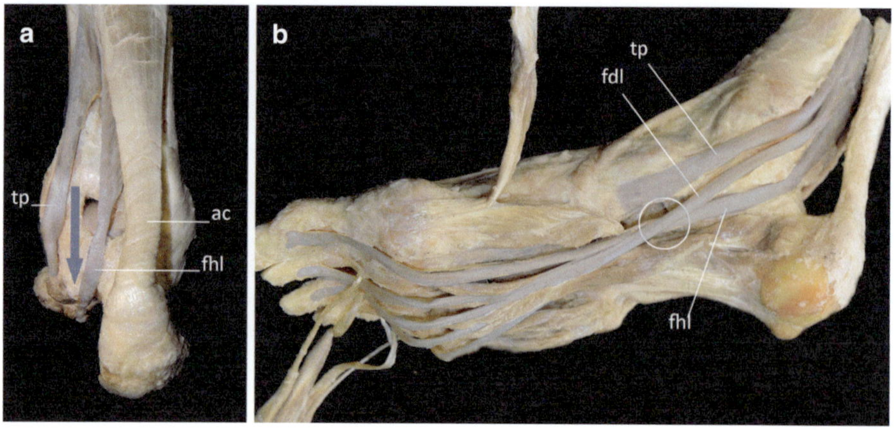

Fig. 2.48 Course of the flexor tendons beneath the medial longitudinal arch, anatomical specimen, (**a**) dorsal view, with a weakened tibialis posterior *(tp)* the load *(blue arrow* with tip on sustentaculum tali) will exert on the flexor hallucis longus tendon (*fhl*) (**b**) medial view, tibialis posterior tendon (*tp*), crossing of the flexor hallucis longus tendon (*fhl*) and the flexor digitorum longus tendon (*fdl*) in the chiasma plantare (*white circle*) just below the talo-calcaneo-navicular joint

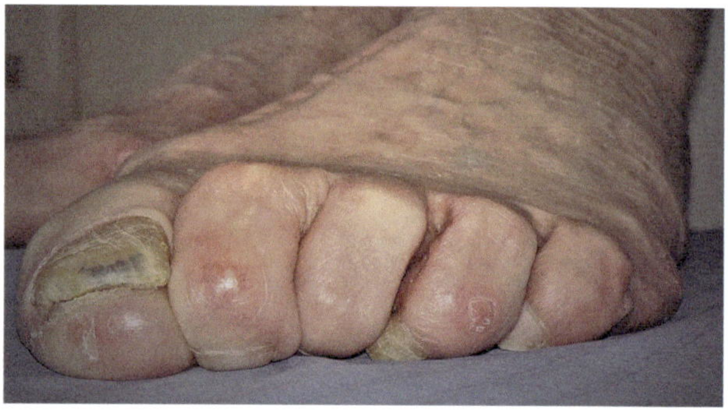

Fig. 2.49 Curled up toes

pressure on the flexor tendons and the plantar aponeurosis, all of which are traversing on the plantar side of the arch (Fig. 2.48).

As a result, all toe joints are hyperflexed. The toes may be 'curled up on the ground' with the nail surfaces pointed towards the ground (Fig. 2.49).

Increased tension of the flexor hallucis longus tendon plantarflexes the IP joint of the great toe, while the first MTP joint is hyperflexed by the extremely tensed plantar aponeurosis. Now, the entire great toe is pressed against the ground with a non-physiological force. Passive dorsiflexion of the first MTP joint, as needed in propulsion, is impossible. This leads to the clinical manifestation of the functional hallux rigidus (Fig. 2.50).

The flexor hallucis longus tendon can be tensed to such an extent that it turns the great toe with its medial side towards the ground. This is important for the development of ulcers at the medial parts of the hallux. (for details see Sect. 7.4.2 and Chap. 7).

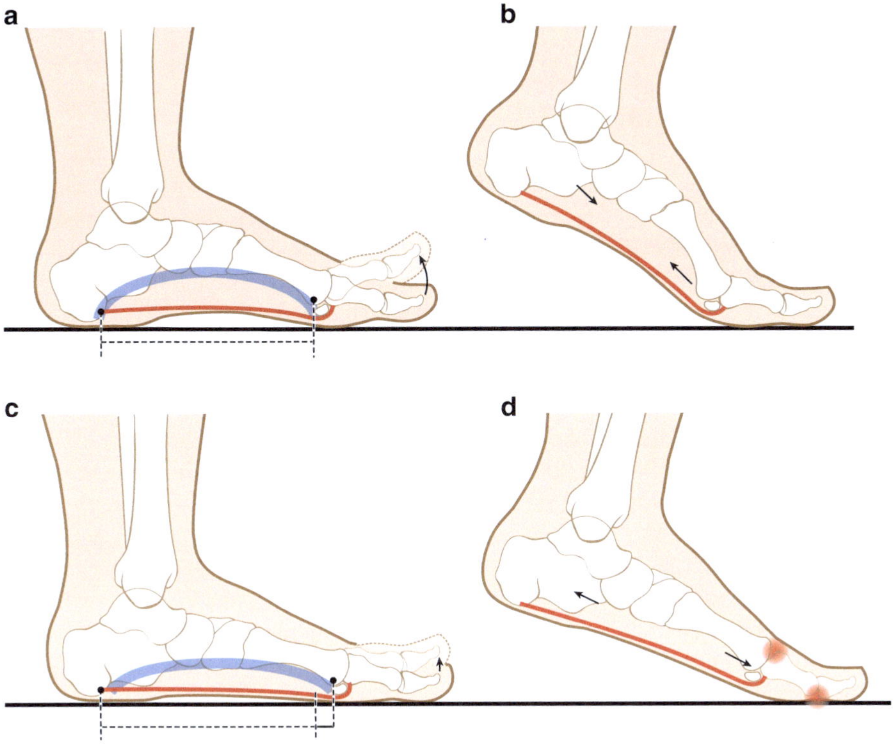

Fig. 2.50 (**a**, **b**) Windlass mechanism, (**c**, **d**) Functional hallux rigidus in case of pes planus ('reversed windlass')

Another aspect of a tibialis posterior dysfunction is the insufficient locking of the lamina pedis. As a result, the foot remains flexible and cannot act as a lever during propulsion. It is not possible to lift the heel and therefore shorter steps must be taken. Forward motion without loading the forefoot to lift the heel can only be achieved by an abduction (movement deviating laterally) of the foot. The hip has to be turned outwards to accomplish walking.

Locking of the lamina pedis is further impeded if the tibialis posterior dysfunction is combined with a pes equinus (shortening of the gastrocnemius and soleus muscle). In order for a pes equinus deformity to reach a plantigrade position at all, the heel must evert, and the forefoot has to deviate laterally. Due to the weakness of the posterior tibialis, the eversion of the calcaneus cannot be counteracted. The body's weight forces the calcaneus to evert further and therefore shifts the Achilles tendon laterally. In this lateralised position, the pull on the Achilles tendon reinforces the eversion rather than inverting the heel. As the weakest point of the medial column, the talocalcaneonavicular joint collapses and 'opens up medially'. Consequently, the forefoot deviates laterally even further.

In severe cases, the tibialis posterior tendon can thin out and tear, leading to a complete collapse of the medial longitudinal arch with extensive biomechanical consequences. In order to detect the above-mentioned deformity, diagnostic X-ray examinations must be carried out on a weight-bearing foot.

2.7.3 Toe Deformities

Thirty-two to 46% of patients in a diabetic foot outpatient clinic is affected by deformities of the 2nd to 5th toes [9, 10]. This is significant both in terms of the number of people affected and the extent of the consequences for each individual. The often simple and definitive correction is not used nearly enough (as of 2018). In most cases, the toes are clawed to a certain degree. The overextension in the MTP joint causes the plantar cushion structures to deviate distally until they are no longer positioned under the MTHs [11].

2.7.3.1 Key Position of the MTP Joints and Zig-Zag Deformity

An imbalance between intrinsic and extrinsic muscle function is seen as the main cause of toe deformities [12, 13]. Plantar flexion of the proximal phalanges in the MTP joints is caused by the plantar aponeurosis and the interossei. This is a prerequisite for the strong extrinsic toe flexors to press the stretched toes onto the ground.

As diabetic polyneuropathy worsens distally, the intrinsic muscles at the sole of the foot are more susceptible to motor neuropathy than the extrinsic muscles of the lower leg [14]. Distal motor neuropathy therefore impairs the ability of the short foot muscles to align the toes, while the functionality of the long toe muscles situated in the lower leg is maintained. The weakness of the short foot muscles, in this case, affects the interossei and leads to instability in the MTP joints. Under load, the proximal phalanges dislocate dorsally and are ‘pulled up’ to the MTHs by the extensor tendon hoods. The MTP joints are overstretched and the attachments of the interossei on the proximal phalanges are shifted from the flexor to the extensor side. This causes the interossei to lose their ability to plantarflex the toes. Their contraction now results in toes that ride on the MTHs. The MTHs are therefore positioned in a more plantar position in the sole of the foot than normal, which is also due to the subluxated toes riding on top. If the foot is loaded, the long flexor tendons are extremely taut around the low-lying MTHs and bend the toes in the IP joints. The result is a zig-zag deformity or ‘claw toe’ (Fig. 2.51). For this position of the toe, the extensors are now ‘too long’ and shrink over time, which fixes the toe in its clawed position.

By hyperextending (overstretching) the MTP joints, the plantar plates become overstretched and thin out. The plantar fat pads (balls of the foot) are connected to the plantar plates and deviate distally under load. This has dramatic consequences for the MTHs, as they are no longer protected during propulsion by their cushion-like structures.

In extreme cases, the plantar plates can weaken in such a way that the proximal phalanges luxate dorsally. In this situation, the tips of the claw toes lose contact with the ground. The plantar plates can even tear. The MTHs then luxate in plantar direction. They pass through the gaps in the plantar plates and lie directly under the skin (Fig. 2.52).

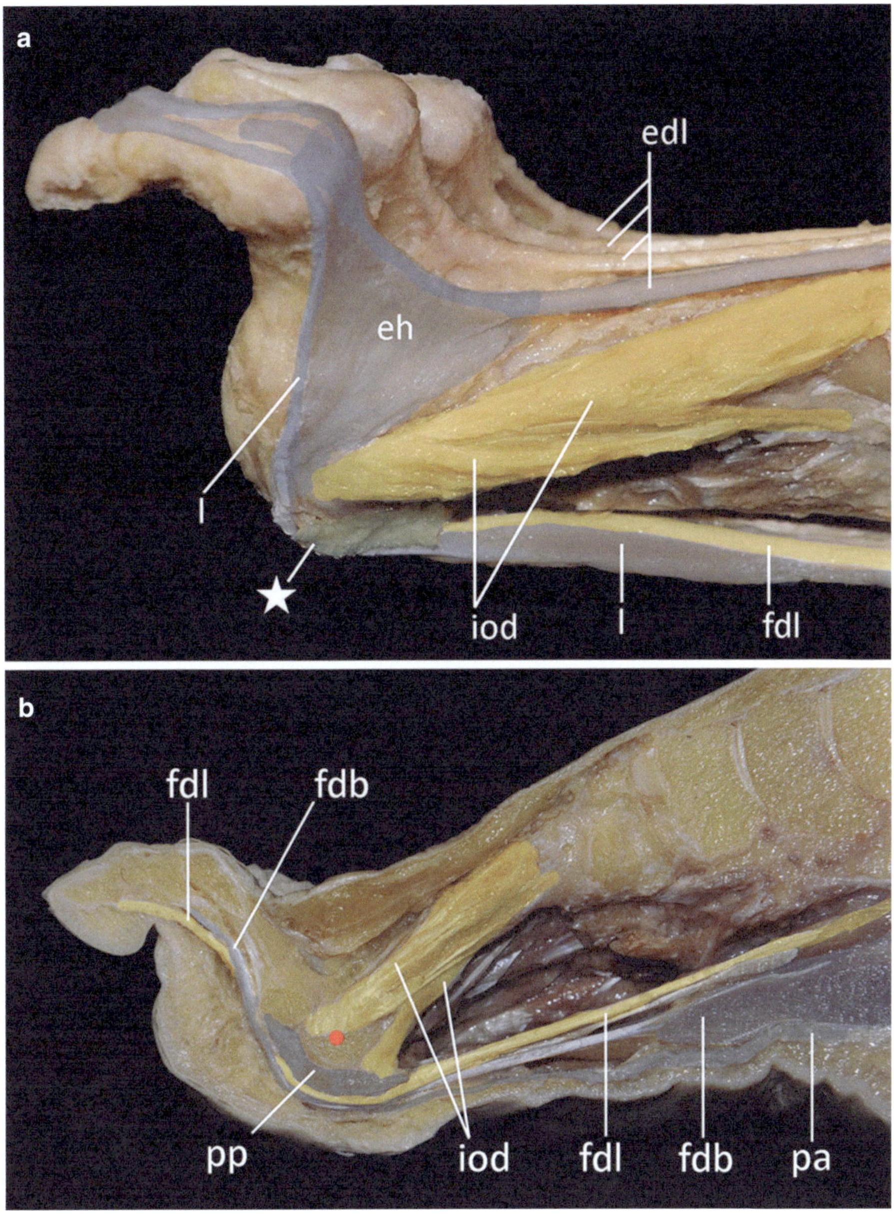

Fig. 2.51 Claw toe (**a**) anatomical specimen of the 2nd toe, tendon of flexor digitorum longus *(fdl)*, extensor digitorum longus *(edl)*, lumbrical *(l)*, extensor hood *(eh)*, interosseous dorsalis *(iod)*, deep transverse metatarsal ligament *(white star)* (**b**) sagittal section through the 2nd ray, medial view, tendon of flexor digitorum longus *(fdl)* and brevis *(fdb)*, interosseous dorsalis *(iod)* lies dorsal of the transverse axis of the 2nd MTP joint *(red dot)*, plantar plate *(pp)*, plantar aponeurosis *(pa)*

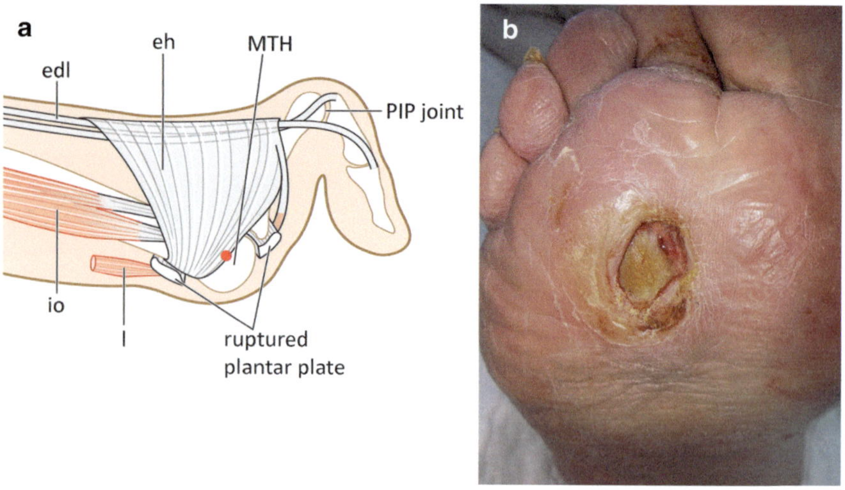

Fig. 2.52 Rupture of the plantar plate (**a**) schematic drawing: metatarsal head *(MTH)*, extensor hood *(eh)*, Extensor digitorum longus *(edl)*, interosseous *(io)*, lumbrical *(l)*, transverse axis of the MTP joint (*red dot*) (**b**) clinical examination: lesion beneath the MTHs

In a pes planus (flat foot), the toes are already hyperflexed in the IP joints during weight transfer in midstance. Unlike claw toes, with flat feet the toes are generally not in a zig-zag position because they are not hyperextended in the MTP joints. Rather all joints are hyperflexed and the toes are 'curled up on the ground'. This makes passive dorsiflexion of the toes during propulsion more difficult or even impossible. In very pronounced cases, the toes curl up so that the nail plates become part of the weight-bearing zone (see also Fig. 2.49).

In the case of a pes cavus (high arched foot), the longitudinal arch is strongly raised and cannot flatten sufficiently under load to tighten the plantar aponeurosis. The reverse windlass mechanism cannot take place and the toes remain hyperextended (overstretched) in the MTP joints. These effects lead to a progressive zig-zag deformity (see also Figs. 2.51 and 2.52).

2.7.3.2 Deformities in the Sagittal Plane

Nomenclature of the various deformities of the lesser toes is quite diverse. In this chapter, a description according to the standard by the authors Redkina and Sikorski is applied [15].

A hammer toe essentially presents with hyperflexion (excessive plantar flexion) of the PIP joint, often with a hyperextension of the DIP joint and a slight hyperextension of the MTP joint (Fig. 2.53a). Lesions mainly occur at the dorsal aspect of the PIP joint.

A claw toe is characterised by hyperextension (excessive dorsal extension) of the MTP joint, while the PIP and DIP joints are plantarflexed. Lesions mainly occur at the tip of the toe (Fig. 2.53b).

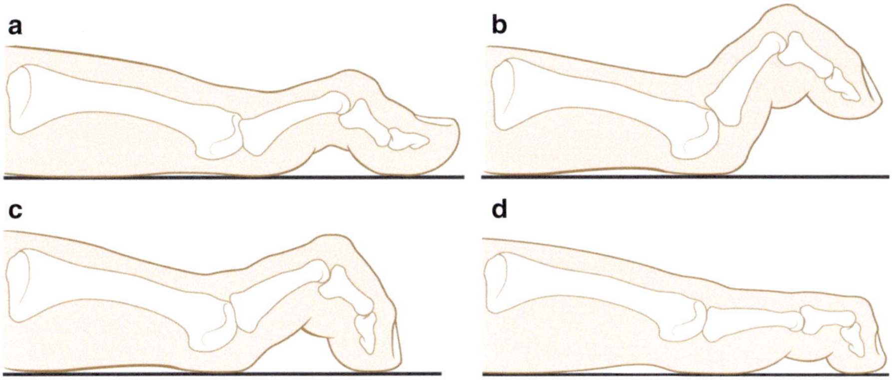

Fig. 2.53 Toe deformities in the sagittal plane (**a**) Hammer toe (**b**) Claw toe (**c**) Claw toe with subluxation of the MTP joint (**d**) Mallet toe

Subluxation of the MTP joint in a claw toe: The extreme weakening of the interossei and the thinning or rupture of the plantar plate allows a subluxation of the toe in the MTP joint, so that the tip of the toe loses contact with the ground, even though the PIP joint is completely plantarflexed. Often, lesions occur on the back of the toe at the level of the PIP joint and under the MTH (Fig. 2.53c).

In a mallet toe, the main anomaly is hyperflexion (excessive plantar flexion) of the DIP joint. It is also known as a distal hammer toe. Lesions can easily develop on the tip of the toe (Fig. 2.53d).

2.7.3.3 Deformities in the Transverse Plane

Hallux valgus and tailor bunions are the most common toe deformities in the transverse plane. They have already been described together with metatarsal deformities.

In patients with a medially deviated (varus) 5th toe, hyperflexion in the PIP and DIP joints is combined with a torsion of the toe. This malformation can be congenital and is often bilateral. Here, the 5th toe usually rests on the 4th and is called 'curly toe' (Fig. 2.54a). In patients with neuropathy and insufficiency of the quadratus plantae or lumbricals, both toes are often turned parallel. The 2nd toe is also frequently affected and combination with a hallux valgus is common (Fig. 2.54b).

2.7.4 Plantarisation

If parts of the foot, which are not designed to bear weight, become non-physiological parts of the weight-bearing area, the authors term this phenomenon '*plantarisation*'. This is of clinical importance because it may increase pressure in areas that are not covered by hairless (glabrous) skin or cushioning tissue structures and will not withstand stress. The risk of ulceration is therefore increased. One-third of all diabetic foot ulcers are located in areas exposed to pressure because of plantarisation.

Fig. 2.54 Toe deformities in the transversal plane (**a**) Curly toe (**b**) Superductus or Infraductus

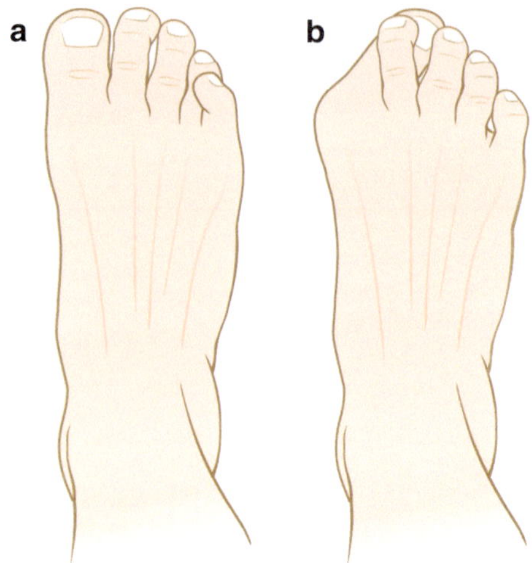

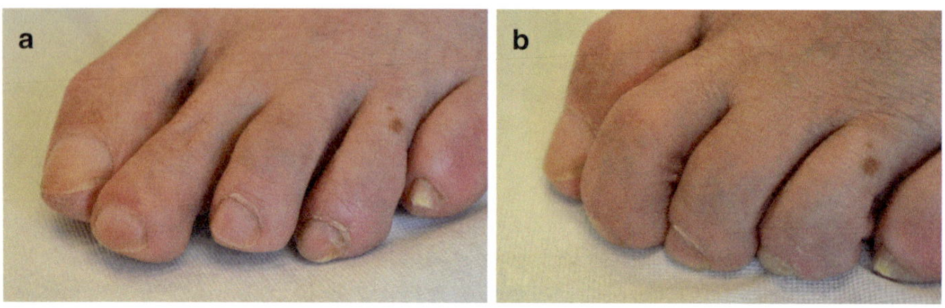

Fig. 2.55 Functional plantarisation in case of a Mallet-toe (**a**) unloaded (**b**) loaded

If the plantarisation can be observed at rest, it is termed *'static'*. If plantarisation does not occur at rest and there is a lesion in an area that suggests plantarisation as the cause of its development, this plantarisation must be provoked in clinical examination (see Chap. 3, Sect. 3.4.1). For this purpose, claw test, push-up test and attentive inspection are used. This inspection includes the observation of the patient's feet while standing and walking and trying to stand on tiptoe. If a plantarisation becomes evident in this situation, it is *'functional'* (Fig. 2.55).

If a 'static plantarisation' is observed, it is necessary to examine the patients foot to see whether the deformity can be corrected manually. If correction is partially possible, the static deformity is 'flexible', otherwise it is 'fixed'. Fixation can be triggered by shrinkage of joint capsules and tendons involved in joints movement or by ossification of joints (*ankylosis*). Surgical interventions on joint capsules and tendons (soft tissue surgery) are usually less time-consuming, less complex and less risky than interventions on the bone.

If plantarisation occurs under load, it is 'functional'. If plantarisation already exists at rest, it is 'static'. 'Static plantarisation' is termed 'flexible' if it can be corrected partially during a manual examination, or 'fixed' if this is not possible.

In the case of a 'static plantarisation' that is 'fixed', the cause of fixation must be determined by a clinical and, if required, radiographic examination. Soft tissue surgery, which is useful in the correction of plantarisation, includes severing, lengthening or transposition of tendons as well as joint capsule releases. The latter refers to a slitting of the plantar or dorsal parts of the joint capsule in order to allow renewed movement. To achieve a satisfactory functional result, fixation often only partially needs to be released.

As a rule, only an ankylosis cannot be corrected at least partially by soft tissue surgery alone.

2.7.4.1 Plantarisation Due to Hyperflexion ('Clawing')

The pathological hyperflexion of the distal phalanx represents the plantarising deformity that determines lesions at the tip of the toes. The tips of the clawed toes become part of the weight-bearing area in the propulsion phase. In this phase, the entire body's weight is carried by a very small area anyway. Due to the deformity, this area decreases further and comprises a bone prominence, which is very easily injured.

2.7.4.2 Plantarisation Due to Torsion ('Twisting')

Torsion is a common phenomenon involving the great toe or the 3rd to 5th toe. The medial side of the great or the lateral parts of the lesser toes is twisted towards the ground.

Torsion of the lesser toes is caused by the flexor digitorum longus. Its tendon runs behind the medial malleolus, passes diagonally in the sole of the foot and attaches to the plantar side of the lesser toes. Its main function is the plantarflexion of the lesser toes, but due to its oblique course, it can also twist the toes with their lateral sides towards the ground. To avoid this rotation, the oblique direction of the tendons is straightened by the quadratus plantae and the lumbricals. If their strength diminishes due to lack of training or peripheral neuropathy, the oblique traction of the flexor digitorum longus muscle prevails and the toes are rotated. Healthy people can also exhibit this phenomenon as the quadratus plantae muscle shows great anatomic variations. Patients with normal protective sensation don't exhibit ulcers but compensate through callus formation and seek help because this overload causes pain.

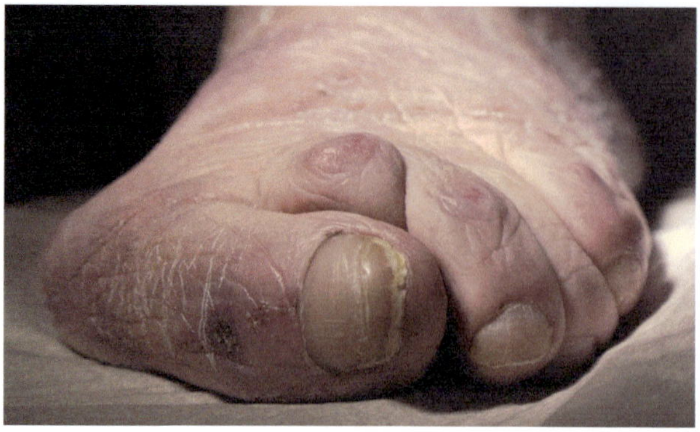

Fig. 2.56 Plantarisation of the medial parts of the great toe

Torsion of the great toe is generated mainly as a result of tension on the long flexor tendon in hallux valgus. Torsion is facilitated by hypermobile joints and a weakened intrinsic musculature of the great toe, which can no longer stabilise the first ray sufficiently. Additionally, a flat foot flattens the longitudinal arch and intensifies the traction on the long flexor tendon. Furthermore, a tibialis posterior dysfunction leads to increased pronation of the first ray by the predominance of the fibularis longus. This causes the rotation of the hallux with its medial side towards the ground. And finally, if the feet are turned outwards (abduction angle > 20°), the propulsion no longer evolves in line with the longitudinal axis of the foot via the tip of the great toe, but via the medial parts of the IP joint (Fig. 2.56). All mentioned phenomena can be mutually reinforcing (see Chap. 7).

> The medial parts of the great toe are, in general, functionally plantarised. The bony prominences without soft tissue padding become part of the weight-bearing area in terminal stance, at a time when the entire body weight is applied to a very small area.

2.7.4.3 Plantarisation Due to Hyperextension ('Overstretching')

With hallux limitus, normal dorsiflexion in the first MTP joint is increasingly restricted until complete stiffness prevents any movement (hallux rigidus). During propulsion, the passive dorsiflexion of the great toe is mandatory. A lack of flexibility in the first MTP joint might be partially compensated by the IP joint. This joint normally does not allow dorsiflexion, but in this case, strong bending forces overstretch the joint and open it up on its plantar side. This leads to a non-physiological strain on the bony components of the IP joint, such as the distal part of the proximal phalanx. In particular, the medial condyle at the head of the proximal phalanx features sharp edges and becomes part of the load bearing area during propulsion. The plantar soft tissue and the skin are not prepared for this stress and may be damaged (Fig. 2.57).

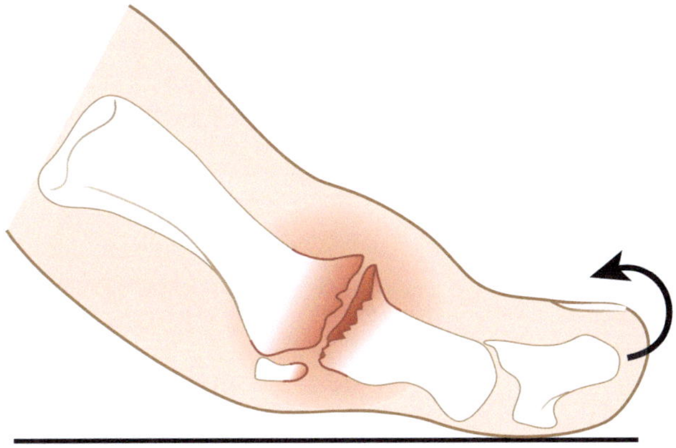

Fig. 2.57 Hallux rigidus, schematic illustration of pathological hyperextension of the distal phalanx due to hallux rigidus during propulsion

Bony protrusions, which physiologically do not reach weight-bearing areas, may become part of these areas by plantarisation. The soft tissue and the skin at this 'inner pressure points' are not prepared for substantial stress and cannot withstand. It is important not to fail to recognise plantarisation because, in general, it can be easily and permanently corrected by surgical measures on tendons and capsules.

2.8 Hairless and Hairy Skin

Areas designed to withstand high and repeated pressure are protected by hairless (glabrous) skin. These areas, such as the plantar surface of the heel, have an epidermal layer nearly ten times thicker than that of normal hairy skin. Hairless skin has also numerous sweat glands while hair and sebaceous glands are not present. The epidermis is tightly intertwined with the connective tissue of the dermis. Papillae of the dermis are arranged in double columns. On the epidermis these double columns are visible as epidermal ridges. The imprint of the ridges ('fingerprint') is person-specific and is used in criminology to identify individuals. Functionally, the ridges enhance adherence to a contact surface. This type of skin does not slide on the underlying musculoskeletal structures and has a better resistance to pressure. Therefore, skin transplants in a weight-bearing area should not be performed, if possible, with split skin (Chap. 21) (Figs. 2.58 and 2.59).

2.8.1 Pressure Ulcer by Repeated Stress

Pressure ulcers are the result of frequently repeated, borderline intensive stress on the same area over long periods of time. Pressure and shear forces arise between bony prominences on one hand and the environment on the other. A significant

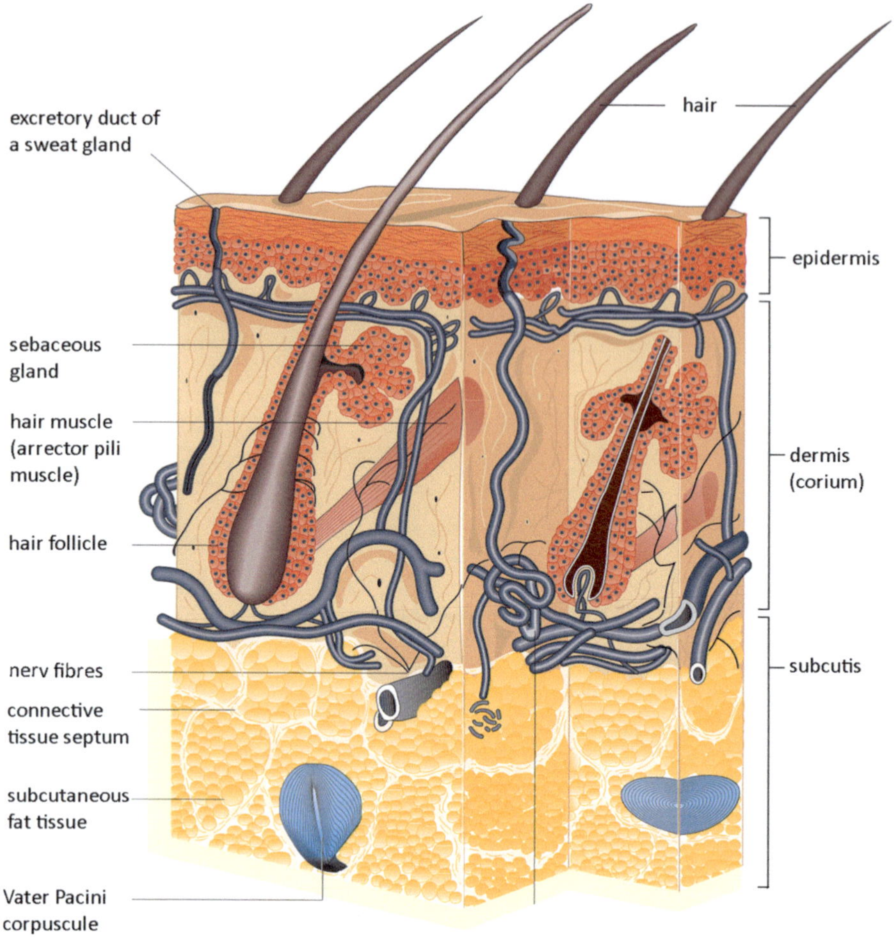

Fig. 2.58 Schematic drawing of hairy skin

prominence stretches the skin located above for 24 h, 365 days of the year. In addition, the skin is easily injured and thus squeezed, crushed, bruised, or scarred. In this situation, it is almost inevitable that damage will occur.

External factors such as shoes or the pavement are, in principle, not the cause of ulceration.

The main cause in the majority of ulcers is the internal condition of the foot that exposes vulnerable prominences. External protection might have been ineffective or insufficient but is generally not the cause.

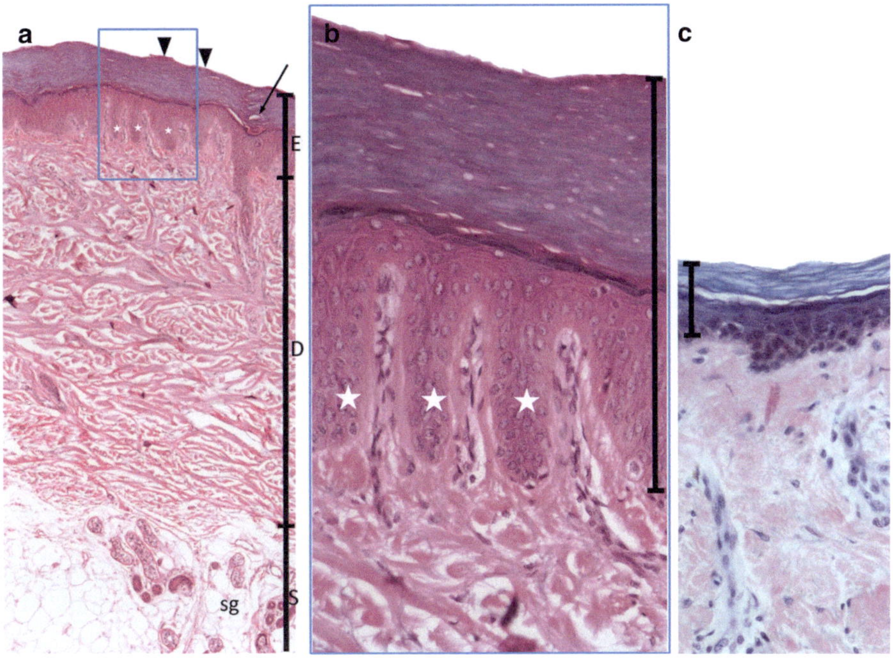

Fig. 2.59 Hairless (glabrous) and hairy skin, histological slices (**a**) layers of hairless skin, histological slice magnification ×40, Epidermis *(E)* with an excretory duct of a sweat gland *(black arrow)* and epidermal ridges *(black arrow heads)*, Dermis *(D)*, Subcutis *(S)* with sweat glands *(sg)* (**b**) hairless skin, magnification ×200, The epidermal basal layers are folded (white stars) and closely interlocked with the dermal papillae between them. (**c**) hairy skin, magnification ×200; In comparison of hairless skin *(b)*, in hairy skin *(c)* the epithelium *(black bar* in **c***)*, as well as the horny layer, are thinner and the interlocking between epithelium and dermis less solid

Skin appendages such as the toenails are particularly delicate. Damage to these appendages due to pressure can be induced without a bony prominence beneath.

When ulcers occur, the subcutaneous fat pad is usually reduced to such an extent that bony prominences are located directly under the skin and the risk of trauma has increased. Atrophy of the fat pad is not only due to monotonous trauma but also to other, still unknown, causes. So, atrophy is also present in non-weight-bearing areas [16–20].

An acute overload may cause redness, blisters and necrosis similar to burns or other factors damaging the skin. A latent overload, repeated hundreds or thousands of times each day, leads to the development of hyperkeratosis and pressure ulcers.

2.8.2 Development of Pressure Ulcers

In the case of chronic overload, the integrity of the skin is initially preserved by thickening the corium which enhances its resistance. Walking on this thickening

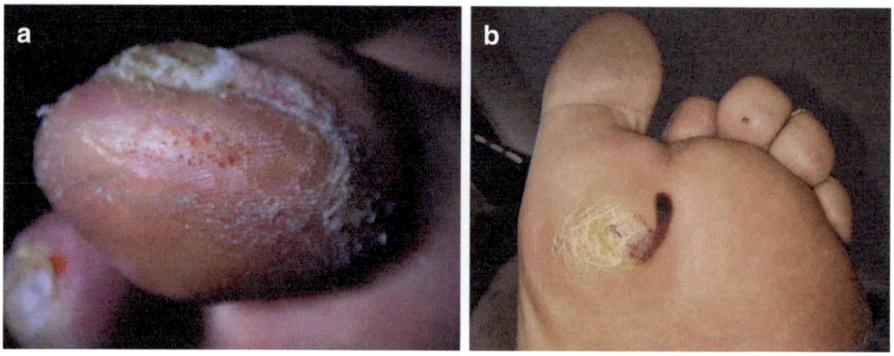

Fig. 2.60 (**a**) Callus with pinpoint haemorrhages (**b**) Haemorrhagic callus

means that the proximal and distal surfaces are compressed or stretched at each step. These forces rise with increasing thickness and overcome the epidermal elasticity. Cracks appear on the surface, while subtle blisters with bleeding arise at deeper levels. These characteristic, pinpoint haemorrhages (Fig. 2.60a) are followed by larger blisters that may join and create *haemorrhages in calluses* (Fig. 2.60b) [21]. The cracks on the surface can make contact with the haemorrhagic areas and allow the invasion of microorganisms. As a consequence, abscesses within and beneath the callus may develop. The cracks may become crusted and close, while the traumatised tissue beneath the callus gives way to further expansion of the abscess. An ulcer develops that resembles a punched hole and is sometimes called '*malum perforans*' (Fig. 2.61).

Apart from this larger, plantar hyperkeratosis called callus or callosity, shear forces (friction) combined with more focused pressure give origin to a deeply penetrating hyperkeratosis. The result is a *corn* which is pressed into deeper tissues by the same pressure that had stimulated the genesis of the hyperkeratosis in the first place. On the surface, the corn becomes only slightly larger (Fig. 2.62) but extends in depth and causes pain.

Prophylactic measures to prevent ulcers mainly aim at interrupting the transition from an uncomplicated hyperkeratosis to the formation of blisters and haemorrhages [22]. The measures usually applied are patient support, podiatry, protective footwear and sometimes other measures of internal or external offloading. These are discussed in the following chapters. The pattern of calluses is a precious clue to discover excessive stress early and easily. These regions under threat call for better offloading by optimisation of footwear or surgical procedures (internal offloading). Which overstressed region has to be addressed in which way is to be decided according to the estimated risk and the probability of successful reduction of this risk.

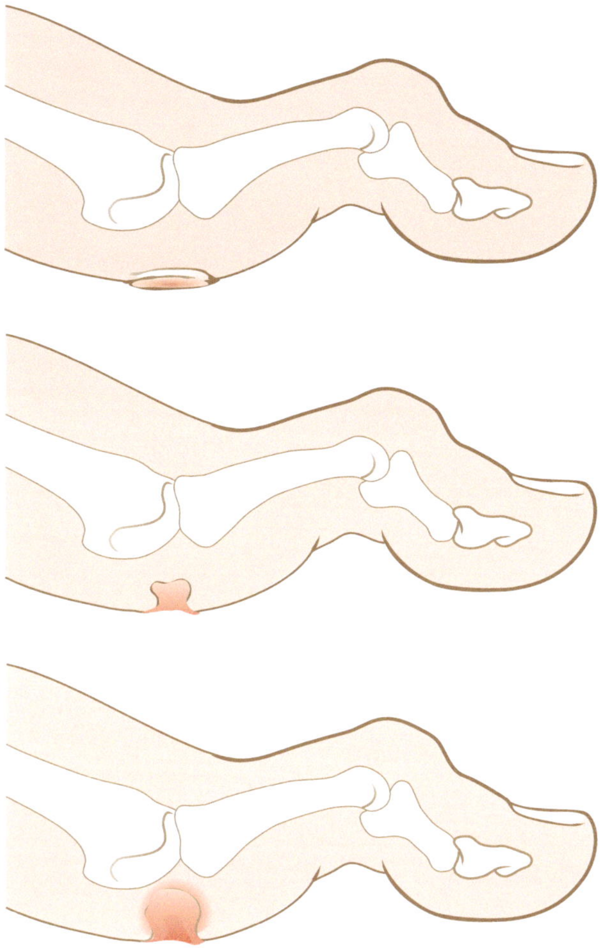

Fig. 2.61 From callus to ulcer

2.9 Recommended Literature

Leslie Klenerman and Bernard A. Wood: The human foot: a companion to clinical studies.

This collaboration between a palaeontologist and an orthopaedic surgeon gives affectionate insights into the evolution of foot and gait. 192 pages, 2006. London: Springer. ISBN: 185233925X

Serge Tixa: Atlas of Palpatory Anatomy of the Lower Extremities : A Manual Inspection of the Surface

This beautiful atlas illustrates a didactic, technical approach in finding the different anatomical structures (bones, ligaments, tendons, muscles and nerves) in the lower extremities. The photos are unique in their presentation of the structures. 220 pages, 1998, McGraw-Hill, ISBN-10: 0070653577

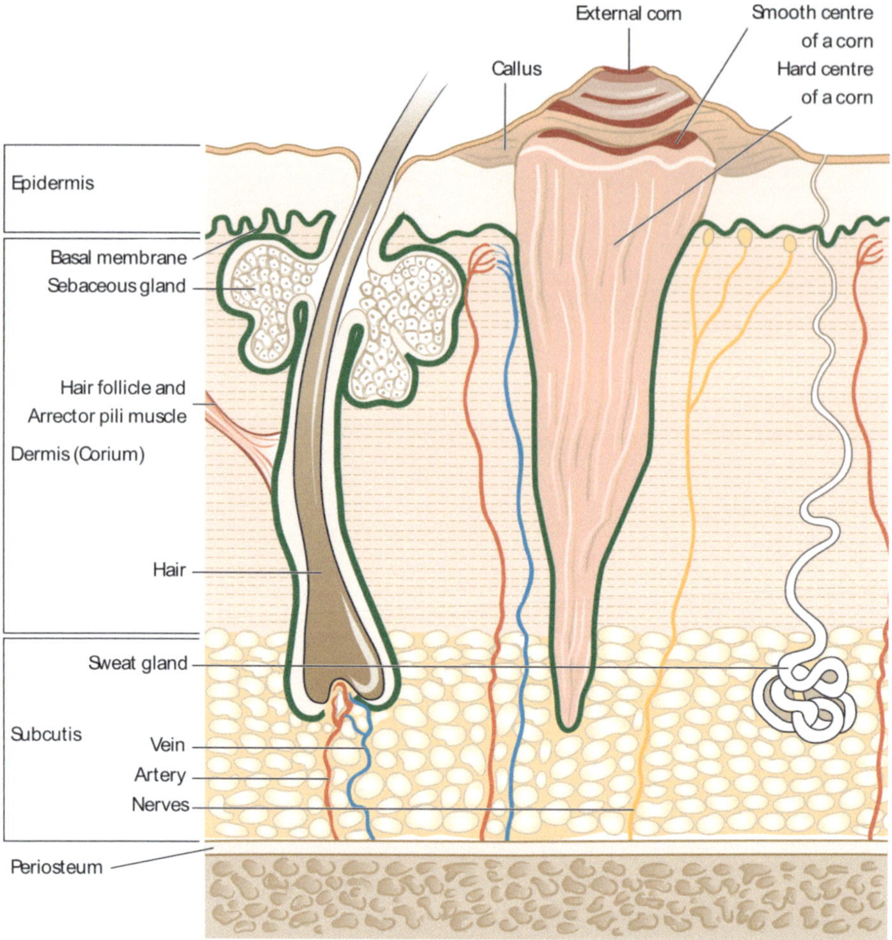

Fig. 2.62 Schematic illustration of a corn

References

1. Wood B, Richmond BG. Human evolution: taxonomy and paleobiology. J Anat. 2000;197(Pt 1):19–60.
2. Klenerman L, Wood BA. The human foot : a companion to clinical studies. London: Springer; 2006.
3. Whitmore I. Terminologia anatomica: new terminology for the new anatomist. Anat Rec. 1999;257(2):50–3.
4. Lang J, Wachsmuth W. Bein und Statik. Praktische Anatomie. Berlin: Springer; 1972.
5. Dullaert K, Hagen J, Klos K, Gueorguiev B, Lenz M, Richards RG, Simons P. The influence of the Peroneus Longus muscle on the foot under axial loading: a CT evaluated dynamic cadaveric model study. Clin Biomech (Bristol, Avon). 2016;34:7–11. https://doi.org/10.1016/j.clinbiomech.2016.03.001.
6. Debrunner HU, Jacob HAC. Der Fuß als Ganzes. In: Debrunner HU, Jacob HAC, editors. Biomechanik des Fußes. Stuttgart: Enke; 1998. p. 7–106.

7. Klaue K. The Foot. London: Springer; 2015.
8. Cavagna GA, Heglund NC, Taylor CR. Mechanical work in terrestrial locomotion: two basic mechanisms for minimizing energy expenditure. Am J Physiol. 1977;233(5):R243–61.
9. Holewski JJ, Moss KM, Stess RM, Graf PM, Grunfeld C. Prevalence of foot pathology and lower extremity complications in a diabetic outpatient clinic. J Rehabil Res Dev. 1989;26(3):35–44.
10. Smith DG, Barnes BC, Sands AK, Boyko EJ, Ahroni JH. Prevalence of radiographic foot abnormalities in patients with diabetes. Foot Ankle Int. 1997;18(6):342–6.
11. Bus SA, Maas M, Cavanagh PR, Michels RP, Levi M. Plantar fat-pad displacement in neuropathic diabetic patients with toe deformity: a magnetic resonance imaging study. Diabetes Care. 2004;27(10):2376–81.
12. Andersen H. Motor dysfunction in diabetes. Diabetes Metab Res Rev. 2012;28 Suppl 1:89–92. https://doi.org/10.1002/dmrr.2257.
13. Bus SA, Yang QX, Wang JH, Smith MB, Wunderlich R, Cavanagh PR. Intrinsic muscle atrophy and toe deformity in the diabetic neuropathic foot: a magnetic resonance imaging study. Diabetes Care. 2002;25(8):1444–50.
14. Andersen H, Gadeberg PC, Brock B, Jakobsen J. Muscular atrophy in diabetic neuropathy: a stereological magnetic resonance imaging study. Diabetologia. 1997;40(9):1062–9. https://doi.org/10.1007/s001250050788.
15. Redkina V, Sikorski A, Beike J. Deformitäten der Kleinzehe - Pathogenese und praxisnahe Nomenklatur. Fuß & Sprunggelenk. 2013;11:95–100.
16. Brash PD, Foster J, Vennart W, Anthony P, Tooke JE. Magnetic resonance imaging techniques demonstrate soft tissue damage in the diabetic foot. Diabet Med. 1999;16(1):55–61.
17. Cheung YY, Doyley M, Miller TB, Kennedy F, Lynch F Jr, Wrobel JS, Paulson K, Weaver J. Magnetic resonance elastography of the plantar fat pads: Preliminary study in diabetic patients and asymptomatic volunteers. J Comput Assist Tomogr. 2006;30(2):321–6.
18. Gooding GA, Stess RM, Graf PM, Moss KM, Louie KS, Grunfeld C. Sonography of the sole of the foot. Evidence for loss of foot pad thickness in diabetes and its relationship to ulceration of the foot. Invest Radiol. 1986;21(1):45–8.
19. Kao PF, Davis BL, Hardy PA. Characterization of the calcaneal fat pad in diabetic and non-diabetic patients using magnetic resonance imaging. Magn Reson Imaging. 1999;17(6):851–7.
20. Waldecker U, Lehr HA. Is there histomorphological evidence of plantar metatarsal fat pad atrophy in patients with diabetes? J Foot Ankle Surg. 2009;48(6):648–52. https://doi.org/10.1053/j.jfas.2009.07.008.
21. Rosen RC, Davids MS, Bohanske LM, Lemont H. Hemorrhage into plantar callus and diabetes mellitus. Cutis. 1985;35(4):339–41.
22. Delbridge L, Ctercteko G, Fowler C, Reeve TS, Le Quesne LP. The aetiology of diabetic neuropathic ulceration of the foot. Br J Surg. 1985;72(1):1–6.

3 Diagnostic Pathways

This chapter describes the steps involved in recording the patient's medical history and performing a physical examination. The order is based on possible procedures for an initial consultation. It focuses firstly on building trust as a necessary basis for good communication and secondly on systematically identifying the causes of DFS.

3.1 Overview

In this book, *the causes of the diabetic foot are divided into conditions and triggers*. This concept assumes that excessive stress on the musculoskeletal system, subcutaneous soft tissue and the skin is part of life. As a result of evolution, warning mechanisms restrict the extension of an injury and repair is provided without permanent impairment. The weakening of this resilience is referred to as *underlying conditions of DFS* (Fig. 3.1). The *triggers* determine where DFS becomes active. If they are not treated properly, they will prolong the existence of the ulcer or lead to its reactivation.

3.2 Some Basic Considerations Regarding Communication

3.2.1 The Basis of Trust Between the Patient and the Therapist

'Good treatment' means to integrate professional skills into the framework of values of the person affected. It is important to show this intention from the beginning and to make conscious use of the 'first impression'. Making eye contact before looking at the foot, paying particular attention to the patient's previous efforts to maintain their health, and involving any family members present at the event helps in building trust. This will make good news credible and unpleasant truths more acceptable later. After presenting oneself, the person providing therapy could

D. Hochlenert et al., *Diabetic Foot Syndrome*,
https://doi.org/10.1007/978-3-319-92055-9_3

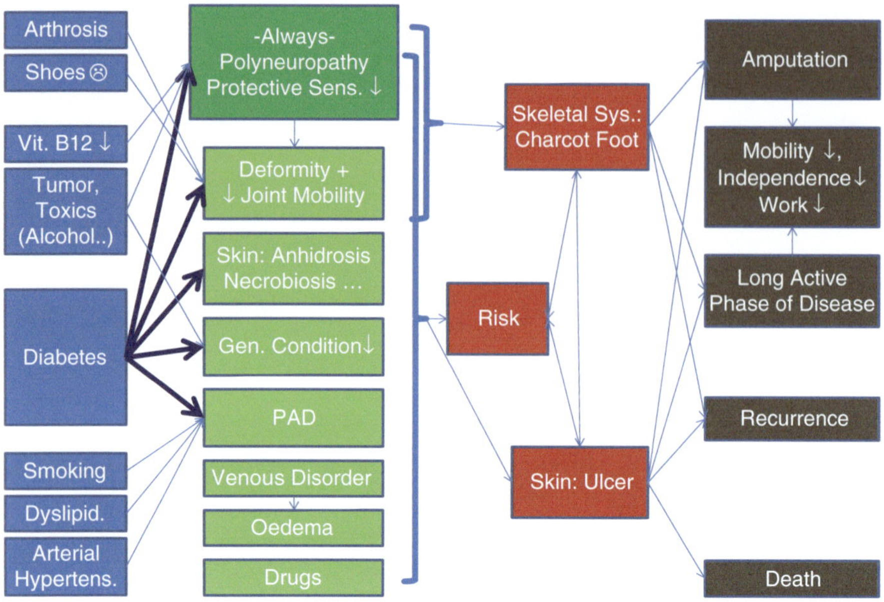

Fig. 3.1 Conditions which reduce resilience (*green*) and their causes (*blue*) as underlying causes for the development of DFS (*red*) and complications of DFS (*brown*)

express a confident and generous smile and *start in an open manner* such as 'Please, tell me.' A slightly more restrictive question would be: 'What has happened?' or 'What brought you here?' or as a second question 'What have you done about this?'. Previous methods of treatment should be dealt with in a non-judgemental way whilst avoiding any remarks which may be taken as criticism.

3.2.2 'Compliance' of the Affected Person and Therapist

One of the most common causes of poor results in non-specialised medical facilities is the unexpected behaviour of people who do not experience pain with the normal intensity. They may ignore instructions to an unusual degree, which can lead to resentment or even aggression on the part of the therapist and is often labelled 'Non-Compliance'. The concepts of 'Compliance' and 'Adherence' express the extent to which a prescribed or agreed course of action is carried out. This assumes a common context, in which a prescription or an agreement between patient and therapist has been made. Ideally, the therapist puts himself in the role of the patient. However, in the case of DFS, this is almost impossible. Those who are unaffected cannot imagine a world without the limitations on our actions due to pain [1]. The only useful way at present is to adjust the expectations of the therapist to the situation. They have to realise that patients with limited sensitivity to pain are not going to obey complex rules which restrict their mobility. It is the task of the therapist to apply simple procedures with as few restrictions as possible on the mobility of the patient. From this it is understood that:

1. **It is inherently impossible to ensure complete, uninterrupted rest for the feet of a person who does not feel pain and is otherwise able to walk.**
2. **Agreements on offloading that allow exceptions are not put into practice as agreed. The limits of the exceptions are tested and extended.**
3. **The affected person is unlikely to discard all the shoes which they have worn in the past and will continue to wear some of them.**

Awareness of these aspects must be included in all therapeutic concepts. Examples:

1. After surgical procedures which require a subsequent period of rest, measures must be taken which make it impossible for the foot to be put under stress.
2. If it is absolutely necessary to use the agreed offloading device without exception, it mustn't be removable.
3. Instructions for wearing offloading devices, if their use is considered to be essential for the success of the therapy, must not include exceptions.
4. If compromises are possible from a medical point of view, testing their limits should be discussed. Otherwise, these tests will take place without being agreed.
5. Surgical measures for internal offloading improve the resilience of the foot which is most needed when protective shoes or devices are not worn. Prophylactic surgical measures should be taken into account whenever the risk is acceptable.

3.2.3 Unrealistic Demands

Some common options in the treatment of people affected by a diabetic foot are impossible to put into practice in the real world for more than a few days. Typical examples of *unrealistic demands* are:

'Get rid of all the shoes you own and wear only the protective shoes which have been prescribed to you from now on.'—This request is unrealistic because only one pair of shoes may be initially available. For most people in developed countries this is not sufficient to ensure mobility at home and outside while maintaining basic standards of hygiene. Later on, when more shoes are available, the affected person has become accustomed to making compromises and no longer considers it necessary to discard the shoes that were used previously. Many people lovingly build up a collection of shoes in the course of their lives, which they think of as a part of their personality. For such people, the thought of being separated from their collection is almost unbearable.

'As long as the ulcer exists, do not walk' or 'walk as little as possible.' —These recommendations attempt to achieve offloading by reducing the number of footsteps. It limits the independence of the patient who in turn becomes dependent on support from others. Also, for many people, mobility is synonymous with vitality. Most importantly, this recommendation contradicts the central requirement of a healthy lifestyle for people with diabetes. Thus, from a more general, patient-centred point of view, it might be wise to not follow such an advice as strictly as the therapist might have expressed.

3.2.3.1 Consequences of Unrealistic Demands

Instructions which require the patient to make an unattainable effort or which they can only partially carry out, create a *barrier* between patient and therapist. Patients fail to appear for follow-up appointments or wear protective shoes only when visiting the clinic.

The compromises the patient has found out are kept in secret and therefore cannot be discussed. The patient does not profit from the experience held by the therapeutic team and the team doesn't learn from the successful compromises the patient has found.

Such unrealistic demands eliminate the learning effect for the therapist, who does not perceive responsibility in case of failure. 'We learn from our mistakes, therefore one is not enough!' is a German saying. When the patient is blamed for 'walking too much again' or 'wearing the wrong shoes again', then the therapists often fail to look for ways of optimising their strategies. And which patient doesn't 'walk too much'? How many do not wear the protective shoes 'yet again'?

Unrealistic goals lead to disappointment, which undermines job satisfaction and may lead to 'burn out'.

3.2.3.2 Alternatives

Instead of using standards with a tendency towards overprotection, it makes sense to *tailor recommendations* to the risks faced by the single patient and to his or her willingness to take risks. This way, recommendations difficult to follow can be reduced to a minimum. Therapists should pro-actively address critical everyday situations. These include going to the toilet during the night, taking showers or baths, going to the public swimming pool or sauna, making the first few steps after getting up in the morning, or encounter exceptional situations such as social events or holidays, especially in warm countries and at the beach. Patients should feel able to discuss openly the compromises which they are prepared to make. If patients test their limits and go beyond them sometimes, the results will help to develop a better workable compromise in the future.

- **No recriminations if the therapy concept fails.**
- **The failure of a concept should, if possible, lead to a change of the therapeutic regimen even if the cause of the failure is the non-adherence of the patient.**
- **Solidarity and empathy should not be cast in doubt as a result of failure. Supporting the patient to use his or her resources in a sensitive way sometimes includes criticism. The patient must know and feel at each moment that the therapist is on his or her side.**

3.3 Underlying Conditions Reducing Resilience

In order to develop the subacute structural breakdown typical of the diabetic foot, conditions which reduce the extraordinary resilience of the foot are necessary. This section resumes the steps in the diagnosis of these prerequisites.

3.3.1 Polyneuropathy

Without a reduction in protective sensation (loss of protective sensation = LOPS), in other words, without a reduction in the sensitivity to pain, the patient would soon seek help and generally be able to behave in an appropriate manner. This would remove the unique and most important feature of the disease. For this, it is crucial to detect a reduction of protective sensation, which in the context of DFS is the relevant consequence of polyneuropathy (PNP). However, the examinations which are typically carried out to detect PNP, identify signals which are transmitted via the thick, myelin sheathed A-fibres of nerves. Pain, on the other hand, is transmitted via the fine unmyelinated C-fibres. In this way, the *investigations to detect polyneuropathy* can produce a nearly normal result despite the patient's reduced sensitivity to pain and actually marked presence of LOPS. A lack of pain, for example during debridement, is proof of reduced pain perception. In this case, the patient has '*small-fibre Neuropathy*' despite normal tests [2, 3]. Liniger et al. investigated the sensitivity to vibration of normal persons and people with DFS in [4]. By performing the tuning fork test, they found that 8 out of 38 ft with DFS showed sensitivity to vibration in the range of healthy normal persons. They concluded that sensitivity to vibration of under 5/8 is associated with an increased risk of DFS even in people at higher age for whom these values are normal. Two ulcerations were found with apparently normal sensitivity to vibration [4] (Fig. 3.2).

- **If an affected person can walk on a plantar wound without great difficulty, a relevant polyneuropathy is proven!**
- **Loss of protective sensation (LOPS) may be present despite normal tests for polyneuropathy!**

Tests for the presence of Polyneuropathy or the loss of protective sensation (LOPS) are carried out and interpreted in many different ways. This is important to bear in mind:

- Tests should be carried out in each medical facility according to a standardised procedure.
- The diagnosis does not depend on the result of a single test but on the whole picture and the possible relevance for the individual patient. Generally speaking,

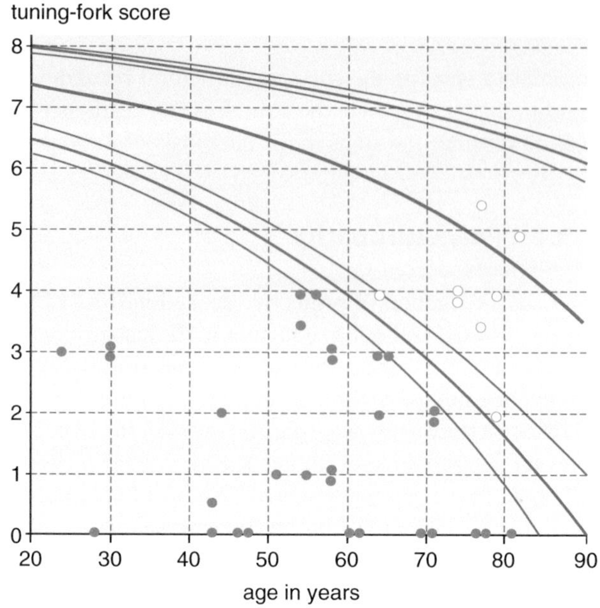

Fig. 3.2 Sensitivity to vibration in first MTH of 38 ulcerated feet in 26 people with diabetes. The open circles describe the sensitivity in a range which is typical for 90% of normal people. Modified according to Liniger et al. [4]

it is essential for people with DFS that the diagnosis of PNP is made without any doubt. When accepted by the patient, necessary aids can be prescribed and will hopefully be applied.

The following is an example of a possible procedure and interpretation.

3.3.1.1 Performing the Tuning Fork Test

1. The vibrating tuning fork is placed on a bone of the wrist. The patient is asked what is felt. The description should correspond to the sensation of vibration. The patient is informed that the following examination of the foot will concern this sensation. Then the patient is asked to close the eyes or to look at the ceiling in order to test only the sensitivity of the feet and not the patient's vision. In order not to falsify the results it is important that the examiner does not reveal their expectations through their tone of voice.
2. The vibrating tuning fork is placed medially on the MTP joint of the hallux. The patient is asked 'Can you feel the vibration here too?' After confirmation, the tuning fork is removed, made to vibrate again and then stopped without the patient noticing. The tuning fork, which is no longer vibrating, is then again placed on the MTP joint of the hallux and the patient is asked again if they can feel the vibration. If the patient affirms, the first step on the wrist must be repeated to exclude the possibility that the patient has not understood the principle. If they have clearly understood the principle but are unable to differentiate between the tuning fork when it is vibrating to the maximum and when it is not vibrating, then the sensitivity to vibration has vanished.

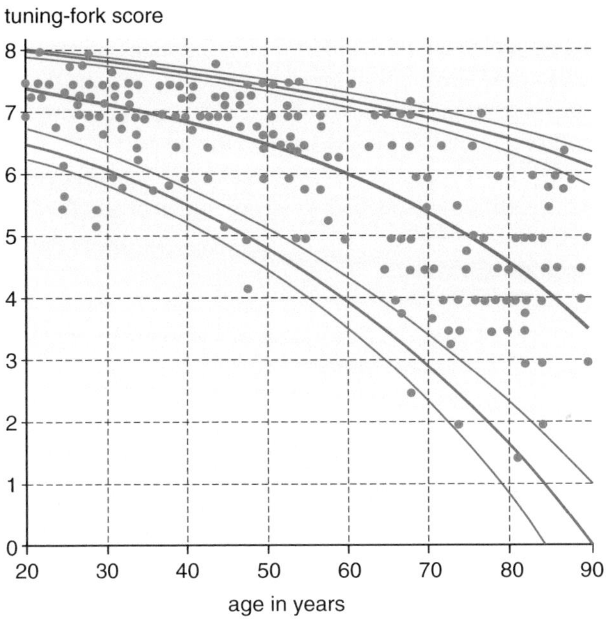

Fig. 3.3 Sensitivity to vibration in 214 neurologically healthy people not affected by diabetes, at the first metatarsal bone. The two thicker lines describe the 90% confidence interval modified according to Liniger et al. [4]

3. The vibrating tuning fork is again placed medially on the MTP joint of the hallux. While the intensity of the vibration is fading out, the patient is asked to indicate the exact moment when the vibration can no longer be felt. The intensity of vibrations which the patient can still feel is expressed in eighths.

Interpretation of the result: up to the age of 30 at least 7/8, from 30 to 40 years of age at least 6/8 and after the age of 40 at least 5/8 should be felt. Most healthy people feel more than 4/8, even at an advanced age [4] (Fig. 3.3).

Possible sources of error: Even those patients who feel no vibration at all realise as a result of the questions being asked that there are vibrations taking place and that they should be aware of them. These patients interpret other types of sensation as vibration and give responses which may simulate absolute normality. For this reason, it is necessary to include other indicators of polyneuropathy (painful or almost painless wounds, callosities, anhidrosis of the skin…) to ensure the plausibility of the examination result [5, 6].

3.3.1.2 Performing the Monofilament Test

The Semmes-Weinstein-Monofilament creates a pressure of 10 g when pressed on the contact surface until the filament bends. This can be felt by a healthy person with minimal callus formation on every part of the skin. Major callus formation can reduce the sensitivity for the monofilament in the absence of a nerve disorder.

The patient is asked to close their eyes or to look at the ceiling. The sole of the foot is then touched for about 1 s using the monofilament causing it to bend to an excursion of about 1 cm. The monofilament is then removed and the patient is asked where they felt this sensation. This is tested at different points, which should include the ball of the hallux, the ball of the 5th toe and the heel.

Possible sources of error: repetitive touches at brief intervals with the monofilament produce a different impulse which is easier to detect and falsify the result [7].

3.3.1.3 Further Examinations

The *Pinprick test* or Cutaneous pressure pain perception threshold (*CPPPT*) examines pain caused by pressure on a small area of the skin. In this way, the actually relevant sensory quality is tested. Different needles are used for this purpose, that should not lead to injury. So-called *von-Frey hairs* consists of glass fibres and are pressed onto the sole of the foot until they bend. The examined person indicates whether nothing, pressure or pointed pain is perceived. For quantitative analysis, glass fibres of different thicknesses are used, applying pressures of 8–512 mN. In one study, 98% of those with diabetic feet were unable to perceive pain [8].

As part of the *Neuropathy Disability Score* (NDS) the examination of the Achilles tendon reflex is recommended [9]. The *Neuropathy Symptom Score* (NSS)[10] standardises symptoms in order to integrate this aspect into assessment and diagnosis. Cold-warm-discrimination, sharp-blunt-discrimination, 2-point-discrimination, measurement of the secretion of the sweat glands and further tests can complete the picture [11].

NDS items	Description
Vibration sensation (128 Hz tuning fork)	0 = present, 1 = reduced/absent
Temperature sensation (cold tuning fork)	0 = present, 1 = reduced/absent
Pin-prick	0 = present, 1 = reduced/absent
Ankle reflex	0 = normal, 1 = present with reinforcement, 2 = absent per side

A score of 6 or more is considered to be abnormal

DNS items	Rate
Unsteadiness in walking	0 = absent, 1 = present
Numbness	0 = absent, 1 = present
Burning, aching pain or tenderness in legs or feet	0 = absent, 1 = present
Prickling sensations	0 = absent, 1 = present

A score of 1 or more is considered to be abnormal

3.3.2 Peripheral Arterial Disease (PAD)

A strong pulse, the presence of an adequate growth of hair on the toes, unrestricted toenail growth and warm skin are signs of intact blood circulation. The growth of adequate amount of hair is known as ‘hairy toe sign’. The amount of hair in other

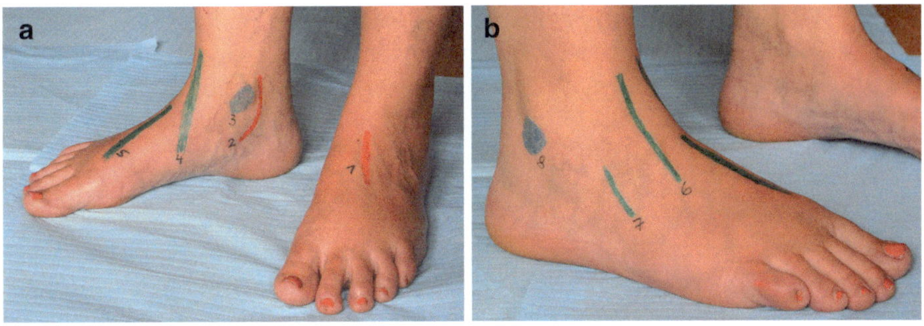

Fig. 3.4 (**a, b**) *1* Arteria dorsalis pedis, *2* Arteria tibialis posterior, *3* Malleolus medialis, *4* M. tibialis anterior tendon, *5* M. extensor hallucis longus tendon, *6* M. extensor digitorum longus tendon, *7* M. fibularis (peroneus) tertius tendon, *8* Malleolus lateralis

parts of the skin has to be taken into account as someone who has no more than fluff on their legs will be unlikely to have dense hair on their toes. However, none of these signs are absolute proof. For this reason, if the clinical signs are unclear a Doppler ultrasound examination must be performed. This provides an estimate of the flow. The sound can be classified as a monophasic, biphasic or triphasic flow. Unfortunately, that this interpretation of the result depends on the investigator's judgement, but with sufficient experience, it is possible to make a good estimate of whether the flow is disturbed or undisturbed. Doppler also allows the determination of the ankle-brachial-index (ABI). If this does not produce sufficient clarity a duplex examination must be carried out. These exams are described more in detail on the following pages.

3.3.2.1 Palpation of the Pulse

The pulsation of the **A**rteria **d**orsalis **p**edis (ADP) can be felt on the instep of the foot. The **A**rteria **t**ibialis **p**osterior (ATP) can be felt behind the inner ankle. Behind the outer ankle the **A**rteria **f**ibularis (AF) can be detected. It is common from middle age onwards that the pulse of the Arteria fibularis is no longer perceptible (Fig. 3.4).

This examination has important pitfalls:

- Firstly, it is possible to feel one's own pulse in the fingertips.
- Secondly, many neuropathic patients show a rhythmic fasciculation of the extensor tendons of the instep. These tendons are responsible for lifting the toes. Their fasciculation can be felt like a typical pulse for some beats.

These pitfalls can be avoided if the examiner is sure to feel at least 10 consecutive beats.

The 10 Beats Rule:
The pulse is trustworthy only if more than ten beats are clearly felt.

3.3.2.2 Dermal Signs and Preliminary Clinical Tests

In the case of a persistent, relevant, circulatory disorder the skin becomes thin and the dermal appendages atrophy. The nails grow slowly and become rippled. The hair on the toes falls out and fails to grow back. The skin becomes cool and in classic cases turns red-blue (livid) (Fig. 3.5a).

Possible pitfalls:

- In the case of a concomitant infection, or when the foot has been kept very warm, the temperature may be normal despite impaired perfusion.
- If the circulatory disorder is of very recent onset, the hair and nails may appear absolutely normal.

For this reason, it is often wise to make use of other clinical examination methods in addition, even if their use is not generally accepted:

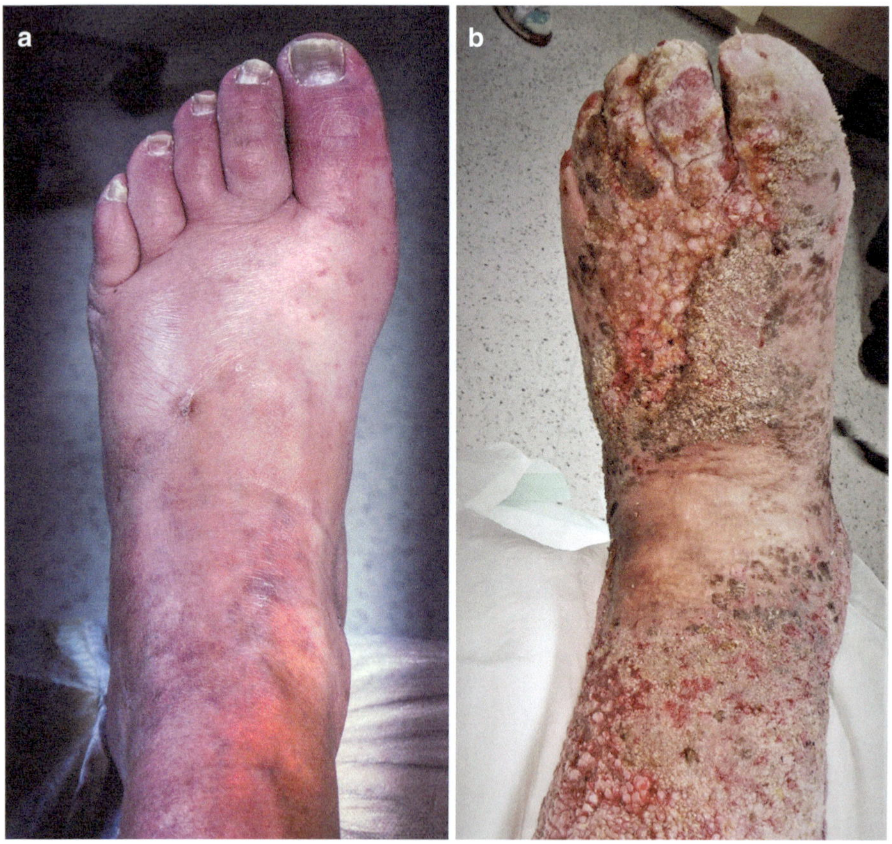

Fig. 3.5 Two typical aspects of morphological changes due to vascular disease: (**a**) chronic angio-neuropathic foot (**b**) chronic lymphatic oedema with ulcers

Capillary refill time (CRT): The skin becomes pale after pressure is applied for a few seconds. The previous colour returns after around 3–4 s. In the case of restricted capillary blood supply this takes longer. This test has been advocated as an indicator of perfusion status in seriously ill patients (shock). Normal values reach from <1 s for children to <3 s in adults and <4.5 s in the elderly [12].

Perfusion pressure tested by lifting the foot: With normal arterial flow, the patient can raise their leg from a lying position and the pulse remains normal. The skin does not turn pale. The circulation is regarded as critically abnormal if the foot pales when raised more than 50 cm and the pulse is imperceptible when a pocket doppler is applied. This effect can be measured more accurately using the *hydrostatic toe pressure* measurement [13, 14]. There are many variations on this examination. The best known in German speaking countries is the Ratschow test. To perform this test the legs are raised and then lowered. The time taken to refill is measured whilst lowering the legs. While the legs are raised the feet are moved, for example, rhythmically plantar- and dorsiflexed or rotated. When lowering the legs, the time taken for diffuse reddening is measured (up to 5 s is normal, >20 s is pathological) as well as the time for filling the veins of the instep (up to 20 s is normal, >60 s is pathological). Concomitant diseases which are associated with a general weakening of the muscles make this examination impossible for many people with DFS [15].

3.3.2.3 Doppler Examination

The patient reclines horizontally and a pocket doppler is applied to search for the site where the arterial pulsation can best be heard in the region of the ADP and the ATP. The angle is as narrow as possible (30–45°), because an upright transducer does not produce a signal. At least 5 mL of gel is required to guarantee an acoustic coupling at a narrow angle. Now the cuff is pumped up around the calf until the pulsating sound disappears. Then the pressure in the cuff is released until the sound can be heard again. The pressure measured in the cuff is documented, and the ankle pressure is taken as the highest reading of either artery.

After the examination, the pressure in both arms is measured according to Riva-Rocci (normal blood pressure measurement) and the higher systolic pressure is used to calculate the quotients. Some guidelines recommend using a Doppler technique to measure the arm pressure instead of using the stethoscope. Various options for calculation have been published [16, 17]. The ankle-brachial-index is the ankle pressure divided by the brachial pressure. In the case of patients on dialysis, taking a blood pressure measurement on the arm with the shunt leads to false results and to an undesired increase in the pressure of the shunt's veins. Under no circumstances should this be done.

When *describing the flow*, there is a differentiation between monophasic, biphasic and triphasic flow. The descriptions relate to the number of flow peaks which can be derived during a heart cycle. The second phase of the heart cycle corresponds to the relaxation of the heart muscle. At the start of this phase, the aortic valve closes and the blood flows back to the heart. If nothing restricts the flow, this short interruption of the flow can be detected in the periphery as it separates the sound of the flow into two parts (biphasic flow). When the sound is not divided into two sounds and no double hissing can be heard, but only a single sound, it is referred to as a monophasic flow profile. The flow behind a constriction is typically monophasic. Using a doppler instrument with a graphic display it may even be possible to detect a reverse flow in the low-flow phase (triphasic flow). The graphic display also enables the calculation of the pulsatility index. This is more conclusive in the detection of a severe vascular disease with concomitant medial arterial sclerosis (Mönckeberg's sclerosis) [18].

Possible sources of error:

- Using an insufficient amount of gel can easily lead to incorrect results.
- In the central part of the interphalangeal space between the first and the second metatarsal bone on the instep, a good signal may often be detected. This signal does not originate from the Arteria dorsalis pedis but from a connecting artery between the dorsal arch and the deep plantar arch. This should not be used to calculate the pressure index. However, this connecting artery is important, because it determines the development of collateral vessels and must be protected during surgery.

3.3.3 Other Factors Which Prevent Wounds from Closure

The other common factors which prevent wounds from closure can be identified asking the medical history or during clinical examination. Occasionally blood tests or skin biopsies are necessary.

- Skin diseases such as Anhidrosis, Necrobiosis lipoidica, Eczema as a result of allergic reactions or infections with bacteria or fungi, autoimmune diseases of the skin and skin tumours.
- Oedema of different origin
- Chronic venous insufficiency
- Diseases of the lymphatic system (Fig. 3.5b)
- Gout with uric acid precipitates in the joints, in fistulas that are connected to the joints and in soft tissue. These precipitates form a white material that resembles toothpaste.
- Concomitant diseases such as *end-stage kidney failure*, particularly those on renal replacement therapy. The importance of early stages of renal disease as an independent risk factor for the emergence of foot lesions is a controversial topic for discussion [19–21]
- Diseases which adversely affect the general condition of the patient such as anaemia, tumours or completely uncontrolled glucose metabolism.
- Medications such as cytotoxic chemotherapy (e.g. *Hydroxycarbamide*), radiotherapy or an immune-modulatory therapy, for example in the case of rheumatic diseases [22].

3.4 Triggers: Catalyst for Structural Breakdown

The factors which reduce resilience and impair wound closure are generally not sufficient to cause an ulcer. Further actions catalysing structural breakdown are required. These triggers determine the area of the foot where the DFU will be located. In the case of ulcers due to subliminal pressure repeated during walking, these are sites located above bony protuberances. The pattern of calluses on the skin gives an early indication of the areas which must bear a greater load than is physiologically intended. If no bony protuberance is involved, the trigger may be an accidental traumatic, thermal or chemical injury. An example of accidental trauma is chiropody performed by the patient on themselves, also known as 'bathroom surgery'.

3.4.1 Examination of the Foot

The actual steps in the examination depend on the individual experience of the examiner and the typical procedures in the medical facility. A foot surgeon whose focus is on reconstructive procedures would examine the patient's feet from a different perspective to a diabetologist searching for the causes of an ulceration. The following explanations are a suggestion for possible steps in the examination.

3.4.1.1 Inspection

A first important impression is given by the patient's *gait* whilst they think they are unobserved, for example, when they are called from the waiting area and walk to the treatment room. The following points are particularly important:

- Are the steps confident, swift and with long strides or are they ataxic, slow and short?
- Is the whole gait cycle completed or is the movement terminated prematurely as in the case of strolling (both sides) or limping (one-sided)?
- At what angle in relation to the direction of walking the foot is placed (angle of abduction). In other words, are the typical movements of the foot during the gait cycle performed along the longitudinal axis of the foot or along a rotated axis involving the medial portion of the hallux? (Fig. 3.6)

The inspection is continued on both bare feet. In order not to overlook anything, a fixed sequence should be adhered to. This includes:

- The dorsum of both the foot and the toes
- The borders
- The back of the heel
- The tips of the toes
- The interdigital spaces
- The sole of the foot

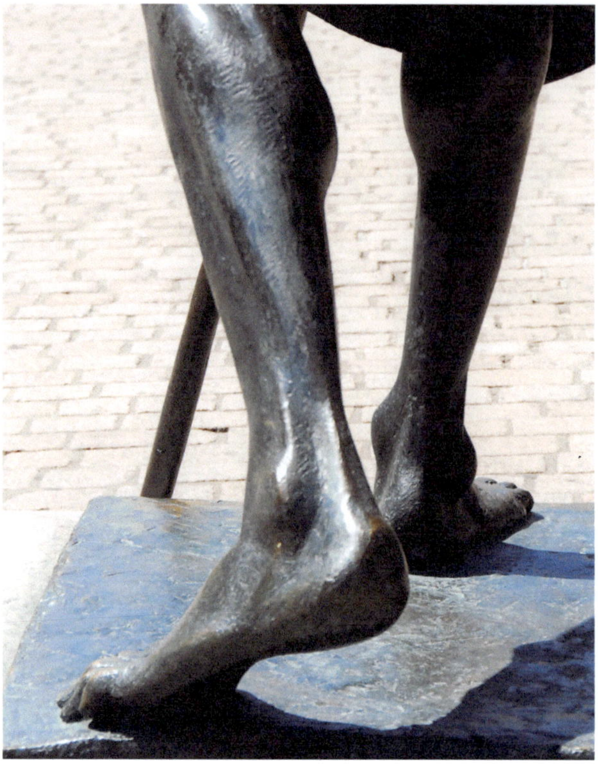

Fig. 3.6 Walking with wide abduction angle, from 'The Pilgrim from Speyer on the Path of St. James' by Martin Mayer 1990 in front of the Cathedral of Speyer

The following aspects are examined:

- The texture of the skin and adnexa (hair and nails).
- Symmetry
- Pattern of calluses
- Deformities
- Lesions

The patient is asked to make a circling movement with the foot. In this way a limitation such as for example a peroneal paralysis can be identified.

3.4.1.2 Palpation

At this point, the aim is to obtain a general impression of the strength, mobility and overall health of the foot and to test specific limitations that do not require provoking measures. The patient is asked to let their feet rest limply.

- The examiner takes the heel of the right foot in the right hand or the left foot in the left hand. This allows a better evaluation when testing the mobility of the hallux later during the examination. *Temperature*, possible *swellings* and areas which are *sensitive to pressure* are noted by palpation with the free hand.

- Then the toes are moved passively. Deformities such as *clawed toes* are classified as *reversible or fixed* (non-rectifiable) plantarisation. In the case of a reversible plantarisation, an intervention on the tendons is often sufficient. In the case of fixed plantarisation the cause of the fixation must first be established. An experienced surgeon, integrating the information derived from conventional X-ray images, can weigh up the options. Fixed deformities, that are not due to anchyloses, can also be treated by soft tissue interventions.
- With the hand on the heel, the examiner sets the position of the heel. In most situations, the heel must be aligned beneath the lower leg in neutral position. It is important to set the position of the heel because this largely affects the mobility of the tarsal joints. Every consideration of their mobility is based on the condition that the heel is orientated in neutral position. The examiner moves the foot to its *maximum dorsiflexion and plantarflexion* in order to find the limits of these movements (Fig. 3.7). When testing the limits of a passive dorsiflexion of the foot, considerable force is sometimes required.
- This is repeated with the heel inverted and with the heel everted. With the heel in neutral position, a maximal dorsiflexion of about 30° is normal. For unimpaired walking, a dorsiflexion of 5–10° is necessary. The range of motion can be limited by an inversion of the heel to such an extent that dorsiflexion might become impossible, even in normal feet.
- With the heel everted, the tarsal joints are relaxed. This allows an abduction and a flattening of the foot and greater dorsiflexion seems to be possible. This movement does not take place in the ankle joint as a normal dorsiflexion would do, but in the tarsal joints. The flattening of the foot thus compensates a short triceps surae. Flattening of the foot also extends the distance that plantar tendons have to bridge and can induce a functional hallux rigidus. *Functional hallux rigidus* can be tested everting the heel with one hand, bringing the forefoot to a dorsiflexion typical of unimpaired gait (about 10°) with the palm of the other hand and simultaneously trying to dorsiflex the hallux to 30° (see Fig. 3.7d).
- As patients are generally unable to relax their muscles immediately, *weakness in the function of the Achilles tendon* can also be identified. The weakness of the dorsiflexors and the fibular musculature (Peroneal Nerve Injury, *Peroneal palsy*, Peroneal paralysis, *drop foot* or foot drop) is tested by asking the patient to deliberately dorsiflex while the examiner tries to block this movement.
- If sufficient dorsiflexion of the foot is not possible (*pes equinus*), it might be useful to determine the contribution of the soleus and gastrocnemius muscles to this limitation. With the knee bent, the foot is brought to an angle as small as possible in relation to the tibia. If the dorsiflexion is not restored in this position of the knee, the Achilles tendon must be palpated. If it is at maximum tension, the cause might be a *shortening of the gastrocnemius and soleus muscle*. If it is not tense, a *stiff ankle joint* might be the cause. In this case, the joint will also be degenerated and enlarged.

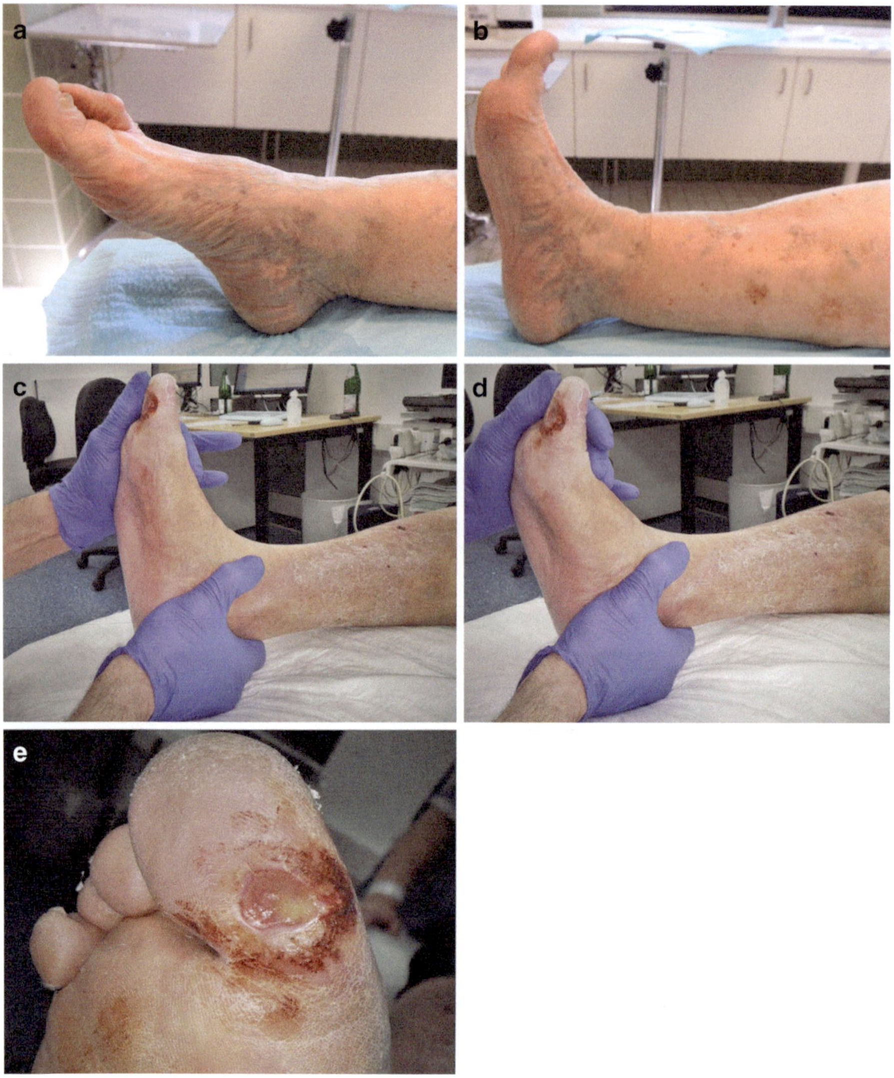

Fig. 3.7 (**a**, **b**) Active range of motion of the foot in plantarflexion/dorsiflexion. (**c**) With the heel in normal (neutral, rectus) position and the forefoot in slight pronation, the foot is plantarflexed due to a short triceps surae and the hallux can be passively dorsiflexed. (**d**) While the heel still is in normal position, the foot is forced in slight dorsiflexion simulating the movement during the gait cycle. This is possible only if the heel is everted, the subtalar plate becomes flexible and allows this movement in the tarsal joints. The whole foot is abduced. This compensations of the consequences of a short triceps surae permits walking but extends the distance to be covered by the FHL tendon. The hallux is now unable to be dorsiflexed corresponding to a functional hallux rigidus. (**e**) Ulcer as consequence of the functional hallux rigidus

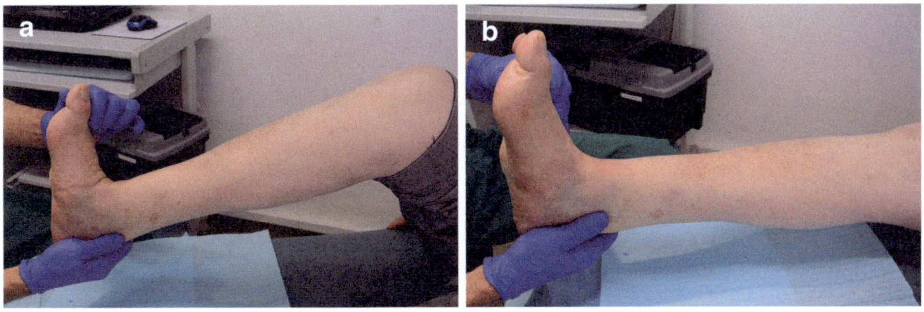

Fig. 3.8 (**a**, **b**) Silfverskjöld—Test

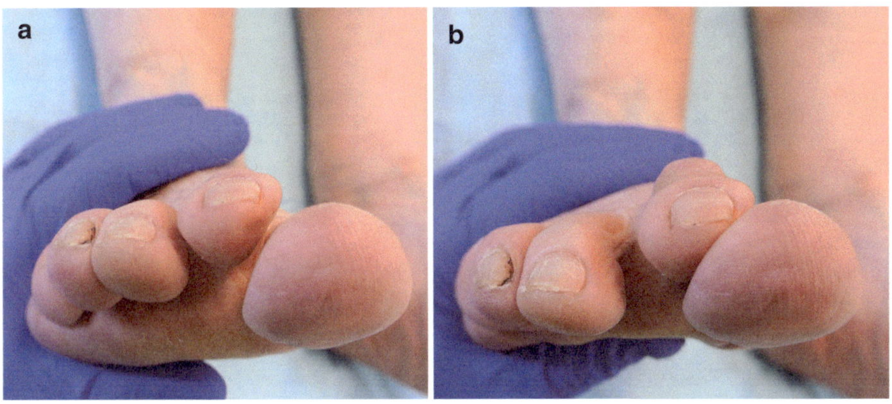

Fig. 3.9 (**a**, **b**) Push-up test

- If bending the knee restores dorsiflexion, the examination continues, and the knee is slowly stretched while the examiner continues to force maximum dorsal extension of the foot. By stretching the knee, the foot is automatically plantarflexed. This so-called *Silfverskjöld test* indicates the *short gastrocnemius muscle* as cause of the pes equinus if the entire plantarflexion is reached only with the fully extended knee. In this case, an intervention on the gastrocnemius muscle is sufficient ('gastroc slide', see Chap. 20, Sect. 20.4.5 for details) [23] (Fig. 3.8).
- A pathological increase in plantar pressure beneath the forefoot is particularly serious in the case of concomitant pes planovalgus or pes cavus because the resulting problems tend to be mutually aggravating. In this case, an examination by an experienced foot surgeon to plan an operative extension before ulcers occur is particularly helpful. Footwear alone is generally not able to compensate for such a problem and off-loading a concomitant lesion might be very difficult.
- Applying pressure proximal to the MTHs tightens the plantar aponeurosis (*push-up Test*) (Fig. 3.9).

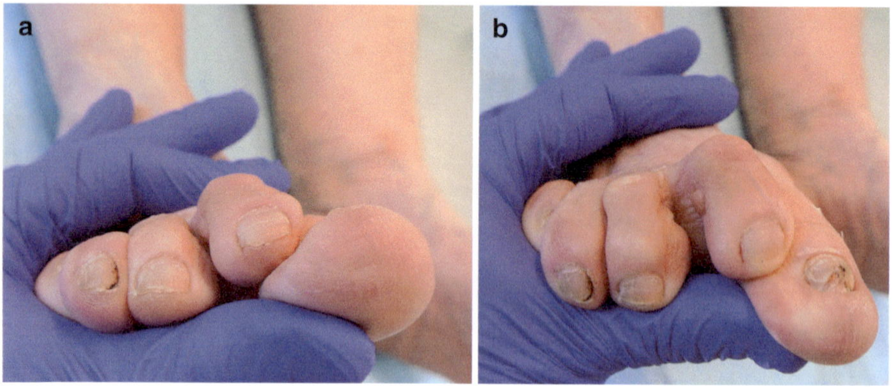

Fig. 3.10 (**a**, **b**) Strength of flexion of the toes

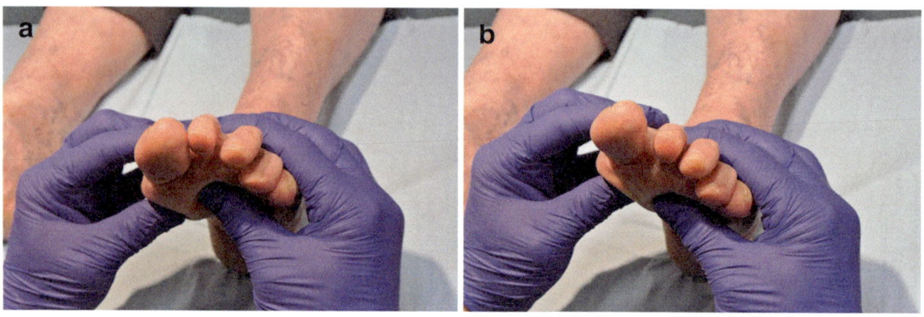

Fig. 3.11 (**a**, **b**) Testing mobility of the first ray

- In this way, the toes stretch physiologically according to the reverse Windlass-Mechanism. The patient might be asked to press the toes against the hand of the examiner in order to estimate their strength and the amount of load they may carry in terminal stance (Fig. 3.10).
- Possible *hypermobility of the first ray* can be identified when the examiner holds ray 2–5 firmly using one hand and the other hand moves the first ray in plantar and dorsal direction (Fig. 3.11). Mobility by more than half the thickness of the metatarsal shaft indicates hypermobility and may allow for harmful movements.

Note: The examiner must hold the feet in their hands!

3.4.1.3 Provoking Functional Deformities

In the next step, pressure in the region of risk is carefully examined. This area is indicated by the pattern of callosities or by wounds. During this phase of the examination, provocative tests are used to search for functional plantarisation. The corresponding lesions are located in areas that do not belong to the physiological contact surface of the foot. The tests are necessary if the location of the ulcer is at a typical site of plantarisation as described below and plantarisation is not evident at inspection.

In the case of a lesion on the *plantar or medial plantar side of the IP joint of the hallux, a hallux limitus or rigidus might be the trigger*. This may be functional and thus unapparent at rest. The hallux becomes rigid due to tension at the FHL tendon in stance. If the test for the functional hallux rigidus has not been performed before (see Sect. 3.4.1.2 and Fig. 3.7d), this is done now.

In the case *of lesions at the tips of the toes or on the lateral side of the fifth toe or on the medial hallux, torsion or clawing might be the triggers.* Possible causes are also narrow shoes which bring pressure to the sides or from the front. However, the most important and frequent trigger in these areas is plantarisation of skin not prepared to bear weight. In order to choose the appropriate therapy, it is essential to differentiate clearly.

Whilst *sitting* the patient presses their bare toes consciously onto the floor and then tries to simulate standing on the MTHs by raising the heel and pressing the forefoot onto the floor (Fig. 3.12). This is repeated when *standing*. The examiner must observe how the patient places the foot on the ground, whether it is abducted or not and if the architecture changes. In this way, it can also be established whether the toes are still in contact with the floor or if the patient is standing on the MTHs only.

The *plantarisation of these areas of skin* is often only apparent if provoked while standing on the tips of the toes or while walking barefoot or by observing an intentional clawing of the toes ('claw test'). Some patients are not able to discontinue an intentional alignment of otherwise functionally misaligned toes. In this case, it is particularly important to observe situations when the patient is distracted. An example could be the moment of first contact with the ground while changing position. If this does not achieve the goal, the patient should be actively distracted using challenging manoeuvres. If no clear distinction is possible, the decision must be made on the basis of the 'claw test'. In this case, the interpretation of the clinical importance of clawing depends on the subjective judgement of the examiner and is only possible with appropriate experience. Deformities of the nail may confirm a suspected plantarisation of the tip of the toe.

3.4.1.4 Claw Test

In the claw test, the patient is asked to bend their toes as much as possible. The functional maximum extension of the plantarisation is revealed. This occasionally shows the impaired capillary filling of the skin in projection on the bony nail bed (Fig. 3.13). As a result of the pathological movement and pressure in terminal stance, calluses and wounds may develop as well as changes to the nails. Microtraumas of the toenails open portals of entry and enables nail mycosis to develop.

Note: Narrow shoes can only be assumed to be the cause of pressure ulcerations at the tips or edges of toes if a plantarisation has been excluded, combining information derived from provocation tests, claw tests, calluses and deformed toenails.

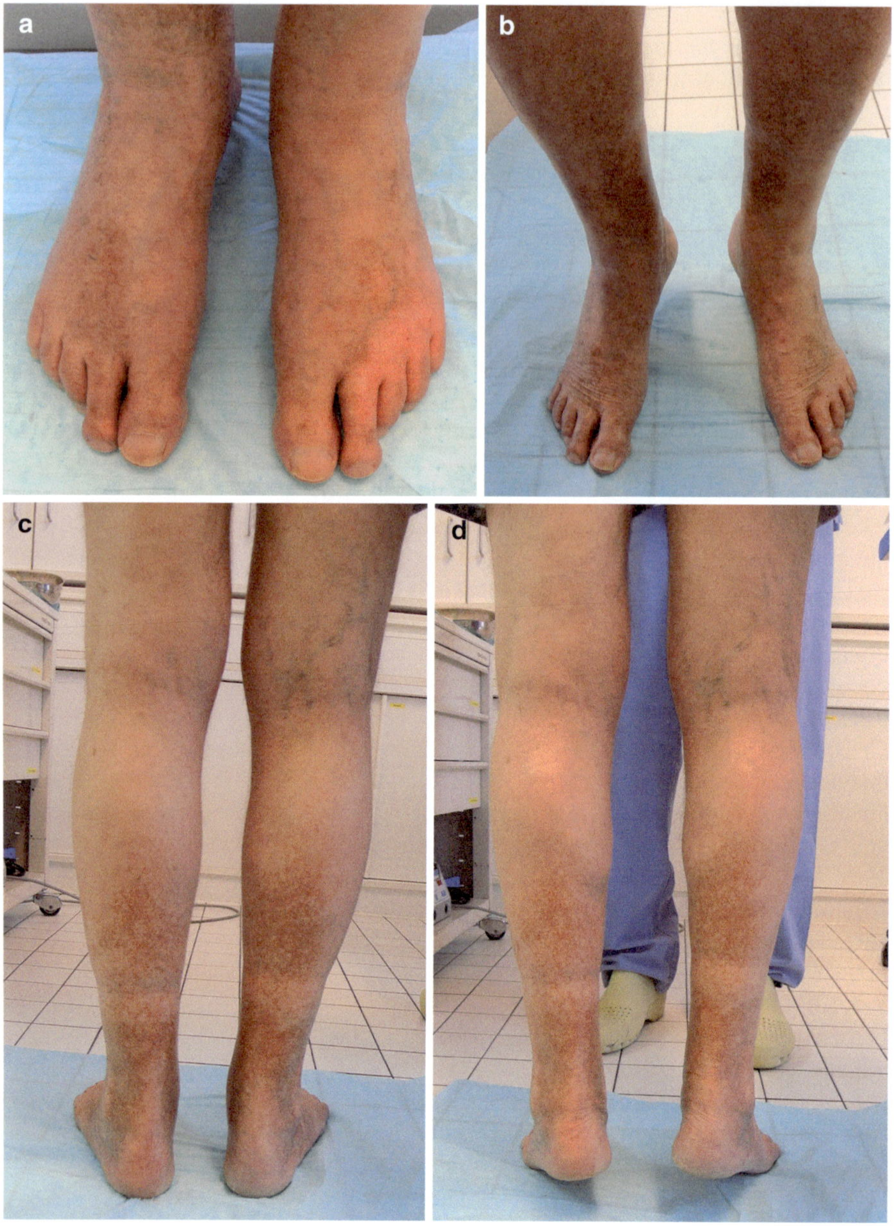

Fig. 3.12 Simulating the pressure of walking when seated (**a**) and when standing in plantigrade position (**c**) and on tip toes (**b** and **d**), note the insufficient action of the quadratus plantae muscle

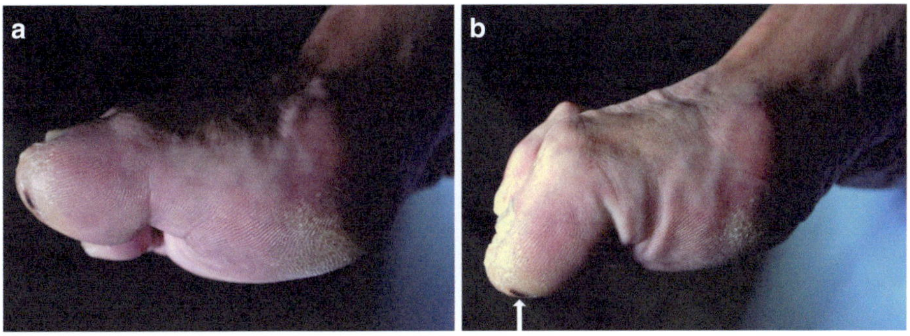

Fig. 3.13 (**a**, **b**) Claw test with hyperflexion in particular of the hallux and plantarisation of the apex

3.4.1.5 Coleman Bloc Test

A particular challenge arises in the detection of the causes of a lesion on the plantar side of the 5th MTH with a concomitant high arched foot. This is usually also combined with shortening of the calf muscle complex (soleus and gastrocnemius muscle). In order to choose the right therapy, it is important to establish whether the high arched foot is flexible or fixed and to what extent the shortening of the calf muscle complex is relevant. The *Coleman Block Test* is a suitable instrument [24]. If the inversion of the heel can be corrected in a position in line with the lower leg (neutral or rectus position of the heel) by means of a diagonal support of the heel and the outer edge of the forefoot, an appropriate insole will probably correct the deformity. This will result in a partially restored flexibility and a relieve of pressure for both the lateral side of the forefoot and the head of the first metatarsal (Fig. 3.14) [25]. If the inverted heel cannot be corrected in the test, an extension of the calf muscle complex or an intervention to rearrange the hindfoot must be considered (Fig. 3.15).

3.4.2 Examination of the Shoes

Shoes protect the feet from traumatising impact and transfer pressure from the feet to the ground. It is recommended that patients who have no protective sensation do not take any steps without wearing shoes. For this reason, the examination of all the shoes worn by a patient is one of the routine procedures for a diabetic foot clinic. For this examination the following questions must be answered:

3.4.2.1 Is There Harmful Content?

Is there anything in the shoes which does not belong there? The most unexpected things have been found in shoes, from drawing pins to bags of gummy bears (Fig. 3.16).

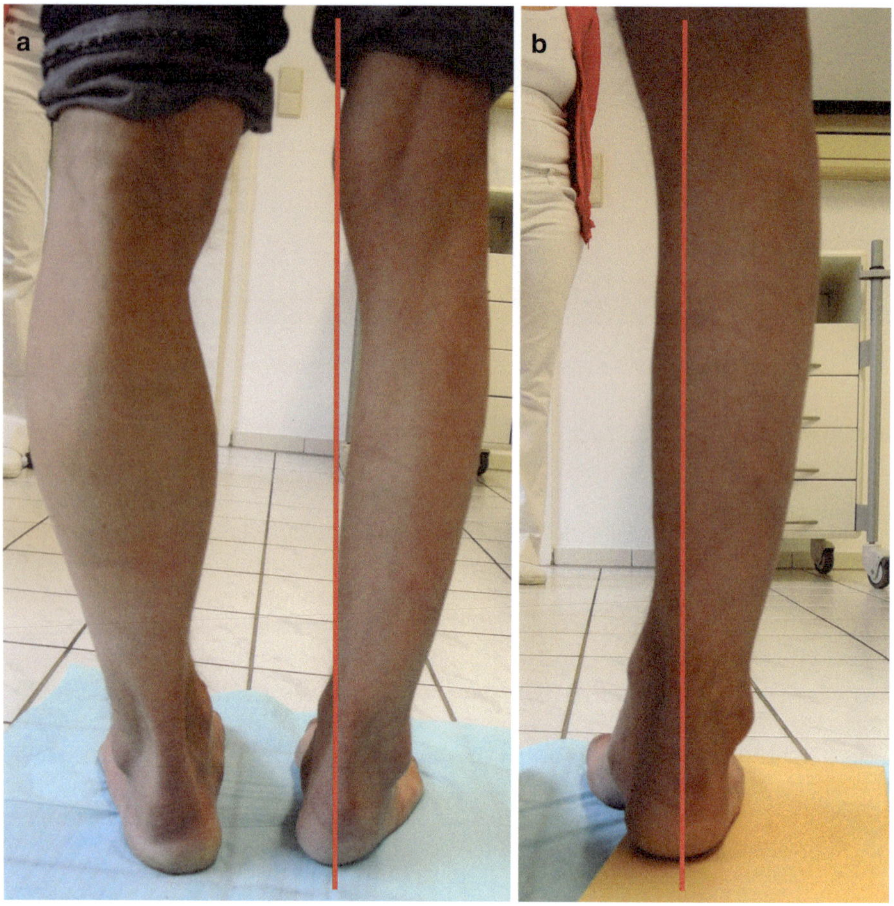

Fig. 3.14 Coleman block test: The diagonal elevation of the lateral margin (**b**) neutralises the varus position (inversion) of the heel (**a**). This means that the supply with corresponding insoles could also correct the position successfully

Some patients insert several insoles into their shoes in the hope of getting positive side effects such as absorption of perspiration. These additional insoles counteract the work of the orthotist and can easily slip and roll up in front of the toes. For this reason, additional insoles might be harmful and this must be discussed with the patient.

Fig. 3.15 (**a–f**) Latero-plantar lesion above the 5th MTH in the case of pes cavus combined with drop foot (pes equinovarus) and concomitant peroneal paralysis. Therapy: percutaneous Achilles tendon lengthening, surgical wound closure by V-Y-flap, immobilisation in TCC for 5 weeks, followed by corrective shoes with modified peroneal splint with integrated cushioning. (**g–h**) Long-term result after 50 months without local recurrences

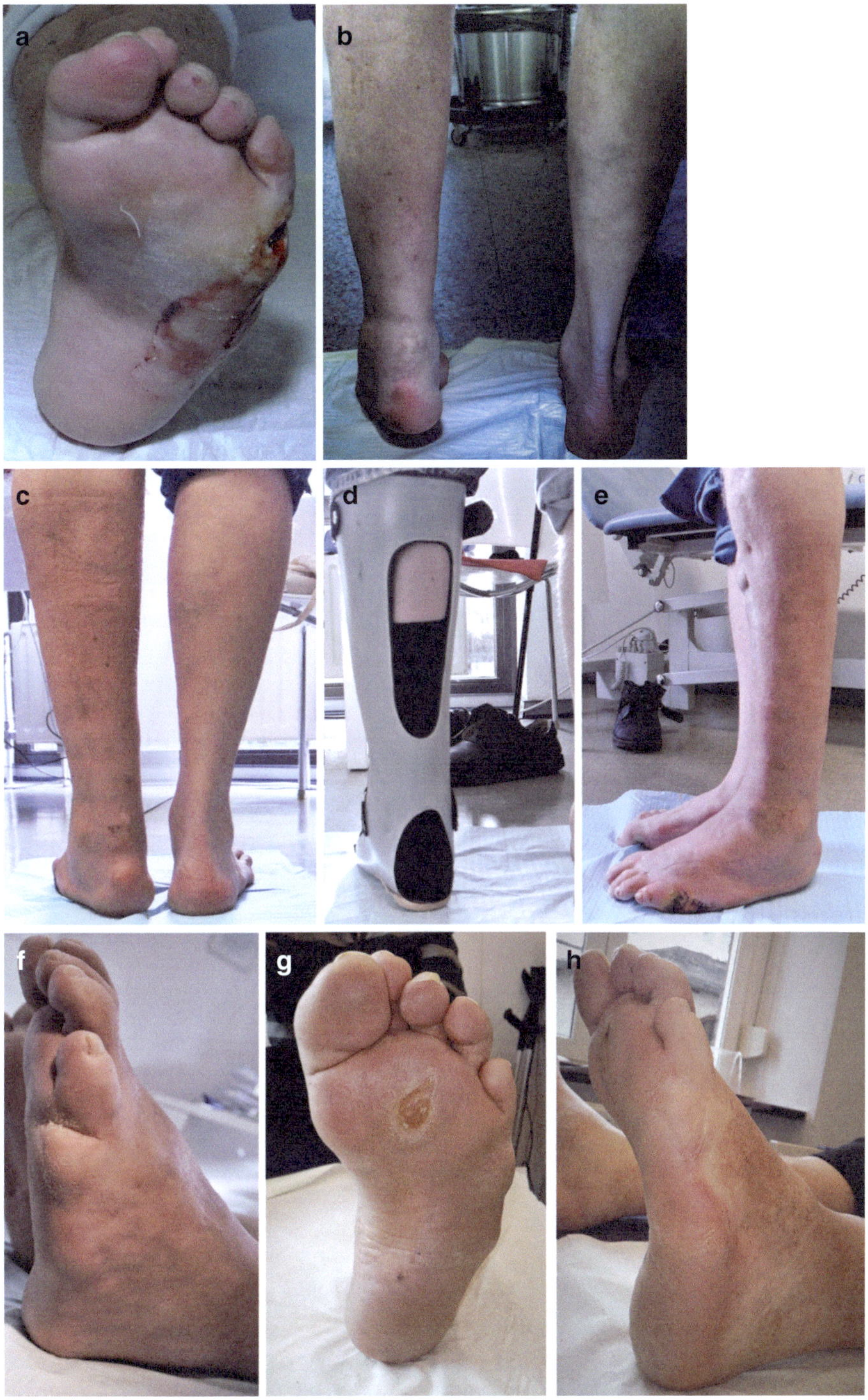
a
b
c
d
e
f
g
h

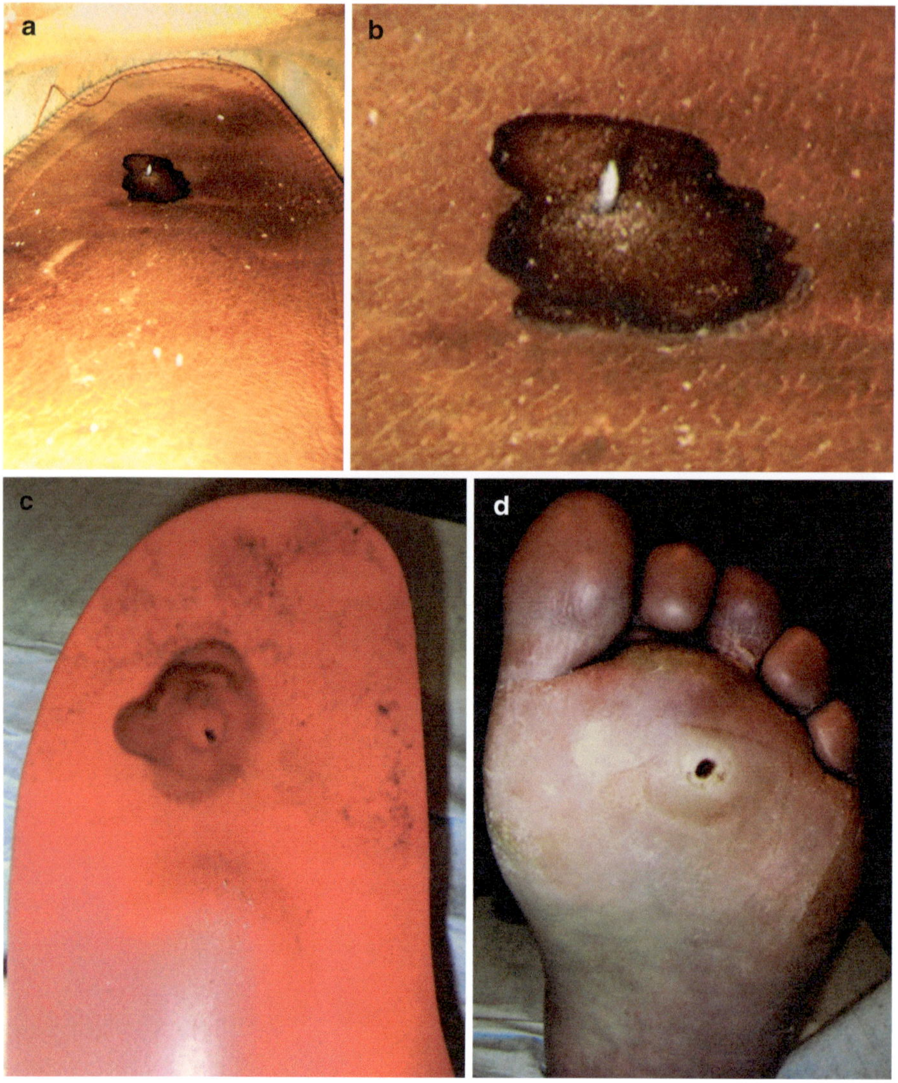

Fig. 3.16 Example for a find in a shoe; (**a**) perforated nail, which was trodden through the sole of the shoe (**b**) and the insole (**c**) into the sole of the foot (**d**), leading to the somewhat atypical location of the plantar lesion

3.4.2.2 Is the Type of Shoe Adequate?

Is the type of shoe suitable to compensate for the phenomenon of overloading? Shoes can vary in a symptom-related escalation of protective functions from very soft shoes to shoes which are similar to prosthetic constructions. Insufficient protective properties are suggested by the presence of hyperkeratosis, by the pattern of calluses and possibly by complaints from the patient if some sensation remains.

Excessive measures may lead to the protective shoes not being worn and the patient will then have to resort to wearing any available shoes with all unwanted consequences. If the patient wears the overprotective shoes consistently then the foot loses its remaining protective mechanisms because these are no longer used and trained. For example, a stiffening of the sole leads to disuse of the remaining intrinsic muscles. Therefore, if the MTP joints are flexible, sole stiffeners should not be used routinely, but only if really necessary. Using unnecessary protective measures, in turn, means that after a while the patient will be unable to walk without these components. *What once was excessive is now needed.*

3.4.2.3 Are the Shoes the Right Size?

The shoe may be too tight for the following reasons:

1. The feet become longer and wider with advancing age. People accustomed to a certain size since youth tend to force their feet into shoes which over the years become tighter and tighter. Due to neuropathy, this is not only painless but might be perceived as comfortable because protopathic perception is restored.
2. When bearing load in terminal stance the foot becomes broader and as a result, the shoe might be 'too narrow'. The sole also becomes longer as it is the outer part of a curve formed by the flexed foot. If this extra length is not considered, the shoe becomes 'too short'.
3. With increasing age and abdominal circumference, it becomes more difficult to reach the feet and to close the shoes correctly. Recommended shoes are held between the instep, the sole and the ball of the heel and are wide and soft at the toe box. When the shoes are not closed properly the feet slide to the front of the wide shoe, which as a result appears to be too short (Fig. 3.17).

It may also be difficult to choose or to manufacture shoes. Reasons for this may be:

1. The instep is not steep enough and it is difficult for the foot to find a grip and prevent the foot from slipping to the front.
2. The feet are much broader than it would be normal at this size. The width of the last is expressed as a letter of the alphabet. From a certain width of the last it becomes more and more difficult to find shoes which are wide enough without being too long. This may be an indication of the need for custom-made shoes.

3.4.2.4 Are the Shoes Intact?

This involves inspection of the uppers, soles, side cushions, and lining material. A little dentist's mirror is ideal for inspecting the lining inside the toe box. Using a mobile phone with integrated camera and flash, photos can be taken to document the damage and help to start a dialogue with the patient. This is how the image in Fig. 3.16a was taken.

If the wear and tear does not equate to the age of the shoes, this may be a reason to question their constant use.

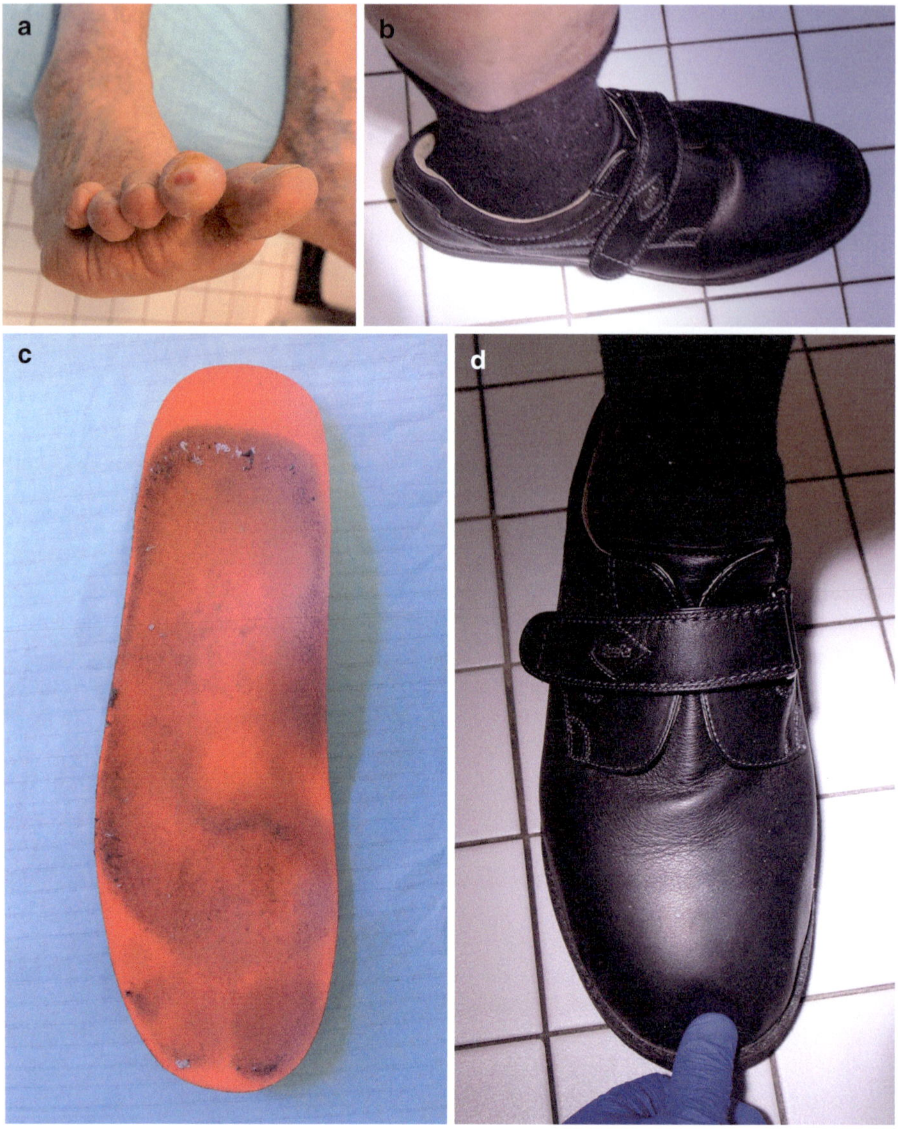

Fig. 3.17 (**a–d**) Example of a shoe in which the patient slides through to the front

After that, the insole is removed and inspected for damage and for worn out material, e.g. whether the resilience of the elastic elements is sufficient.

Finally, the shoe is felt from the inside to determine whether the lining is still fully intact. It has to be ensured that no stitches or anything else protrudes and might be felt from the inside.

3.4.3 Unspecific Traumas

The causative objects of injuries such as cuts and punctures are either sharp object in the shoe or on the floor. For this reason, a meticulous examination of all shoes is an essential part in the search for triggers of a wound occurring in non-weight-bearing areas. Also, in the case of injuries caused by traumatic impact the patient may have been walking around without protective shoes and bumping into the bed-post, chair legs or other obstacles. This results in bruised tissue, which depending on the severity may lead to necrosis. A discussion with the family as to the potential cause of the trauma, taking into consideration of the location of the trauma, may assist in identifying the cause or the trigger for the wound. In this way, potentially recurring causes may be neutralised. For example, screws on wheelchairs or walking frames and bedposts can be softened using upholstering materials.

3.4.4 Thermal Damage

In general, burns are more common than frostbite. The actual source of the damaging burn often remains a mystery to the afflicted person. Days after the causal event, blisters or ulcers can be seen which are easily put down to other causes. In some cultures, the most common cause during the winter are *hot-water bottles*. The key question for the first step into investigating the cause of heat injury in winter is: 'Do you own a hot-water bottle?' (Fig. 3.18). Further all conceivable sources of heat are possible. In winter it could be for example radiators, in summer hot tarmac or the hot sand on a holiday beach.

In the case of frostbite, the cause is often clearer to the patient. Hunters, for example, may stand too long in the snow waiting for prey.

The following characteristics are typical of injuries resulting from heat or cold:

- The pattern of distribution corresponds to the contact area of the source of heat and is not related to areas that are prone to bear an excessive load.
- Several toes and sometimes both feet are simultaneously affected.
- All wounds are at the same stage, which implies that they were caused at the same time.

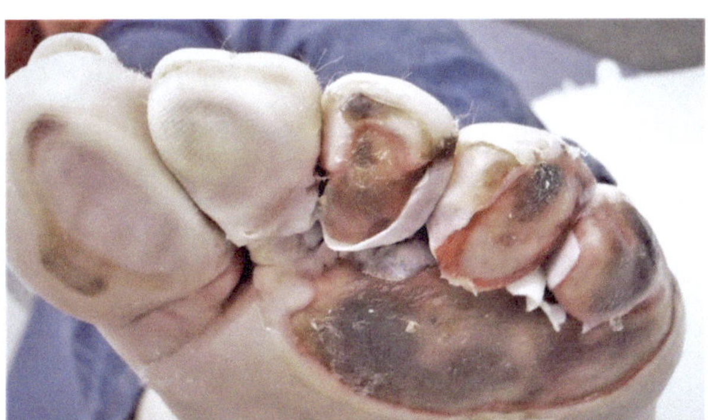

Fig. 3.18 Burns from a hot-water bottle: many localisations, which correspond to a contact area, but no typical load-bearing pressure

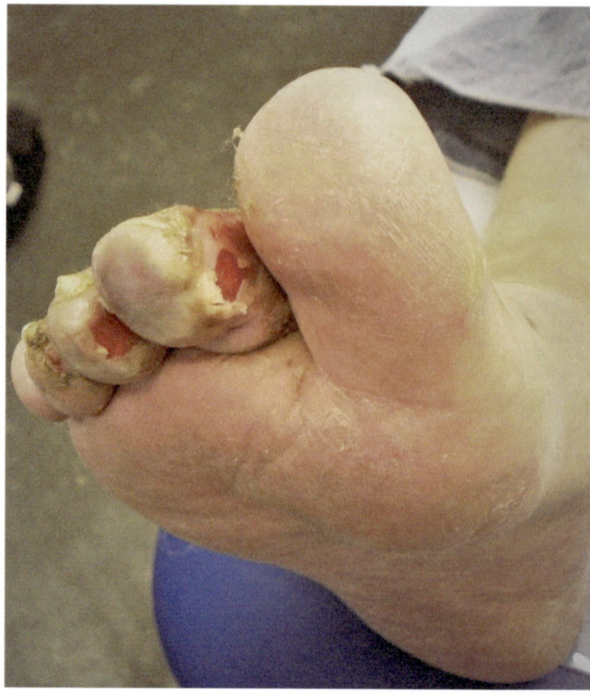

Fig. 3.19 6 days after acetic acid had been accidentally poured over the feet while the affected person was wearing sandals. The acid was intended to serve as weedkiller

- The wounds at first may appear harmless. The tissue is damaged down to deeper layers than usually seen with pressure ulcers. Early on this tissue still appears rosy and firm, so that the depth of the necrosis is often underestimated in the first place.

3.4.5 Chemical Damage

Chemicals can damage the skin of the feet. Among these are salicylates or other products which are used in ointments or baths for the removal of calluses. Other examples are aggressive liquids such as weedkillers (Fig. 3.19).

3.5 Recommended Lecture

Kaj Klaue: The Foot; From Evaluation to Surgical Correction

Springer-Verlag Berlin Heidelberg, 2015, ISBN 978-3-662-47696-3. This book resumes the views of a dedicated surgeon on examination and pathology as well as on surgical therapy of foot disorders in general. The assets are the coherence of the content and the many well-selected pictures.

Solomon Tesfaye, Andrew Boulton: Diabetic Neuropathy

Oxford Diabetes Library, 1st Edition (2009), ISBN-13:9780199551064. This book summarizes key points in the diagnosis and appropriate management of the various clinical presentations of diabetic neuropathy.

References

1. Brand P, Yancey P. The gift of pain. Michigan: Zondervan; 1994.
2. Ali Z, Carroll M, Robertson KP, Fowler CJ. The extent of small fibre sensory neuropathy in diabetics with plantar foot ulceration. J Neurol Neurosurg Psychiatry. 1989;52(1):94–8.
3. Hoitsma E, Reulen JP, de Baets M, Drent M, Spaans F, Faber CG. Small fiber neuropathy: a common and important clinical disorder. J Neurol Sci. 2004;227(1):119–30. https://doi.org/10.1016/j.jns.2004.08.012.
4. Liniger C, Albeanu A, Bloise D, Assal JP. The tuning fork revisited. Diabet Med. 1990;7(10):859–64.
5. Meijer JW, Smit AJ, Lefrandt JD, van der Hoeven JH, Hoogenberg K, Links TP. Back to basics in diagnosing diabetic polyneuropathy with the tuning fork! Diabetes Care. 2005;28(9):2201–5.
6. Thivolet C, el Farkh J, Petiot A, Simonet C, Tourniaire J. Measuring vibration sensations with graduated tuning fork. Simple and reliable means to detect diabetic patients at risk of neuropathic foot ulceration. Diabetes Care. 1990;13(10):1077–80.
7. Mueller MJ. Identifying patients with diabetes mellitus who are at risk for lower-extremity complications: use of Semmes-Weinstein monofilaments. Phys Ther. 1996;76(1):68–71.
8. Chantelau EA. Nociception at the diabetic foot, an uncharted territory. World J Diabetes. 2015;6(3):391–402. https://doi.org/10.4239/wjd.v6.i3.391.
9. Young MJ, Boulton AJ, MacLeod AF, Williams DR, Sonksen PH. A multicentre study of the prevalence of diabetic peripheral neuropathy in the United Kingdom hospital clinic population. Diabetologia. 1993;36(2):150–4.
10. Yang Z, Chen R, Zhang Y, Huang Y, Hong T, Sun F, Ji L, Zhan S. Scoring systems to screen for diabetic peripheral neuropathy. Cochrane Database Syst Rev. 2014. Reviews (3). https://doi.org/10.1002/14651858.cd010974.
11. Tesfaye S, Boulton AJ, Dyck PJ, Freeman R, Horowitz M, Kempler P, Lauria G, et al. Diabetic neuropathies: update on definitions, diagnostic criteria, estimation of severity, and treatments. Diabetes Care. 2010;33(10):2285–93. https://doi.org/10.2337/dc10-1303.
12. Schriger DL, Baraff L. Defining normal capillary refill: variation with age, sex, and temperature. Ann Emerg Med. 1988;17(9):932–5.
13. Hiller B. The hydrostatic measurement of systolic toe blood pressure: a preliminary validation of the method. Vasa. 1998;27(4):229–32.
14. Jachertz G, Stappler T, Do DD, Mahler F. The pole-pressure test: an easy alternative in patients with ischemic legs and incompressible arteries. Vasa. 2000;29(1):59–61.
15. Lawall H, Huppert P, Rümenapf G, Deutschen Gesellschaft fur Angiologie und Gefassmedizin. Leitlinie Periphere arterielle Verschlusskrankheit (PAVK), Diagnostik, Therapie und Nachsorge. 2015:S3.
16. Diehm C, Kareem S, Diehm N, Jansen T, Lawall H. Does calculation of ankle brachial pressure index need revision? Vasa. 2005;34(2):123–6; discussion 127.
17. Schroder F, Diehm N, Kareem S, Ames M, Pira A, Zwettler U, Lawall H, Diehm C. A modified calculation of ankle-brachial pressure index is far more sensitive in the detection of peripheral arterial disease. J Vasc Surg. 2006;44(3):531–6. https://doi.org/10.1016/j.jvs.2006.05.016.
18. Janssen A. Pulsatility index is better than ankle-brachial doppler index for non-invasive detection of critical limb ischaemia in diabetes. Vasa. 2005;34(4):235–41.
19. Hurley L, Kelly L, Garrow AP, Glynn LG, McIntosh C, Alvarez-Iglesias A, Avalos G, Dinneen SF. A prospective study of risk factors for foot ulceration: the West of Ireland Diabetes Foot Study. QJM. 2013;106(2):1103–10. https://doi.org/10.1093/qjmed/hct182.
20. Margolis DJ, Hofstad O, Feldman HI. Association between renal failure and foot ulcer or lower-extremity amputation in patients with diabetes. Diabetes Care. 2008;31(7):1331–6. https://doi.org/10.2337/dc07-2244.
21. Ndip A, Lavery LA, Boulton AJ. Diabetic foot disease in people with advanced nephropathy and those on renal dialysis. Curr Diab Rep. 2010;10(4):283–90. https://doi.org/10.1007/s11892-010-0128-0.

22. Quattrone F, Dini V, Barbanera S, Zerbinati N, Romanelli M. Cutaneous ulcers associated with hydroxyurea therapy. J Tissue Viability. 2013;22(4):112–21. https://doi.org/10.1016/j.jtv.2013.08.002.
23. Jerosch J, Heisel J. Operative Therapie von Fuß und Sprunggelenk: Fußchirurgie in Klinik und Praxis 1. Aufl. Köln: Deutscher Ärzte-Verlag; 2008.
24. Coleman SS, Chesnut WJ. A simple test for hindfoot flexibility in the cavovarus foot. Clin Orthop Relat Res. 1977;123:60–2.
25. Stinus H. Neue Ansätze in der konservativen Versorgung des Hohlfußes. Paper presented at the Gesellschaft für Fusschirurgie - Association for Foot Surgery; 2013.

Therapeutic Pathways: Conditions

4

Causal therapy of a diabetic foot tries to restore the reduced resilience and to prevent the repetition of triggers. In this chapter, current treatment concepts for the most important conditions which reduce resilience (polyneuropathy and peripheral arterial disease) are described. Because infection might be an important aggravating factor, it is also considered in this chapter. Specific measures to reduce the effect of triggers are closely related to the type of the entity and are described some chapters ahead.

4.1 Overview

Polyneuropathy is the most common single component of all the paths leading to a DFS [1]. In addition, ischemia and infection are major components of the processes which might end in amputation [2, 3].

4.2 Polyneuropathy (PNP)

According to our current state of knowledge, a *loss of protective* sensation due to polyneuropathy cannot be restored. In order to prevent ulceration in people with diabetes-related polyneuropathy, therapeutic measures compensate for the loss of protective sensation. This is achieved through measures such as offloading (see in each of the chapters on entities, especially the subheadings external and internal offloading), regular podiatrist care and improving behavioural aspects. In the event of an imbalance between repeated trauma and protection, tissue damage ensues. Therapy then focuses on restoring the balance by enhancing protection.

Many patients with a DFS suffer not only from a loss of sensitivity (*negative signs/symptoms*) but from mixed forms of polyneuropathy, where so-called *positive symptoms* dominate the patient's experience of the disease [4]. These are

D. Hochlenert et al., *Diabetic Foot Syndrome*,
https://doi.org/10.1007/978-3-319-92055-9_4

marked by sensations which torment the patient in the absence of the typical trigger. For example, the feet might appear cold, but objectively they are warm. Pharmacological treatment should follow the guidelines for painful distal symmetrical polyneuropathies [5].

Apart from pure neuropathic problems due to diabetic neuropathy, unilateral symptoms may also occur. One-sided sensations of pain appear to affect people with diabetes frequently and may aggravate an already existing neuropathy. These symptoms often appear to be a result of *nerve compression (= entrapment) syndromes*. When nerves and muscles in narrow places are compressed, the result may range from painful irritation to paralysis. In some cases, intervention to decompress the affected nerve segments can provide major relief of pain [6]. Evidence that this form of therapy might have a significant influence on the natural course of the disease and consequently the long-term risk of ulceration or re-ulceration are based only on a small number of limited studies [7, 8], and this proposal is disputed [9].

4.3 Peripheral Arterial Disease (PAD)

The degree of severity of PAD is generally classified according to clinical aspects e.g. in the Fontaine classification. The indication for arterial revascularisation is also categorised according to clinical aspects: In Fontaine stage II (claudication) revascularisation can be performed, in stages III (rest pain) and in stage IV (Necrosis) revascularisation must be performed, if possible. With increasing severity of PAD the outcome worsens [10]. In addition, the outcome of revascularisation is significantly worse in stage IV than in stage II or III [11]. It's undisputed that people with diabetes and PAD benefit from an arterial revascularisation [12, 13]. However, people with diabetes and a loss of sensation in their legs and feet usually become symptomatic only in stage IV when ulcers and necrosis appear. This is due to the fact that generally they feel neither claudication nor rest pain.

Note: The widely used Fontaine Classification may not be applicable to DFS. Certainly, it cannot be used to decide on an indication for revascularisation in patients with diabetes or other causes of neuropathy.

A distinctive feature of PAD in people with diabetes is the pattern of vessels affected as the *arteries of the lower* leg are commonly compromised and consequently the ischemia affects the foot much more than the muscles of the lower leg [14, 15]. For this reason, not claudication but 'diabetic' gangrene appears as the main clinical symptom of critical ischemia of the leg in people with diabetes and neuropathy. In order to improve the prognosis for those patients, leading experts call for new strategies to be implemented: 'a new approach and classification in neuro-ischaemic individuals both with regard to clinical practice and science/research is badly needed' [16]. In a recent classification, risk assessment of the threatened extremity is based on wound criteria, the degree of severity of the ischemia and of a possible co-existent infection of the foot (WIFi) [17]. People with DFS are explicitly included in the target populations in this classification. The assessment of the degree of ischemia is based not on symptoms such as pain but on haemodynamic measures such as ABI, systolic ankle pressure, toe pressure or transcutaneous oxygen pressure ($TCPO_2$).

For this reason, in patients with DFS the following points are important:

1. Awareness of co-existent neuropathy
2. Precise and comprehensive investigation of the blood vessel status
3. Correct assessment of the prognostic implications of the examination results for the leg and for the patient

In this case, a *step-by-step plan for basic diagnosis* and follow-up may be helpful as a guide to treatment [18]. The clinical examination is followed by measuring the occlusion pressure in the arteries of the foot and calculating the ankle-brachial index (ABI). This was described comprehensively in Chap. 3. An ABI below 0.9 suggests the presence of PAD, a result ≤ 0.4 suggests severe PAD or critical ischemia of the extremities [19]. Frequently, the ABI in people with diabetes is not applicable due to sclerosis of the medial wall leading sometimes to even elevated ABI above 1.4 [20]. The ABI may also be elevated within the normal range and therefore a normal ABI does not exclude PAD in these patients. Assessment is possible with the help of an analysis of doppler waveforms or a hydrostatic toe pressure test ('*pole pressure test*') [21]. If the results of these tests suggest severe ischemia, the blood vessels should be investigated using imaging techniques. Further investigative procedures include colour-coded duplex sonography, contrast-enhanced magnetic resonance imaging (CE-MRI), magnetic resonance angiography (MRA) or computed tomography angiography (CTA) of the vessels of the pelvis and the leg and digital subtraction angiography (DSA), possibly in readiness for an immediate intervention on the compromised vessels. Adequate hydration before and after the angiography is obligatory in order to prevent contrast medium nephropathy. Caution is advised if the patient has moderate to severe renal insufficiency and either DSA or MRA is planned [22, 23]. Individual cases should be discussed with the radiologist performing the test. In these cases, CO_2 may be used as a contrast medium [24]. Imaging of the arteries of the foot, ideally in two planes, is essential for sufficient planning of the therapy, although it is not yet standard practice.

Conservative medical treatment of patients with diabetes and critical limb ischemia offers little hope of success when the goal of treatment is to be curative and not just palliative. At best it can bridge the time until revascularisation, or minimise the limitations on the patient caused by the ulcer in the case of unreconstructable blood vessels or incomplete success of a revascularisation [25, 26]. Revascularisation should be pursued and can be endovascular, interventive or may be performed as 'hybrid intervention' (a combination of open surgery with endovascular measures [27]. However, flexibility in the scale of indications and surgical tactics and the low threshold to perform a revascularisation are more important than the choice of revascularisation method or the perfect operating technique. In other words, not every patient with diabetes and arterial constrictions requires cruro-pedal reconstruction of the lower leg arteries. Many patients with diabetes, particularly if older, have multi-level constrictions or occlusions, where reconstruction is first central (pelvis, upper leg) and where peripheral reconstruction need only be performed when foot ulcers fail to close. For patients with mild to moderate PAD and only minor skin defects, a conservative treatment approach may be justified, provided that the findings are closely monitored. The same applies to patients with multimorbidity, even those with severe PAD and extensive defects, whose treatment is seen as palliative. Interdisciplinary communication is vital in order to achieve the ideal treatment result taking into account the cost and the process-related risks for the patient.

It is still not clear whether it is better to act on the basis of the best available blood vessel or in accordance with the concept of *angiosomes* in order to achieve the best result of revascularisation for the indication DFS [28]. The angiosome concept assumes that every block of tissue on the lower leg and the foot is supplied by a specific artery of the lower leg. In the case of ulcerations, repair can best be achieved by recanalisation of the artery which supplies that particular angiosome [29, 30] (Fig. 4.1a, b). One argument against this concept is that these angiosomes reflect only the anatomy of unaffected blood vessels and it is not clear to what extent this applies in the case of a diabetic foot [31]. In comparative studies no differences

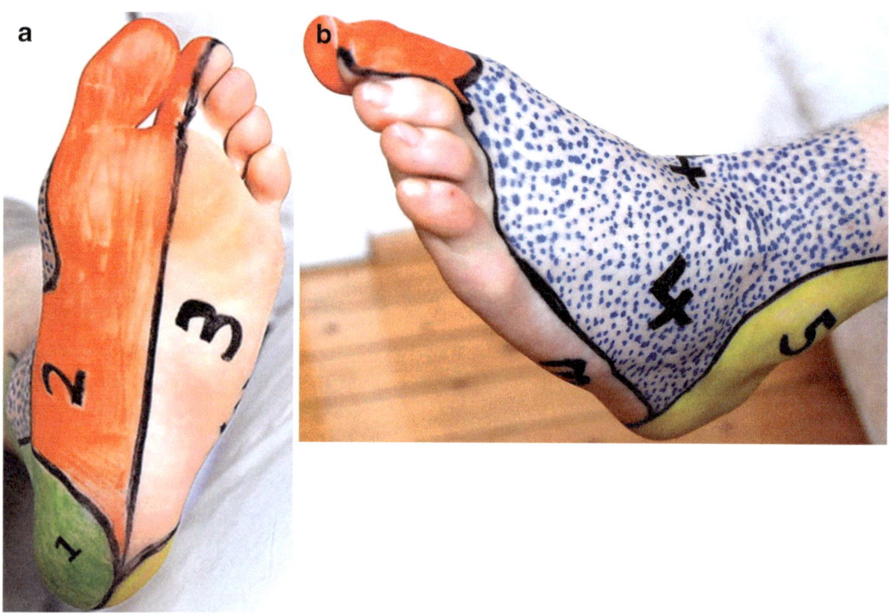

Fig. 4.1 Arterial supply of the foot (**a**, **b**) *1(green)*: Rami calcanei mediales of the Arteria tibialis posterior (ATP), *2 (red)* Ramus plantaris medialis of the ATP, *3 (not coloured)* Ramus plantaris lateralis of the ATP, *4 (blue dots)* Arteria dorsalis pedis; *5 (yellow)* Arteria fibularis, by courtesy of Prof. Rümenapf

could be found between ulcers which were supplied by direct or indirect revascularisation [32] or between applications of pedal and peroneal revascularisation where both vessels were available [33].

An amputation in a region with insufficient blood supply is the start of the dreaded 'salami technique'.

4.4 Infection

Besides ischemia, infection is the most important factor threatening the tissues. The diagnosis of infection is clinical. Validated classifications of diabetic foot infection (PEDIS and Infectious Diseases Society of America (IDSA)) categorise the degree of severity according to the presence and extent of local signs of inflammation, the extent to which deeper layers of tissue are involved, and the existence of systemic signs of infection.

In this text distinctions are made between infections as follows:

1. mild
2. moderate
3. severe, limb-threatening
4. life-threatening

Diagnosis: Conventional X-ray serves as a basic investigative technique for detecting fractures, gas in the tissues, foreign bodies, and the extent of osteomyelitis. However, osteitis is often missed on a normal X-ray examination, especially in early stages. Other imaging techniques (computer tomography, magnetic resonance tomography), various scintigraphic methods (three-phase bone scintigraphy, leukocytic scintigraphy) and particular laboratory investigations (leukocyte count, C-reactive protein, procalcitonin) are additionally applied depending on the clinical investigation.

Antibiotic treatment of uninfected neuropathic foot lesions has no benefits in terms of the onset of remission or its duration [34]. In addition, the non-indicated, prophylactic use of systemic antibiotics not only leads to unnecessary costs but encourages the growth of resistant bacteria. In uncertain cases, offloading the affected part of the foot leads often to relieve of the inflammation that has been thought to be an infection.

When appropriate clinical indicators are present, 'empirical' antibiotic treatment of DFS is initially commenced. In this case, the antibiotic is chosen bearing in mind the most likely bacterial pathogens and the resistance found typically in this facility. For this purpose, annual statistics on the spectrum of bacteria found and their resistance can be provided by the microbiological laboratory.

In general, it is preferable to use tissue samples, fine needle aspiration samples or at least swabs from the depth of a wound rather than superficial swabs. This material for microbiological investigation [35] might be able to guide antibiotic therapy. For epidemiological purposes, i. e. to identify carriers of multi-resistant bacteria, superficial swabs are also helpful. The quality of the procedure for obtaining microbiological samples in a facility can be estimated from the frequency of isolation of only one, or at the most two pathogens, according to the concept that the invasive agents usually belong to only one or very few species. In regions close to the surface there are other microorganisms which take advantage of the wound situation without actually sustaining the wound or becoming invasive.

The duration of antimicrobial treatment is determined by the depth and extent of the microbial invasion. Whilst a treatment duration of 1–2 weeks is usually sufficient when only soft parts are infected, a long-term therapy lasting many months may be necessary for the purely conservative treatment of an infected bone (osteomyelitis) [36].

The indication for *in-patient treatment* is based on a holistic approach. This includes the general condition, the degree of infection, the extent of circulatory damage, the necessary medication and surveillance and the practicality of offloading. In-patient treatment is generally also indicated by the severity of the infection, depending on the individual case [37]. The following criteria indicate in-patient treatment analogous to the interface description of the Cologne Foot Network [38]:

- The necessity for complete bilateral immobilisation
- The necessity for strict immobilisation for patients living alone (Exception: a high degree of adherence to the therapy, guaranteed domestic care)
- The necessity for parenteral antibiotic therapy, where this cannot be provided in a community setting
- The absence of a minimal awareness of the problem (from Wagner 2b on or in the case of deterioration)
- Condition after contralateral major amputation and presence of a problem which might become serious
- Major co-existent condition which cannot be managed quickly enough on an outpatient basis

In the case of extensive infections of soft parts and also when deeper tissue structures are affected (tendons, fasciae, bones and joints) surgery is often unavoidable (compartment drainage, extensive debridement, minor amputation) [39].

4.5 On Time = Immediately

When the central measures of offloading, anti-infective therapy (medicinal, surgical) and reperfusion are not applied in time, a rapid loss of tissue and amputations are to be expected [39].

References

1. Reiber GE, Vileikyte L, Boyko EJ, del Aguila M, Smith DG, Lavery LA, Boulton AJ. Causal pathways for incident lower-extremity ulcers in patients with diabetes from two settings. Diabetes Care. 1999;22(1):157–62.
2. Pecoraro RE, Reiber GE, Burgess EM. Pathways to diabetic limb amputation. Basis for prevention. Diabetes Care. 1990;13(5):513–21.
3. Prompers L, Schaper N, Apelqvist J, Edmonds M, Jude E, Mauricio D, Uccioli L, et al. Prediction of outcome in individuals with diabetic foot ulcers: focus on the differences between individuals with and without peripheral arterial disease. The EURODIALE Study. Diabetologia. 2008;51(5):747–55. https://doi.org/10.1007/s00125-008-0940-0.
4. Veves A, Manes C, Murray HJ, Young MJ, Boulton AJ. Painful neuropathy and foot ulceration in diabetic patients. Diabetes Care. 1993;16(8):1187–9.
5. Tesfaye S, Boulton AJ, Dickenson AH. Mechanisms and management of diabetic painful distal symmetrical polyneuropathy. Diabetes Care. 2013;36(9):2456–65. https://doi.org/10.2337/dc12-1964.
6. Siemionow M, Alghoul M, Molski M, Agaoglu G. Clinical outcome of peripheral nerve decompression in diabetic and nondiabetic peripheral neuropathy. Ann Plast Surg. 2006;57(4):385–90. https://doi.org/10.1097/01.sap.0000221979.13847.30.
7. Aszmann O, Tassler PL, Dellon AL. Changing the natural history of diabetic neuropathy: incidence of ulcer/amputation in the contralateral limb of patients with a unilateral nerve decompression procedure. Ann Plast Surg. 2004;53(6):517–22.
8. Nickerson DS, Rader AJ. Low long-term risk of foot ulcer recurrence after nerve decompression in a diabetes neuropathy cohort. J Am Podiatr Med Assoc. 2013;103(5):380–6.
9. Cornblath DR, Vinik A, Feldman E, Freeman R, Boulton AJ. Surgical decompression for diabetic sensorimotor polyneuropathy. Diabetes Care. 2007;30(2):421–2. https://doi.org/10.2337/dc06-2324.
10. Morbach S, Furchert H, Groblinghoff U, Hoffmeier H, Kersten K, Klauke GT, Klemp U, et al. Long-term prognosis of diabetic foot patients and their limbs: amputation and death over the course of a decade. Diabetes Care. 2012;35(10):2021–7. https://doi.org/10.2337/dc12-0200.
11. Taylor SM, Cull DL, Kalbaugh CA, Senter HF, Langan EM III, Carsten CG 3rd, York JW, et al. Comparison of interventional outcomes according to preoperative indication: a single center analysis of 2,240 limb revascularizations. J Am Coll Surg. 2009;208(5):770–8.; ; discussion 778–780. https://doi.org/10.1016/j.jamcollsurg.2009.01.025.
12. Apelqvist J, Elgzyri T, Larsson J, Londahl M, Nyberg P, Thorne J. Factors related to outcome of neuroischemic/ischemic foot ulcer in diabetic patients. J Vasc Surg. 2011;53(6):1582–1588.e1582. https://doi.org/10.1016/j.jvs.2011.02.006.
13. Faglia E, Clerici G, Losa S, Tavano D, Caminiti M, Miramonti M, Somalvico F, Airoldi F. Limb revascularization feasibility in diabetic patients with critical limb ischemia: results from a cohort of 344 consecutive unselected diabetic patients evaluated in 2009. Diabetes Res Clin Pract. 2012;95(3):364–71. https://doi.org/10.1016/j.diabres.2011.10.033.
14. Faglia E. Characteristics of peripheral arterial disease and its relevance to the diabetic population. Int J Low Extrem Wounds. 2011;10(3):152–66. https://doi.org/10.1177/1534734611417352.
15. Jude EB, Oyibo SO, Chalmers N, Boulton AJ. Peripheral arterial disease in diabetic and nondiabetic patients: a comparison of severity and outcome. Diabetes Care. 2001;24(8):1433–7.
16. Apelqvist JA, Lepantalo MJ. The ulcerated leg: when to revascularize. Diabetes Metab Res Rev. 2012;28(Suppl 1):30–5. https://doi.org/10.1002/dmrr.2259.
17. Mills JL Sr, Conte MS, Armstrong DG, Pomposelli FB, Schanzer A, Sidawy AN, Andros G, Committee the Society for Vascular Surgery Lower Extremity Guidelines. The Society for Vascular Surgery Lower Extremity Threatened Limb Classification System: Risk stratification based on Wound, Ischemia, and foot Infection (WIfI). J Vasc Surg. 2013;59(1):220–34.e1–2. https://doi.org/10.1016/j.jvs.2013.08.003.

18. Bauer H, Germann G, Gries FA, Imig H, Morbach S, Riepe G, Rothe U, et al. Nationale VersorgungsLeitlinie Typ-2-Diabetes: Präventions- und Behandlungsstrategien für Fußkomplikationen (Langfassung). Accessed 2006.
19. Hirsch AT, Criqui MH, Treat-Jacobson D, Regensteiner JG, Creager MA, Olin JW, Krook SH, et al. Peripheral arterial disease detection, awareness, and treatment in primary care. JAMA. 2001;286(11):1317–24.
20. Emanuele MA, Buchanan BJ, Abraira C. Elevated leg systolic pressures and arterial calcification in diabetic occlusive vascular disease. Diabetes Care. 1981;4(2):289–92.
21. Smith FC, Shearman CP, Simms MH, Gwynn BR. Falsely elevated ankle pressures in severe leg ischaemia: the pole test—an alternative approach. Eur J Vasc Surg. 1994;8(4):408–12.
22. Katzberg RW, Haller C. Contrast-induced nephrotoxicity: clinical landscape. Kidney Int Suppl. 2006;100:S3–7. https://doi.org/10.1038/sj.ki.5000366.
23. Thomsen HS. Nephrogenic systemic fibrosis: a serious late adverse reaction to gadodiamide. Eur Radiol. 2006;16(12):2619–21. https://doi.org/10.1007/s00330-006-0495-8.
24. Rolland Y, Duvauferrier R, Lucas A, Gourlay C, Morcet N, Rambeau M, Chaperon J. Lower limb angiography: a prospective study comparing carbon dioxide with iodinated contrast material in 30 patients. AJR Am J Roentgenol. 1998;171(2):333–7. https://doi.org/10.2214/ajr.171.2.9694446.
25. Bendermacher BL, Willigendael EM, Teijink JA, Prins MH. Medical management of peripheral arterial disease. J Thromb Haemost. 2005;3(8):1628–37. https://doi.org/10.1111/j.1538-7836.2005.01368.x.
26. Lumsden AB, Rice TW. Medical management of peripheral arterial disease: a therapeutic algorithm. J Endovasc Ther. 2006;13(Suppl 2):Ii19–29.
27. Rümenapf G, Dentz J, Nagel N, Morbach S. Neue Konzepte zur interdisziplinären Versorgung von Patienten mit neuroischämischem diabetischem Fußsyndrom (DFS). Gefässchirurgie. 2012;17(5):327–33. https://doi.org/10.1007/s00772-012-1017-4.
28. Neville RF, Attinger CE, Bulan EJ, Ducic I, Thomassen M, Sidawy AN. Revascularization of a specific angiosome for limb salvage: does the target artery matter? Ann Vasc Surg. 2009;23(3):367–73. https://doi.org/10.1016/j.avsg.2008.08.022.
29. Alexandrescu V, Hubermont G. The challenging topic of diabetic foot revascularization: does the angiosome-guided angioplasty may improve outcome. J Cardiovasc Surg. 2012;53(1):3–12.
30. Taylor GI, Pan WR. Angiosomes of the leg: anatomic study and clinical implications. Plast Reconstr Surg. 1998;102(3):599–616; discussion 617–598
31. Reekers JA, Lammer J. Diabetic foot and PAD: the endovascular approach. Diabetes Metab Res Rev. 2012;28(Suppl 1):36–9. https://doi.org/10.1002/dmrr.2258.
32. Varela C, Acin F, de Haro J, Bleda S, Esparza L, March JR. The role of foot collateral vessels on ulcer healing and limb salvage after successful endovascular and surgical distal procedures according to an angiosome model. Vasc Endovasc Surg. 2010;44(8):654–60. https://doi.org/10.1177/1538574410376601.
33. Bergamini TM, George SM Jr, Massey HT, Henke PK, Klamer TW, Lambert GE Jr, Banis JC Jr, Miller FB, Garrison RN, Richardson JD. Pedal or peroneal bypass: which is better when both are patent? J Vasc Surg. 1994;20(3):347–55; discussion 355–346.
34. Chantelau E, Tanudjaja T, Altenhofer F, Ersanli Z, Lacigova S, Metzger C. Antibiotic treatment for uncomplicated neuropathic forefoot ulcers in diabetes: a controlled trial. Diabet Med. 1996;13(2):156–9.
35. Mutluoglu M, Uzun G, Turhan V, Gorenek L, Ay H, Lipsky BA. How reliable are cultures of specimens from superficial swabs compared with those of deep tissue in patients with diabetic foot ulcers? J Diabetes Complicat. 2012;26(3):225–9. https://doi.org/10.1016/j.jdiacomp.2012.03.015.
36. Lipsky BA, Peters EJ, Berendt AR, Senneville E, Bakker K, Embil JM, Lavery LA, Urbancic-Rovan V, Jeffcoate WJ, Foot International Working Group on Diabetic. Specific guidelines for the treatment of diabetic foot infections 2011. Diabetes Metab Res Rev. 2012;28(Suppl 1):234–5. https://doi.org/10.1002/dmrr.2251.

37. Lipsky BA, Peters EJ, Senneville E, Berendt AR, Embil JM, Lavery LA, Urbancic-Rovan V, Jeffcoate WJ. Expert opinion on the management of infections in the diabetic foot. Diabetes Metab Res Rev. 2012;28(Suppl 1):163–78. https://doi.org/10.1002/dmrr.2248.
38. Hochlenert D. Qualitätsbericht Netzwerk Diabetischer Fuß Köln und Umgebung 2006; 2007.
39. Yan J, Liu Y, Zhou B, Sun M. Pre-hospital delay in patients with diabetic foot problems: influencing factors and subsequent quality of care. Diabet Med. 2013. https://doi.org/10.1111/dme.12388.

5 Entities: A System of Diabetic Foot Ulcers

The detailed delineation of entities in the next 12 chapters is preceded by a description of the methods, discussion of basic aspects and overviews. One overview separately covers the lesions on the hallux, since about 30% of all diabetic foot ulcers occur there. If entities occur on several toes, they are described in detail at the hallux. In the descriptions concerning other toes, only the differences are mentioned to avoid unnecessary repetition.

5.1 Why a Classification Based on Location?

The location of an ulcer is easy to establish and important because it is not a matter of chance, where an ulcer develops. In fact, *a rough separation of typical causes can be made at a glance:*

- *Pressure* ulcers are
  - located above bony prominences and are
  - typically surrounded by hyperkeratosis showing a previous continuous overload at this particular region.
- Ulcers due to accidental *trauma* have the following characteristics
  - They are not necessarily located in weight-bearing areas, but appear at random, for example, on the dorsum of the foot.
  - In typical cases, these ulcers do not have hyperkeratosis at the edges.
  - Sometimes they have an atypical shape that indicates the cause of the trauma.
- *Venous ulcers* are situated in the region of the malleoli.
- *Decubitus* ulcers present at the calcaneal tuberosity at the rear part of the heel.
- *Thermal damage* shows some very clear characteristics:
  - Ulcers tend to be extensive.
  - The surface of the ulcer corresponds to the contact area between the source of heat (or cold) and the foot. The severity depends on exposure time and

D. Hochlenert et al., *Diabetic Foot Syndrome*,
https://doi.org/10.1007/978-3-319-92055-9_5

intensity, so that ulcers can be found in both weight-bearing and non-weight-bearing sites.
- If there are several lesions, for example, at both feet or several toes, each lesion will be at the same stage of the healing process because they started at the same time.

In this book, the causes of diabetic foot ulcers are divided into conditions (=pre-requisites) and triggers. *Conditions* weaken the resilience of the foot and make ulcers possible. *Triggers* determine the localisation where the weakened foot is damaged. The conditions cannot be cured and the majority cannot even be improved. Thus, the treatment of the diabetic foot is mainly concerned with the lifelong avoidance of triggers.

A system for triggers is meaningful as it is a clinically oriented classification of the most common causes that need to be addressed in daily routine.

Precise localisation allows ulcers of the diabetic foot to be divided into pathobiomechanically defined subsets. This is possible as in each location only one or few triggers typically induce ulcers. If there is more than one, a simple clinical examination is able to differentiate between them. In addition, it has been possible to define the typical pattern of underlying conditions at each location. The probability of underlying PAD, for example, can be further refined. These localisation-based subunits are therefore relatively homogeneous. The authors call them *entities*. With the help of these entities, it is possible to standardise necessary tests and therapeutic decision making. The known properties of the entities provide further information that can be integrated into the prognosis. From an educational point of view, it becomes easier to understand the otherwise apparently infinite combinations of possible causes and consequences. And hopefully, it will lead to more focused discussions and further developments.

The formation of 'entities' uses a systematic link between location and cause to standardise the resulting therapeutic options and to add prognostic information.

5.2 Material and Methods

In order to provide quality control for contracts between insurance companies and members of networks for the diabetic foot, photos and data of 12,473 cases of an active diabetic foot were gathered to form part of the DFS Register [1]. The analysis of the figures to describe this system was performed in a series of steps. 10,037 of these were eligible for analysis of the regions. 1424 photos where the location was not possible to determine, were not usable. A further 790 with photos concerning the lower limb and 222 cases that had not been followed up, so that there was no intermediate result after 6 months or a final result at the time of remission, were also not included. Of the 1424 cases, in which it was impossible to determine the region, in 363 cases the photo could not be interpreted due to technical imperfections of the photo. In 37 cases the lesions were too advanced to determine where they had originated. In 796 cases it was not possible to determine the localisation with sufficient clarity and in 228 cases the location could be recognised, but did not belong to the 50 predefined areas. Ulcers of the lower leg will be considered in Chap. 18.

In 10,037 eligible cases, the photos could be assigned to 50 locations at the lower extremity. For each of these 50 locations, the basic risk factors and results were determined based on the analysis of treatments in the DFS Register. In this register, single episodes of the disease are recorded and the most important lesion in terms of prognosis is photographed and documented at the initial visit. The results were determined at the time of transition to remission and refer to the whole treatment process regardless of the possible occurrence of other ulcers. The addition of problems that had nothing to do with the documented ulcer confuses the differences, which nevertheless remain discernible.

In a second step, the localisations with similar patterns were grouped in 22 Entities.

5.3 Presentation of Statistical Information Regarding the Entities

The 22 entities are presented here in 12 chapters. For the sake of intuitive visual understanding, the different characteristics of the entities are shown as numbers and additionally in *bar charts* in decreasing order of frequency. In order to make the information easier to access, the number of bars has been reduced from 22 to 16 by merging similar entities. In each chapter, the entity being discussed has a coloured bar. All other entities are depicted in grey.

The *figures* are displayed in full in the tables beside the graphic. To allow more rapid orientation, the numbers of the worst entities in terms of prognosis are highlighted in red and those with less negative prognosis in green. The colour is used to mark the most extreme quintile. This means that the total number of cases grouped in the most extreme 20% is determined and if the cases belonging to the entity fit entirely in this group, the number is coloured. E.g., in Table 5.1 the bone impairment has no red number as the group with the worst characteristics is the group with toe lesions. But since this group makes up more than 20% of all cases, no group is entirely in the last quintile and no group is coloured.

One particular issue is the illustration of the *duration* of the active phase of the disease in a meaningful fashion. The mean duration is approximately twice as long as the median time, which is the time needed by the central patient in a rank with

Table 5.1 Characteristics of active episodes of the disease with main manifestation in different regions. The midfoot in this table includes the MTHs

	Mean	Toes	Midfoot	Ankle	Heel
Frequency		57.8%	28.5%	4.3%	9.4%
Bone impairment	15.0%	14.9%	13.7%	9.8%	14.6%
PAD	41.7%	39.8%	36.5%	**44.3%**	**52.7%**
Revascularisation	9.5%	8.9%	7.7%	**11.3%**	**12.2%**
Amputations below Ankle	7.9%	7.8%	7.5%	2.4%	2.5%
Amputations above Ankle	1.9%	1.5%	1.6%	**1.7%**	**3.4%**
Days until remission, mean	182	159	203	**324**	**213**
Days until remission, median	87	70	103	**147**	**106**
Duration more than 180 days	27.8%	21.6%	32.4%	**44.7%**	**34.6%**
Reactivation in the following year	40.5%	38.5%	46.4%	31.4%	32.5%

increasing duration. This is because extreme distortions at the top cannot be counterbalanced by equally extreme deviations at the lower end of the variability. In other words, a time until remission of zero days or less is not possible, but a time of 4 years can occur. Therefore, we outlined the median time and the probability of duration longer than 180 days. We considered that from a patient's perspective, being ill for more than 6 months is also a relevant impairment that calls for distinct recognition.

In this book, the authors deliberately do not refer to amputations below the ankle joint as 'minor amputations'. The expression is inappropriate because it plays down an important intervention in the life of a person with diabetes. They are very heterogeneous and some are perceived by people affected as mutilating. They include functionally devastating losses of important parts of the foot. And finally, these amputations are often unnecessary and are increasingly common. Therefore, the authors decide not to use a trivialising term.

5.4 Comparison of Lesions on the Toes, Midfoot, Heel and Ankle

The causes and consequences of ulcers on the toes, the midfoot including the MTHs, the heel and the ankle are different (Table 5.1).

The ulcers in scars (entity 22) have been excluded from this analysis because ulcers in this group are located in all of the regions analysed. The total number of episodes in this calculation is therefore 9461. The region most frequently affected by diabetic foot ulcers (DFU) is the area of the toes. These episodes take less time and require more amputations below the ankles than episodes predominantly occurring in other regions. Recurrences are most common if the dominant lesion is located at the midfoot. In case of lesions at the ankle, the episodes are more protracted and heel lesions are most frequently associated with PAD and major amputations. These differences are in line with prior publications [2–6].

The large number of analysed cases enables the differentiation of lesions in a large but nevertheless manageable number of sub-groups that are as homogeneous as possible. This makes it possible to recognise differences between areas that are located close together, which was not possible in previous analyses.

5.5 An Overview of the Hallux

Nearly 60% of all ulcers in DFS are located on the toes and of these approximately half are at the hallux (Fig. 5.1).

From a biomechanical point of view, at the end of terminal stance the main load is carried by the hallux and the 2nd MTH [7]. The freedom of movement of the hallux is limited by necessities due to the movement of the body's centre of gravity at constant speed. The leg under or behind the centre of gravity is pressed onto the ground which restricts its ability to swivel. This forced movement enhances the stress and the monotony with which forces are repeated.

The first metatarsal bone is relatively mobile in its joint with the tarsal bones and is held by muscular strength. There are primarily three mechanisms which contribute to some parts of the skin being exposed to abnormal pressure (see also Chap. 2, Sect. 2.7.4). Hyperflexion of the IP joint or hyperextension of this joint or torsion of the entire toe may cause plantarisation of some part of the hallux. If hyperflexion is the only cause, the lesion will arise at the tip of the toe. If only torsion occurs, the medial aspect of the joint will be the inner pressure point. Finally, if the overextension is the only mechanism, the plantar aspect of the IP joint will present the lesion.

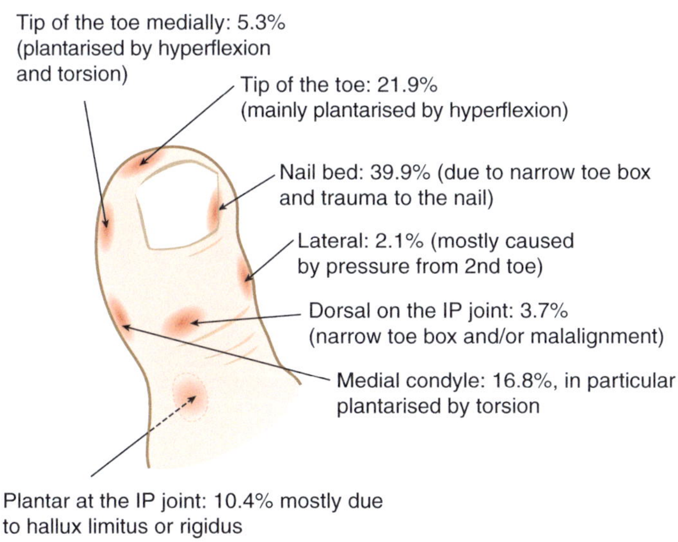

Fig. 5.1 Lesions and their distribution on the big toe, the percentage refers to the entire group of lesions at the hallux

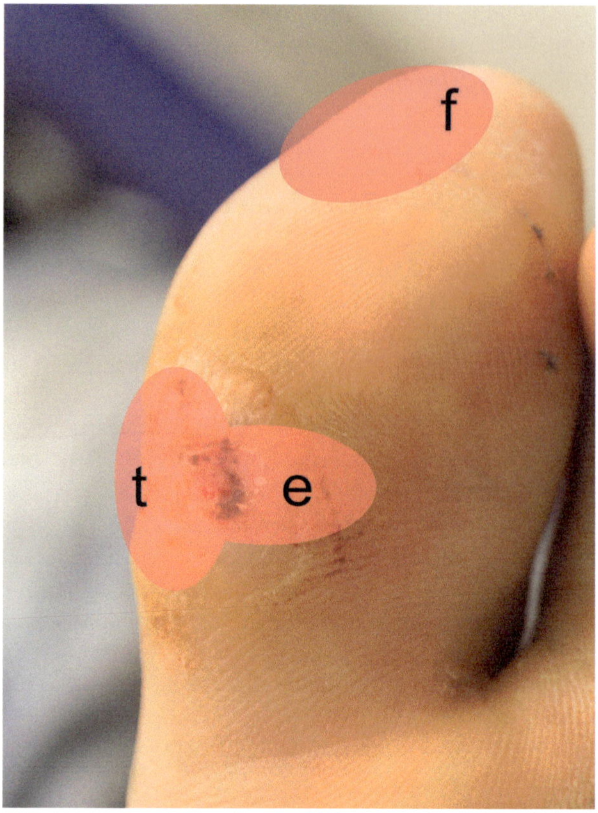

Fig. 5.2 Modalities of plantarisation determine the site of the lesion, *e* hyperextension (hallux rigidus), *t* torsion, *f* hyperflexion (claw toes)

A combination of two mechanisms will change the site slightly. For example, the combination of hyperflexion and slight rotation will lead to an overload at the medial aspect of the apical tuberosity (Fig. 5.2).

The high risk of injury to the hallux is explained by physiologically high pressures that in many cases of deformity are enhanced and meet less resilient tissue due to plantarisation. At the same time, the hallux and its metatarsal joint are of crucial importance for the integrity of the biomechanics of the whole foot. Thus, all necessary efforts should be applied to avoid its amputation.

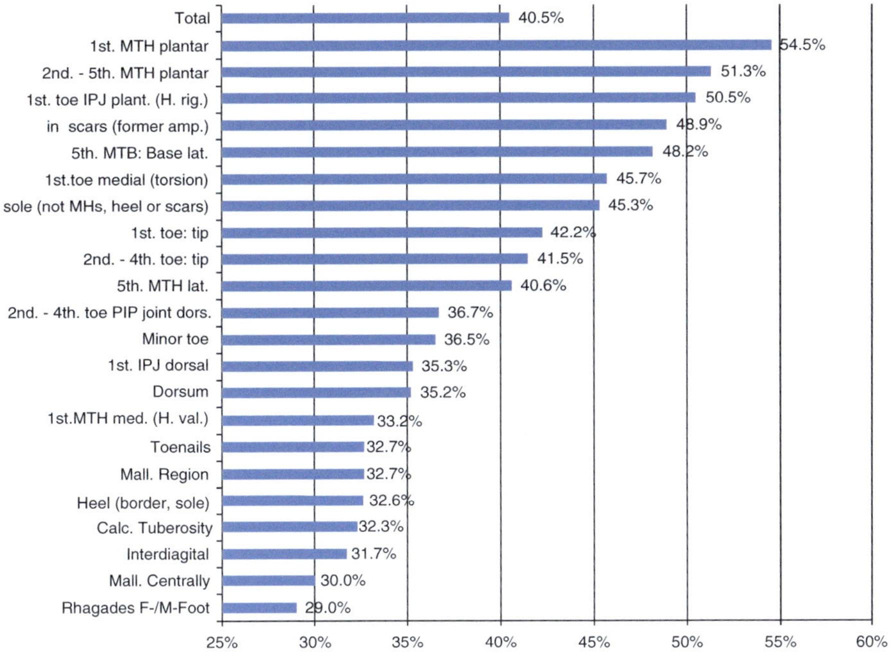

Fig. 5.3 Reactivation in the different entities

5.6 Influence of the Entity on Reactivation Rates

High rates of ulcer reactivation following wound closure are a major challenge. Known risk factors are able to predict only a small part of these events, while the influence of the location has not been analysed in a higher resolution and therefore is not used as effectively as it would be possible. During the year of prevention post ulcer closure, 1499 patients died or were lost to follow up. The reactivation rate within 1 year of the remaining 8538 treatments after wound closure was calculated (Fig. 5.3).

Entities with higher reactivation rates are typically related to biomechanical problems difficult to correct without surgery. Access to surgery is still a critical topic. Compensation with the help of shoes depends on the uninterrupted adherence to therapy, another critical topic.

This might show the need to enhance efforts once ulcers in physically active patients occur in zones of high risk.

References

1. Risse A, Grafenkamp T, Hüppler M, Wimmer J, Birgel B. Wundtherapie bei diabetischem Fußsyndrom. Diabetologe. 2010;6(7):587–96. https://doi.org/10.1007/s11428-010-0613-8.
2. Apelqvist J, Castenfors J, Larsson J, Stenstrom A, Agardh CD. Wound classification is more important than site of ulceration in the outcome of diabetic foot ulcers. Diabet Med. 1989;6(6):526–30.
3. Apelqvist J, Larsson J, Agardh CD. The influence of external precipitating factors and peripheral neuropathy on the development and outcome of diabetic foot ulcers. J Diabet Complicat. 1990;4(1):21–5.
4. Dubsky M, Jirkovska A, Bem R, Fejfarova V, Skibova J, Schaper NC, Lipsky BA. Risk factors for recurrence of diabetic foot ulcers: prospective follow-up analysis of a Eurodiale subgroup. Int Wound J. 2012;10(5):555–61. https://doi.org/10.1111/j.1742-481X.2012.01022.x.
5. Pickwell KM, Siersma VD, Kars M, Holstein PE, Schaper NC, Consortium on behalf of the Eurodiale. Diabetic foot disease: impact of ulcer location on ulcer healing. Diabetes Metab Res Rev. 2013;29(5):377–83. https://doi.org/10.1002/dmrr.2400.
6. van Battum P, Schaper N, Prompers L, Apelqvist J, Jude E, Piaggesi A, Bakker K, et al. Differences in minor amputation rate in diabetic foot disease throughout Europe are in part explained by differences in disease severity at presentation. Diabet Med. 2011;28(2):199–205. https://doi.org/10.1111/j.1464-5491.2010.03192.x.
7. Debrunner HU, Jacob HAC. Biomechanik des Fußes. Bücherei des Orthopäden. Stuttgart: Enke; 1998.

Tips of the Toes (1–2) 6

Lesions at the tip of the toes are frequent and their treatment is probably one of the best examples of the advantages of integrating internal and external offloading.

The tip of the hallux (1) may be subject to a very strong plantarflexion and to a torsion, the latter of which is described in detail in the next chapter. These characteristics separate lesions at the tip of the hallux from those at the 2nd to 4th toe (2). Here forces are lower and torsion is less important.

The lesions at the tip of the minor toe represent the particularities of the minor toe and therefore are depicted together with the other lesions of the minor toe as entity 10.

6.1 Overview

Ulcers at the tip of the toes (Figs. 6.1 and 6.2) develop in two different modes:

- *Plantarisation* of the tip of the toes due to hyperflexion of the distal phalanx. This is common in hammer toes, claw toes or mallet toes. It might be evident at rest or may need provocative tests to be diagnosed (functional plantarisation). The degree of plantarisation can often be observed during the clawing test (see Fig. 3.14).
- *Traumatic contact* with the toe cap because the shoe is too short or not properly closed. The foot thus slides forward until the tips of the toes limit further progression (see Fig. 3.16a–d). Sometimes this is the case in people with wheelchairs, who push the wheelchair backwards while the foot is otherwise completely without load.

D. Hochlenert et al., *Diabetic Foot Syndrome*,
https://doi.org/10.1007/978-3-319-92055-9_6

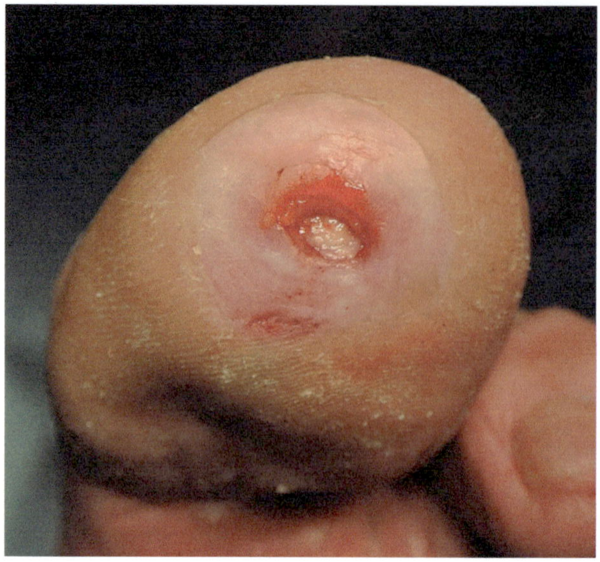

Fig. 6.1 Lesion at the tip of the hallux

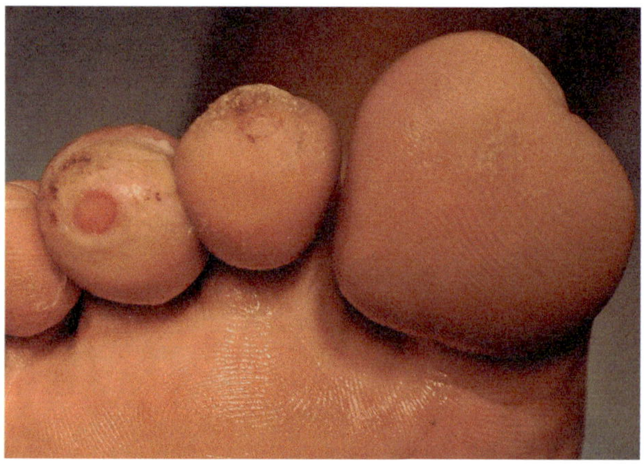

Fig. 6.2 Lesion at the tip of the 3rd toe which on this foot is the longest

6.2 Pathobiomechanics and Pressure Points

1. The *top of the apical tuberosity* is the internal pressure point. It is barely protected. Whilst beneath the toes' pulp a thick cushion separates the bone from the contact surface, at the tip of the toes there are only a few millimetres of soft tissue. Furthermore, the apical tuberosity is situated immediately beneath the nail bed (Fig. 6.3) and therefore is easily compromised by contiguous damage to the nail bed.
2. A second structure at the tip of the toe, prone to suffer from exaggerated pressure, is the *toenail* (Fig. 6.4). The nail bed itself is delicate and easily trauma-

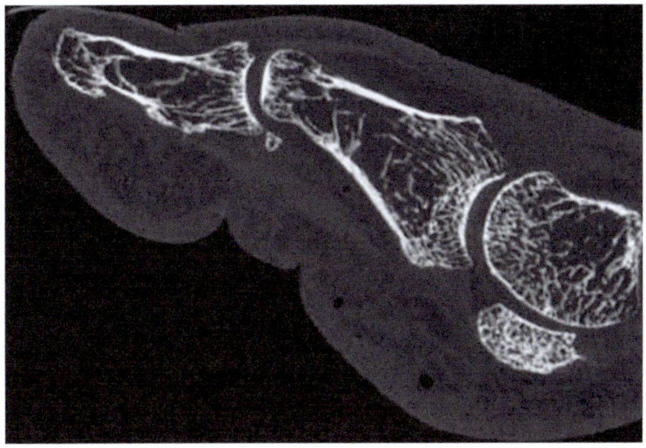

Fig. 6.3 Soft padding of the distal phalanx of the hallux shown in the sagital fine sliced CT scan

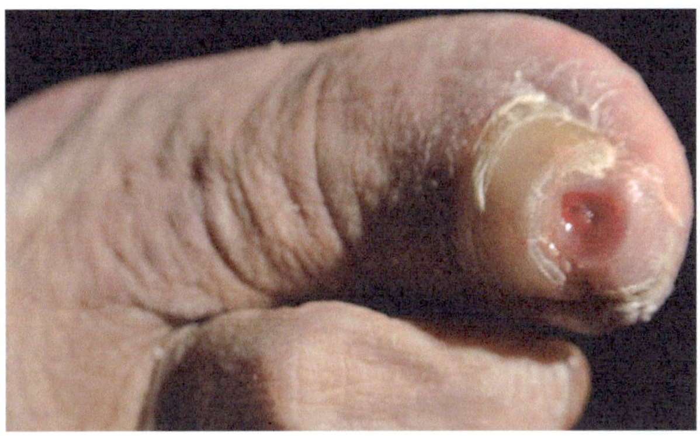

Fig. 6.4 Subungual lesion exposed after partial removal of the nail

tised by pressure exerted from the front side. A long and thickened nail may facilitate trauma as:

- The nail is exposed to stronger pressure.
- The nail can easily be levered off distally.
- Ulcers beneath the nail may be overlooked over long periods of time.

The external pressure point in the case of plantarisation is the inner sole of the shoes. In the case of traumatic impact against the tip of the shoe, the external pressure is exerted by the material of the toe box. This has more dramatic consequences if a rigid cap is integrated into the material at the front of the shoes. This cap is standard in the production of normal shoes as it maintains the smoothness of the leather, making it appear flawless. It might be more dangerous than beneficial in shoes made for people with neuropathy. Wrinkling of the leather may also be avoided by using soft leather and careful sewing [1].

6.3 Tests to Perform

If the deformity is not visible at rest, *tests to provoke functional clawing* must be performed as part of the routine. Determining possible clawing is the aim of the push-up test, the claw test, the functional test in stance and provocation by elevation of the heel (see Chap. 3, Sect. 3.4.1.3).

Lesions at the tips of the toes should be considered to be caused by plantarisation unless clawing is ruled out by integrating information derived from these tests as well as calluses and deformities of the nail.

Additionally, the tests to detect a dysfunction of the Achilles tendon including the *Silfverskjöld test may be performed.* A problem at the tip of the toes will only occasionally need surgical correction by lengthening of the Achilles tendon, but awareness of this condition may complete the picture.

These tests are described in detail in Chap. 3.

6.4 Statistics

Lesions at the tips of 2nd to 4th toe display different characteristics when compared to the hallux and therefore form a separate entity (Fig. 6.5). In addition, the lesions on the big toe are shown separately, depending on whether the nail bed is affected or not.

The figures are shown in Fig. 6.5. The following consequences can be drawn from these figures:

- Lesions at the tip of the hallux, especially if the nail bed is involved, are associated above average with PAD, revascularisation and amputation below the ankle. They easily reach the bone and the frequency of bone involvement in lesions where the nail bed is affected is twice as high as in lesions where there is no nail bed involvement. This is in line with the anatomical proximity. In the case of a PAD, an excessively long, thickened nail could trigger a need for repair in everyday strain for which the existing blood supply is insufficient.
- Lesions at the tips of the 2nd to 4th toe pass more rapidly into remission. Nevertheless, the rate of amputation below the ankle is amongst the highest of all entities, suggesting that many amputations are unnecessary but are often the preferred method in order to reach a quick and final solution [2].

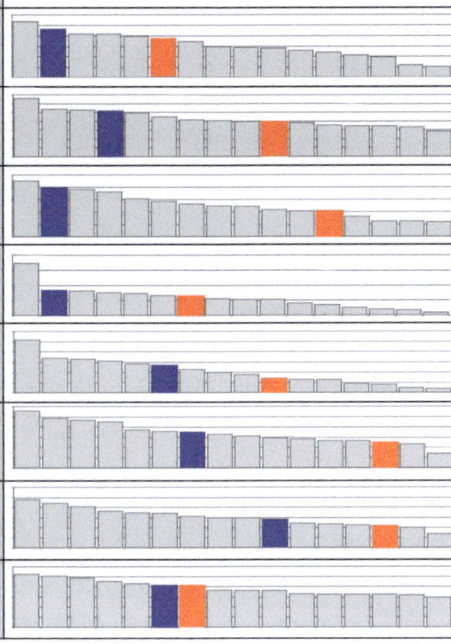

	Tip of hallux	Tip of hallux, nail bed involv.		Tip of 2nd to 4th toe
		no	with	
Frequency	6.1%	3.7%	2.4%	10.3%
Bone involvement	23.3%	18.6%	30.1%	18.8%
PAD	51.7%	51.0%	52.8%	39.5%
Revascularisation	15.8%	14.3%	18.1%	8.3%
Amputation below ankle	11.7%	11.5%	11.9%	9.0%
Amputation above ankle	2.7%	1.3%	4.9%	1.4%
Days until remission	103	97	112	73
Duration > 180 days	28.3%	27.0%	30.5%	20.3%
Reactivation following year	42.2%	41.9%	42.7%	41.5%

Fig. 6.5 Benchmark chart of lesions at the tips of the toes. The tip of the hallux is represented in blue, the tips of the 2nd to the 4th toe are shown in orange and the other entities in grey. They are all ranked in decreasing height

6.5 Principles of External Offloading

6.5.1 Plantarisation of the Hallux

In the case of plantarisation as the trigger for a lesion at the tip of the hallux, several measures can be used that are also suitable for other lesions of the hallux. The following measures can be useful:

1. *Avoid plantarisation* by preventing the toe from clawing
   - Use of a cushion as a spacer in the flexion fold of the IP joint (extends the IP joints of the toe). This is generally only useful for the treatment of ulcers.
   - Use of orthoses as spacers to extend the IP joints of the toe and additionally to keep it aligned.

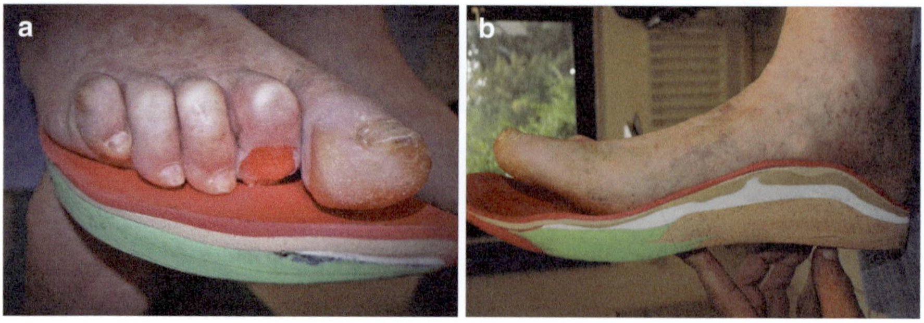

Fig. 6.6 (**a**) Injury at the tip of the 2nd (clawed) toe and its dorsum (**b**) probably due to a ridge at the insole, the same insole seen from the medial side

- Introduction of a 'ridge' on the insole to allow grabbing of the toes. Its use is disputed, however, because of possible increased pressure in a later situation, which is not necessarily foreseeable at the moment of delivery. It also may reduce the tolerance of the shoe for changes in conditions. To decrease the probability of damages secondary to such 'ridges', it has been proposed to add a safety distance between the bony prominence and the prominence of the insole of at least 1 cm (Fig. 6.6)

2. Allow *more distance between the shoe and the tip* of the hallux to reduce the duration and the intensity of the pressure
   - Rocker bottom sole
   - Stiff sole
   - Reduce the elevation of the tip of the shoe (less toe spring) and of the heel of the shoe (less heel spring)
   - High toe box without a stiffened cap to provide room to accommodate the deformity.
   - Elevation of the proximal parts of the hallux and the forefoot increases the distance between the tip and the ground.
3. Changing the position of the foot to a slight *supination/inversion* increases the load on the outer margin of the sole.
   - Supports of the medial arch

An effective offloading of the plantarised tip of the hallux might be difficult to achieve as the clawing may become so drastic that it overcomes each increase in distance.

6.5.2 Plantarisation of the 2nd to the 4th Toe

The external offloading of the plantarised tip of the 2nd to the 4th toe is often easier:

- A spacer placed in the flexion fold of the toe's IP joints extends the toe and creates a distance between the tip of the toe and the sole. This spacer might consist of rolls of felt (Fig. 6.7) held in place by tape.

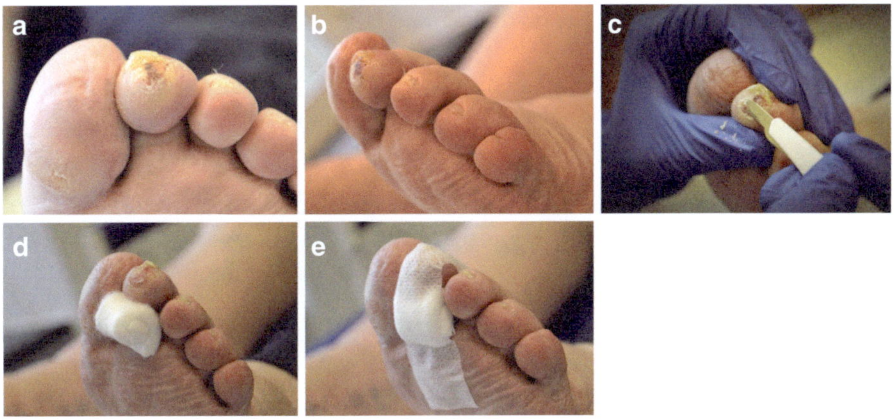

Fig. 6.7 (**a**, **b**) Lesion at the tip of the 2nd toe (**c**) treated by debridement (**d**, **e**) and securing a spacer in the flexion-fold

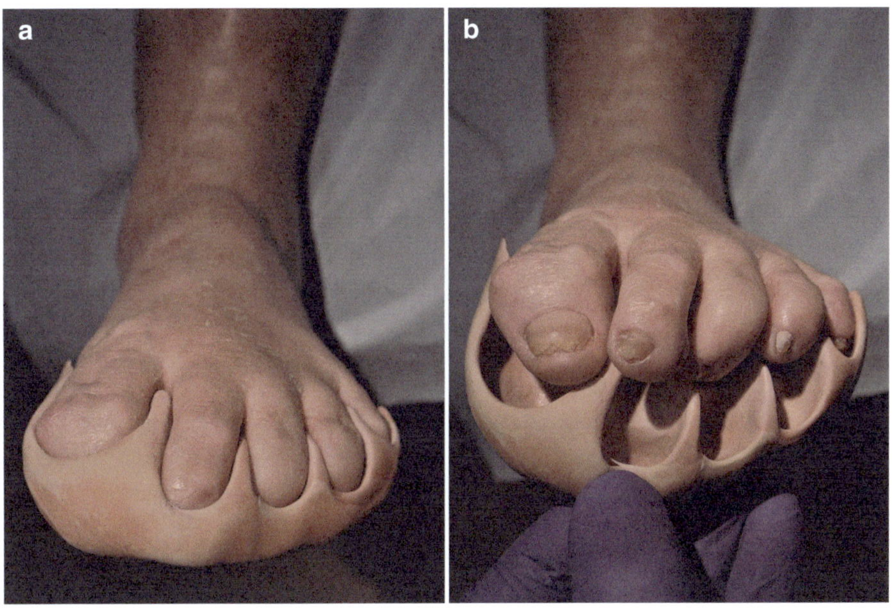

Fig. 6.8 (**a**, **b**) Orthosis

- A qualified podiatrist might also apply an orthosis made of two compounds of silicone that extends the distal phalanx and creates a distance between the tip of the toe and the sole (Fig. 6.8). An orthosis might be able to maintain the toe straightened.

6.5.3 Traumatic Contact with the Toe Box

If plantarisation is ruled out and the trigger is certainly determined as the traumatic contact of the tips of the toes against the inner lining of the tip of the shoe (= toe box), other measures are useful:

1. *Avoid contact* with the tip of the shoe:
   - Create space distally, e. g. by increasing the length of the shoe (about half the thickness of the patient's thumb in addition to the length of the foot).
2. Allow for *non-hazardous contact* with the tip of the shoe:
   - Do not use toe caps.
3. *Prevent the foot from sliding* forward in the shoe:
   - The design of the shoe should prevent the foot from sliding forward if the shoe is closed properly.
   - The closing system of the shoe should be easy to use.
   - Training of the patient in using the shoe and closing it properly.
   - Shoes with a shaft that is higher than the ankle hold the foot tighter, thus preventing the foot from sliding.

6.6 Principles of Internal Offloading

Surgical measures for internal offloading are useful to correct plantarisation permanently:

- The *tenotomy of the long flexor tendon* (Fig. 6.9) is an effective procedure for all toes. It has been well studied, is generally easy to perform with low risks and puts an end to plantarisation [3–9]. This form of tenotomy has been referred to as an 'office procedure' [6] to emphasise the easy application by means of a phlebotomy cannula (see details in Chap. 20, Sect. 20.4.1 with detailed description). In order to decide on the indication in the presence of a PAD, a holistic approach is required, since prolonged trauma on the ulcer usually requires more additional blood supply than the limited traumatism of the intervention.
- In case of a partial fixation due to a stiffened capsule, the capsule can be slit, a procedure that is called 'capsulotomy' or 'capsule release', and can be performed in the same procedure as the tenotomy (see Chap. 20, Sect. 20.4.3).
- In the case of fixed deformity due to anchylosis, a more extensive procedure such as an arthrodesis of the PIP joint or the more complex Hohmann-OP are possible (see also Chap. 20, Sects. 20.4.3 and 20.5.1.2).
- If the bone of the distal phalanx is involved, the resection of any necrotic bone is useful (see Chap. 20, Sect. 20.5.1.1). The access is through the wound after excision of its edges. The flexor hallucis longus tendon (FHL) or the flexor digitorum longus tendon (FDL) is cut and the necrotic bone is removed in the same first intervention. After a short period of offloading and antibiotics, signs of infection in the site of the resection can be expected to clear and the wound can be closed in a second intervention.

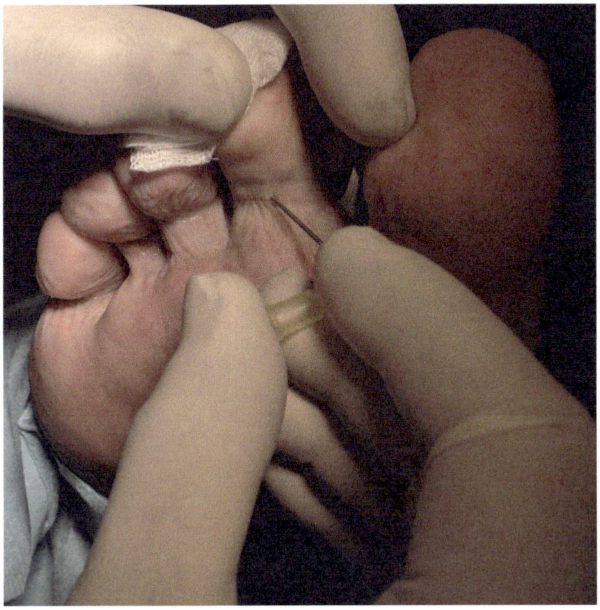

Fig. 6.9 Tenotomy of the flexor digitorum longus tendon of the 2nd toe at the right foot

Time of remission may be up to four times longer if the bone is compromised. In patients operated at the hallux with Wagner 1 or 2 wounds the average is 13 days, in case of Wagner 3 wounds it is 49 days [4]. Therefore, this intervention may be taken into consideration at an early stage.

6.7 Summary

- **Lesions at the tips of the toes are frequent. They are mostly due to plantarisation, less frequently due to traumatising contact with the tip of the shoe.**
- **Lesions at the hallux involving the toenail are among the most dangerous lesions in the field of the diabetic foot. Treatment of PAD is often required in this case.**
- **The hallux is crucial for intact gait and its amputation should be avoided whenever possible.**
- **Offloading is easy to achieve and many amputations are probably unnecessary.**

- **A tenotomy of the long flexor tendons is extremely beneficial. It accelerates wound closure, avoids amputation and prevents recidivism.**
- **At the time of the diagnosis of the ulcer, flaws concerning the shoes are also often discovered. On closer examination, they are often found not to be the predominant cause. Plantarisation must therefore be ruled out as a routine step in the examination. This is necessary in order to avoid overlooking the opportunity of a tenotomy of the FDL or FHL tendon and its many advantages for the patient.**

6.8 Case Report

69-years old male patient in retirement, living alone, diabetes mellitus Type 2 for 15 years, polyneuropathy but no significant PAD, other comorbidities: obesity, in the last two years 3 ulcers at the tip of the hallux on the right foot. Now lesion UT 3B with osteitis of the apical tuberosity (Fig. 6.10).

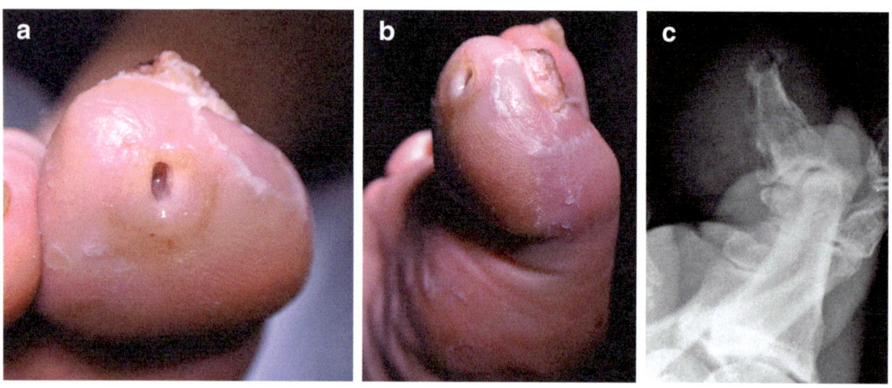

Fig. 6.10 (**a**–**k**) Tenotomy of the FHL tendon, simultaneous removal of the apical tuberosity, adapting suture and later secondary wound closure after of signs of infection had disappeared, antibiotic therapy corrected by testing, operation in an outpatient clinic with conduction anaesthesia. Offloading device is a therapeutic shoe, days 0–27 and (**l**) after 8 months

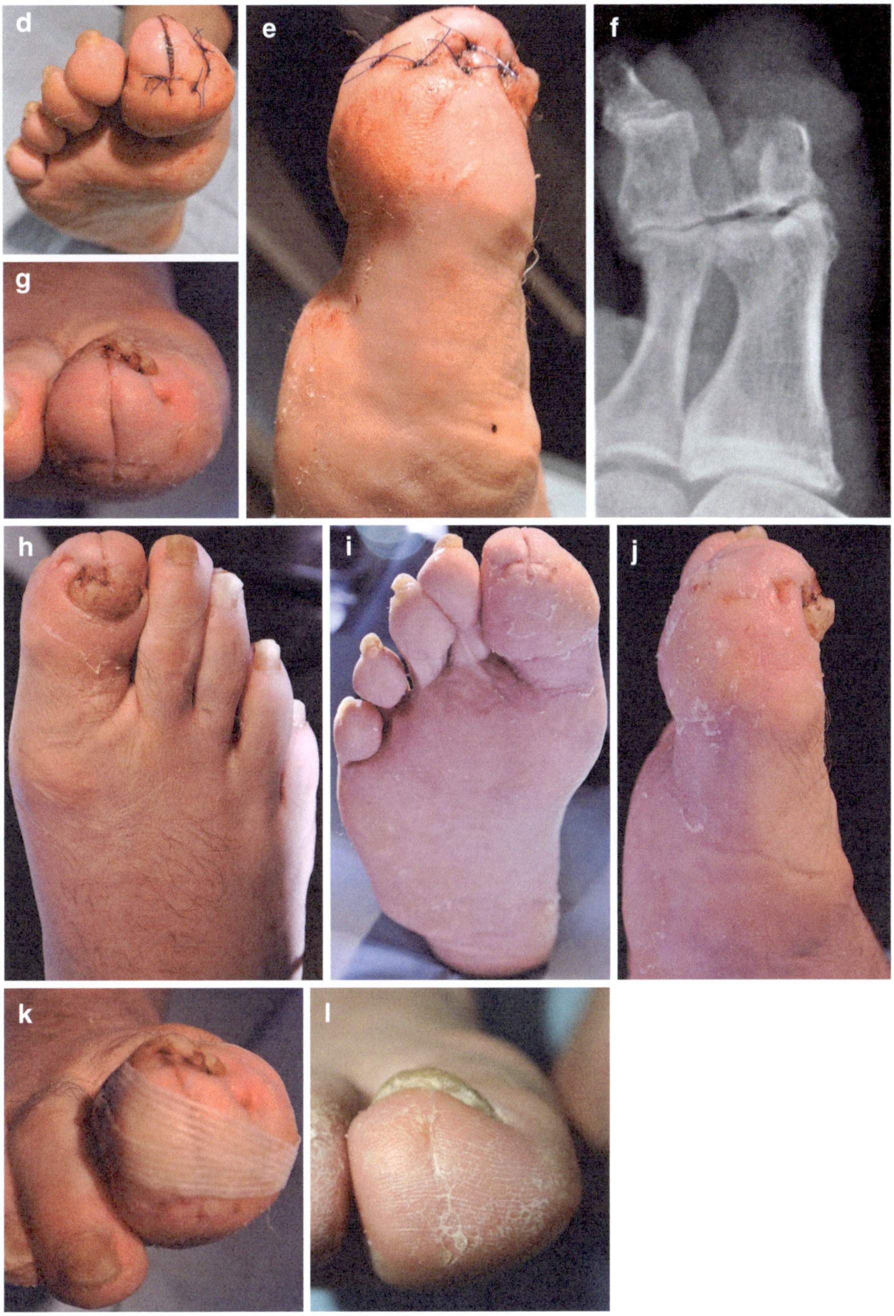

Fig. 6.10 (continued)

References

1. Tovey FI. The manufacture of diabetic footwear. Diabet Med. 1984;1(1):69–71.
2. Ince P, Abbas ZG, Lutale JK, Basit A, Ali SM, Chohan F, Morbach S, Mollenberg J, Game FL, Jeffcoate WJ. Use of the SINBAD classification system and score in comparing outcome of foot ulcer management on three continents. Diabetes Care. 2008;31(5):964–7.
3. Kearney TP, Hunt NA, Lavery LA. Safety and effectiveness of flexor tenotomies to heal toe ulcers in persons with diabetes. Diabetes Res Clin Pract. 2010;89(3):224–6. https://doi.org/10.1016/j.diabres.2010.05.025.
4. Engels G, Stinus H, Hochlenert D, Klein A. Concept of plantarization for toe correction in diabetic foot syndrome. Oper Orthop Traumatol. 2016;28(5):323–34. https://doi.org/10.1007/s00064-016-0453-9.
5. Laborde JM. Neuropathic toe ulcers treated with toe flexor tenotomies. Foot Ankle Int. 2007;28(11):1160–4. https://doi.org/10.3113/FAI.2007.1160.
6. Lountzis N, Parenti J, Cush G, Urik M, Miller OF III. Percutaneous flexor tenotomy—office procedure for diabetic toe ulcerations. Wounds. 2007;19(3):64–8.
7. Pollard JP, Morrison PJ. Flexor tenotomy in the treatment of curly toes. Proc R Soc Med. 1975;68(8):480–1.
8. Tamir E, McLaren AM, Gadgil A, Daniels TR. Outpatient percutaneous flexor tenotomies for management of diabetic claw toe deformities with ulcers: a preliminary report. Can J Surg. 2008;51(1):41–4.
9. van Netten JJ, Bril A, van Baal JG. The effect of flexor tenotomy on healing and prevention of neuropathic diabetic foot ulcers on the distal end of the toe. J Foot Ankle Res. 2013;6(1):3. https://doi.org/10.1186/1757-1146-6-3.

Torsion of the Hallux (3)

7

Lesions situated at the medial margin of the hallux (Fig. 7.1) are almost always due to plantarisation of the medial side of the toe. Even if they point strictly medially, it is in general not the upper of the shoe which is responsible for the pressure that

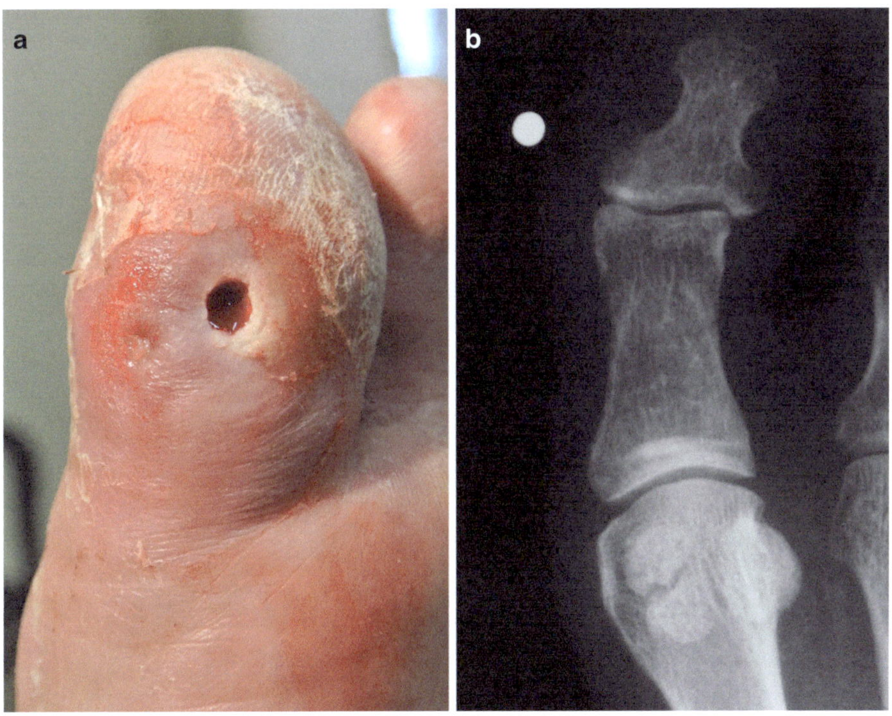

Fig. 7.1 (**a**) Three out of four lesions at the medial outline of the hallux are situated above the IP joint (**b**) Labelling the ulcer by use of a pellet. The ulcer is due to the pressure exerted by the basis of the distal phalanx of the hallux. As an additional finding there is a congenitally divided medial sesamoid bone

D. Hochlenert et al., *Diabetic Foot Syndrome*,
https://doi.org/10.1007/978-3-319-92055-9_7

caused the ulcer, but the toe is rotated with the medial side towards the sole. This plantarisation is based on several pathobiomechanical processes that offer different treatment options.

7.1 Pathobiomechanics and Pressure Points

There are three bony prominences at the medial edge of the hallux that may become the inner pressure point of an ulcer:

First: The *medial basis of the distal phalanx* and **second:** the *medial condyle of the proximal phalanx of the hallux* (Fig. 7.1b). In the region of the IP joint, there are two adjacent medial prominences that belong to each of the articulating bones. It is often only during the course of an operation that it becomes apparent which of both is the cause.

Third: The *medial edge of the apical tuberosity* (Fig. 7.2). The tip is barely protected by soft tissue.

In healthy people, these prominences are not part of the weight-bearing area and therefore, they are not protected adequately by soft tissue. Due to plantarisation, they carry an excessive load with respect to what they are designed to resist. The movement, which is responsible, is a torsion of the toe (Fig. 7.3). This torsion may be *accompanied by more or less clawing of the toe or overextension of the IP joint.* If this clawing prevails, the lesion is situated above the medial edge of the apical tuberosity. If, in contrast, the torsion prevails, the lesion will arise above the medial parts of the IP joint. And if the overextension of the IP joint prevails, the lesion will arise more centrally beneath the IP joint.

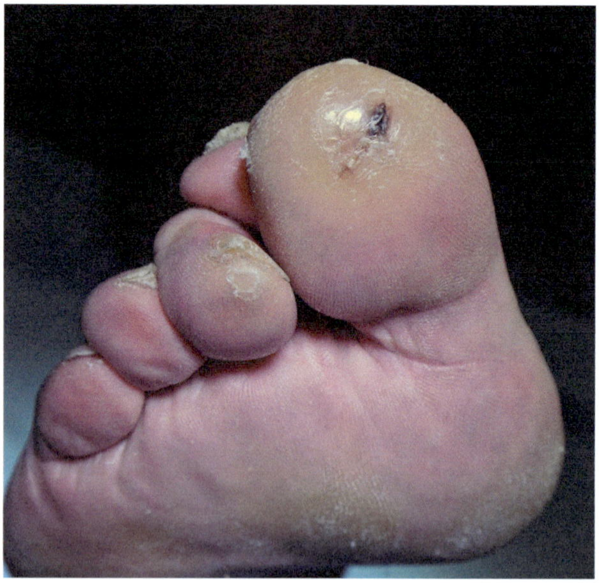

Fig. 7.2 Ulceration at the tip of the hallux medially

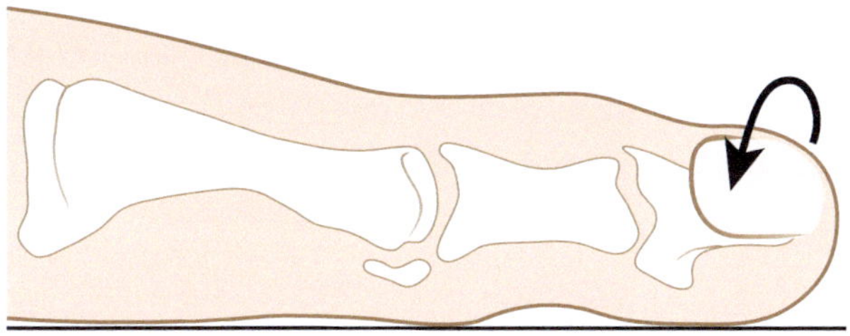

Fig. 7.3 Plantarisation of the medial hallux due to torsion

Several pathobiomechanical phenomena contribute to this malposition. Some are responsible for allowing a rotatory movement, some lead to excessive tension of the tendons. In addition, an excessive abduction of the foot adds further load to the medial margin.

1. Why is the hallux allowed to make a rotatory movement?
   - The bony framework of the first *MTP joint is built as an ellipsoidal joint* and only by the action of ligaments it is forced to the limited range of motion of a hinge joint. These ligaments may become overstretched and allow the movements of an ellipsoidal joint to occur.
   - A *hallux valgus deformity* is regularly present and enhances the stretching of the ligaments in the MTP joint. The deformity itself is often associated with a rotary displacement of the hallux.
   - The first tarsometatarsal joint is often *hypermobile* which means that its ligaments are also less tight than normally. They give way to a rotatory movement of the whole first ray (see Chap. 2, Sect. 2.5.2.3) bringing its medial side into a slightly more plantar position (see Figs. 2.17 and 2.18). It also allows an abduction of the first metatarsal, which is often more noticeable.
   - In case of instability of the medial column (insufficiency or rupture of the tibialis posterior tendon), *the medial arch flattens*. The forefoot then slightly rotates in a pronated position. This rotatory movement rotates the attached hallux as well, bringing its medial parts into a more plantar position.
   - In some cases, the tendon of the *abductor hallucis* muscle attaches not only to the proximal phalanx but also to the distal phalanx. Together with the medial displacement of the first MTH, this tendon is dislocated to the plantar side and contributes to a rotatory movement and a plantarflexion of the hallux (Fig. 7.4).
2. Why do the tendons seem to be too short?
   - Diabetes may, in fact, *shorten* tendons due to molecular alterations of the collagen fibres. Muscles may also shorten due to other still unknown mechanisms and add pull to the respective tendon.
   - The distance that has to be covered by the tendons at the plantar side of the hallux lengthens.
   - This is due to the *flattening* of the medial arch and the added pressure of the navicular that is prominent beneath the arch and adds tension to the FHL tendon (Fig. 7.5).

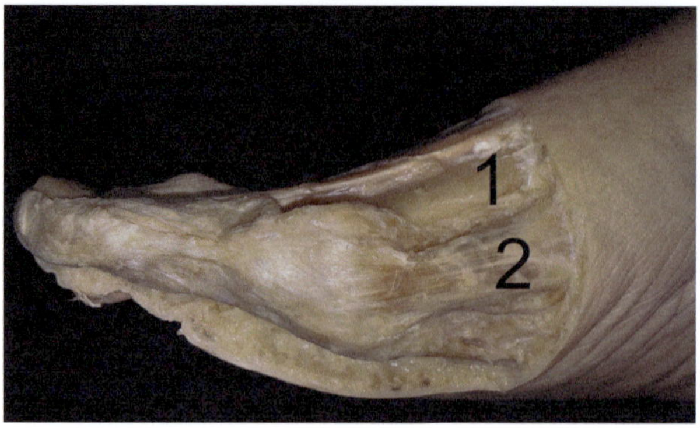

Fig. 7.4 The tendon of the M. abductor hallucis (2) is located more at the plantar side of the first metatarsal bone (1) and the MTH than on the dorsal side. Therefore this muscle not only abducts the hallux but is primarily a strong plantar flexor of the first MTP joint. In the case of a hallux valgus, this plantar flexion effect is intensified and the toe is additionally rotated

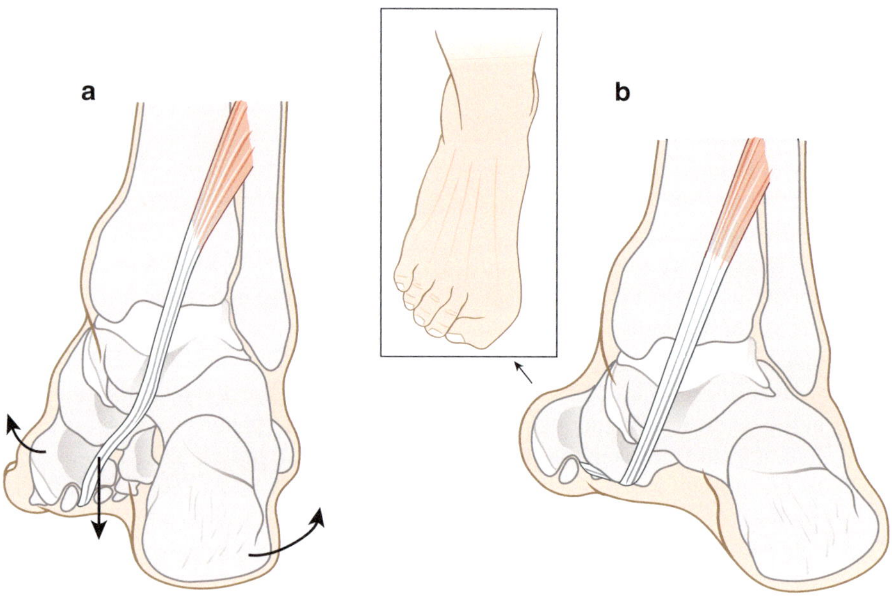

Fig. 7.5 Schematic representation of the course of the FHL tendon. Flattening of the medial column with an increase of the traction of the tendon and resulting deformity of the hallux due to torsion

- Load drives the cornerstones of the medial arch apart until the tension of the plantar fascia blocks this movement. This distance has to be covered also by the FHL tendon. The analogous effect, which tightens the plantar fascia due to what is called '*windlass mechanism*' (see Chap. 2, Sect. 2.5.4.3), also adds traction to the FHL tendon in terminal stance.

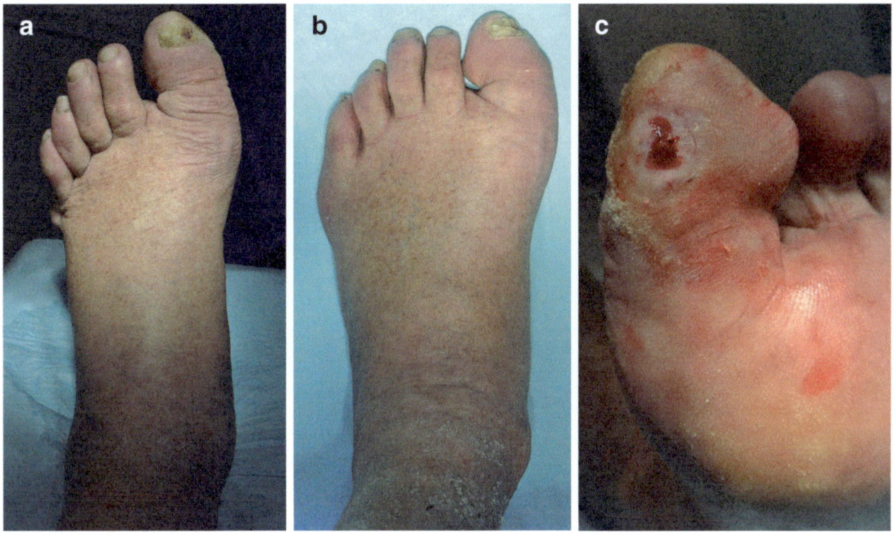

Fig. 7.6 (**a**–**c**) Clinical appearance of the bowstring-effect under load

3. How does this tension rotate the hallux?
   - The so-called '*bowstring-effect*' (Fig. 7.6) vividly depicts how tension on the FHL tendon bends the medial arch and vice versa. The bones of the medial arch are regarded as the bow and the FHL tendon is positioned not contiguous to the metatarsal bone but more laterally and represents the string. A hallux valgus deformity is not needed. In contrast to a real bow, the tendon is not fixed to the extremity of the arch but continues and becomes the flexor tendon of the distal phalanx. When the bow is put under stress, a strong traction on the tendon forces the hallux to perform a flexion with non-physiological intensity. Because the ground doesn't give way, a simultaneous torsion is the only possibility to permit such a strong flexion.
   - The *FHL tendon* inserts at the plantar side of the obliquely positioned distal phalanx. Traction results not only in flexion but also in rotation and further adduction of the hallux (Fig. 7.7).
4. Plantarisation of the medial side of the hallux is also caused by an *abducted foot*. An abducted foot uses the plantarised medial side of the hallux in terminal stance and not the central part of the distal phalanx. In many people with flat feet, the foot is abducted ('placed outwards') and thus, the foot angle is wide. Why is this? The heel of a person with flat feet is everted, the articulations of the hindfoot and the midfoot therefore are not locked and the foot is too flexible to work as a rocker. To move forward, the person must position this unstable foot in such a way that movement is possible, which involves habitually abducting the foot even more than the flattened foot itself would require.

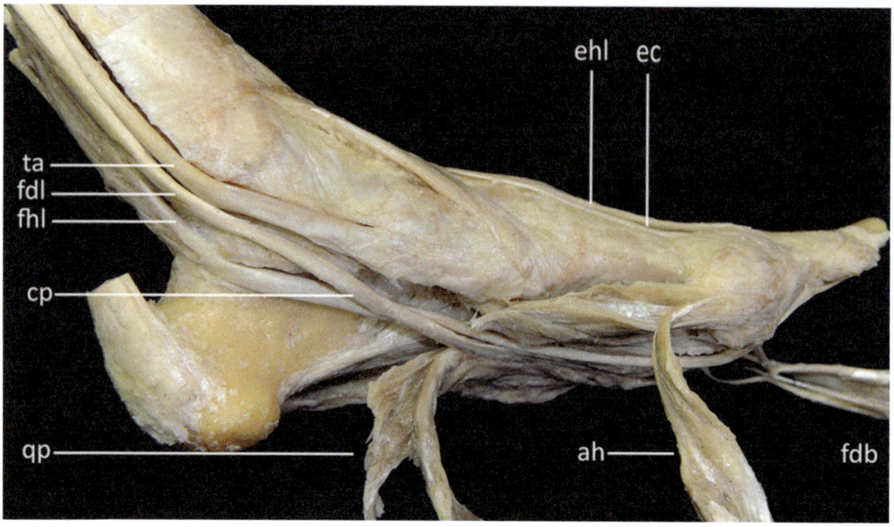

Fig. 7.7 Course of the tendons on the medial side in the anatomical preparation. *ta* tendon of the M. tibialis anterior, *ehl* tendon of the M. extensor hallucis longus, *ec* M. extensor capsularis of the first MTP joint, *tp* tendon of the M. tibialis posterior, *fdl* tendon of the M. flexor digitorum longus, *fhl* tendon of the M. flexor hallucis longus, *cp* Chiasma plantare (cross-over of the tendons of the M. flexor digitorum longus and the tendon of the M. flexor hallucis longus), *qp* M. quadratus plantae, *ah* M. abductor hallucis, *fdb* M. flexor digitorum brevis (qp, ah and fdb are proximally detached)

7.2 Tests to Perform

Generally, the torsion of the hallux is a functional deformity. When the foot is at rest, it can only be suspected. Therefore, *provocative tests* (see also Chap. 3, Sect. 3.4.1), such as the push-up test, the claw test, the functional tests in stance and further provocation by elevation of the heel, are even more important here than it is the case with the other entities. When performing these tests, people might not be able to be sufficiently spontaneous in their movements and therefore fail to reveal the plantarisation. For the sake of correct understanding of the mechanism and the therapeutic options, particular attention must be paid to movements that people make when they are distracted. This might be when changing position or taking a few steps. In some cases, testing goes on for up to 5 minutes until some tell-tale movement reveals the deleterious motion as it would occur during a walk.

Lesions of the medial side of the hallux are predominantly due to plantarisation and should be regarded as such unless plantarisation is not ruled out by these tests.

		Hallux medial all	Hallux condyle	Hallux tip medial
Frequency		6.1%	4.6%	1.4%
Bone involvement	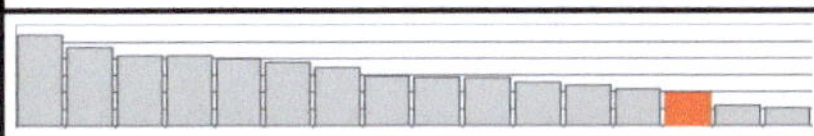	9.7%	8.9%	12.2%
PAD	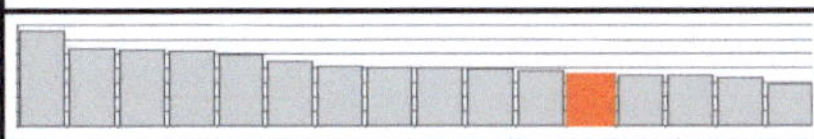	35.4%	33.6%	41.2%
Revascularisation	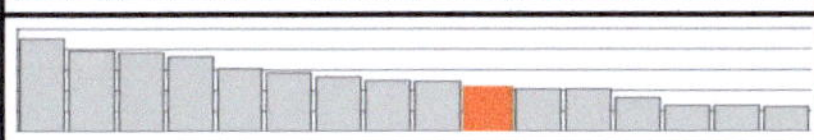	8.7%	7.6%	12.1%
Amputation below ankle	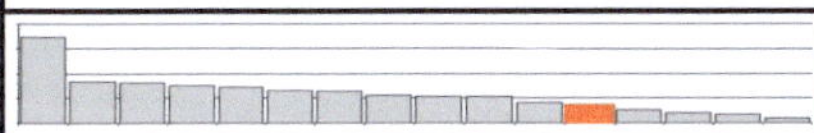	5%	4.4%	6.8%
Amputation above ankle	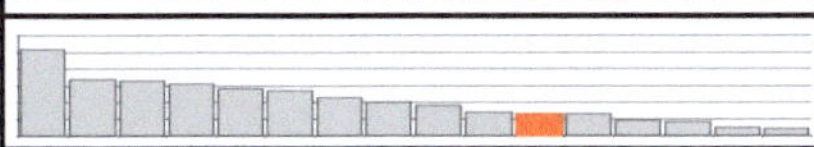	1.3%	1%	2%
Days until remission	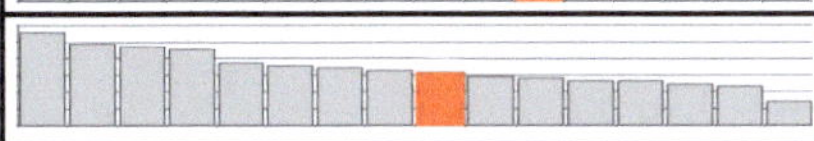	93	88	99
Duration > 180 days	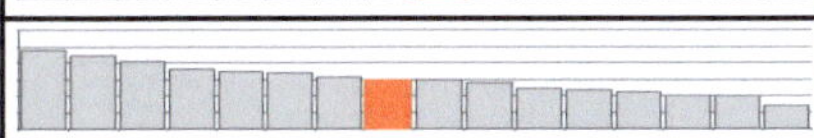	30%	28.8%	33.8%
Reactivation following year	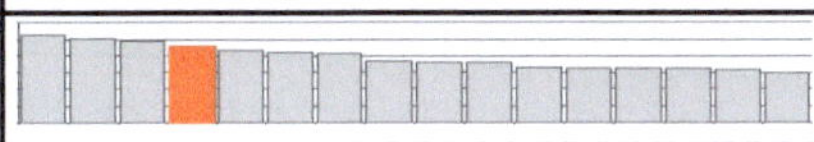	45.7%	46.1%	44.4%

Fig. 7.8 Benchmark figures of lesions of the medial side of the hallux (orange) in a rank of all entities in decreasing height

It is necessary to *observe the patient while walking* in order to assess the angle and the functional impairment caused by flat feet.

Additionally, the testing for short triceps surae, possibly including the *Silfverskjöld test may be performed* (see Chap. 3, Sect. 3.4.1) to detect a dysfunction of the Achilles tendon leading to an overload of the forefoot or aggravation of a flat foot.

7.3 Statistics

The data in Fig. 7.8 shows the often purely neuropathic nature of these lesions. Bone involvement is rare. In line with this, amputations are rare but reoccurrence of an ulcer is frequent.

7.4 Principles of External Offloading

The following goals should be borne in mind when applying the constructive elements listed. The illustration of the use of felted foam demonstrates the first two principles (Fig. 7.9).

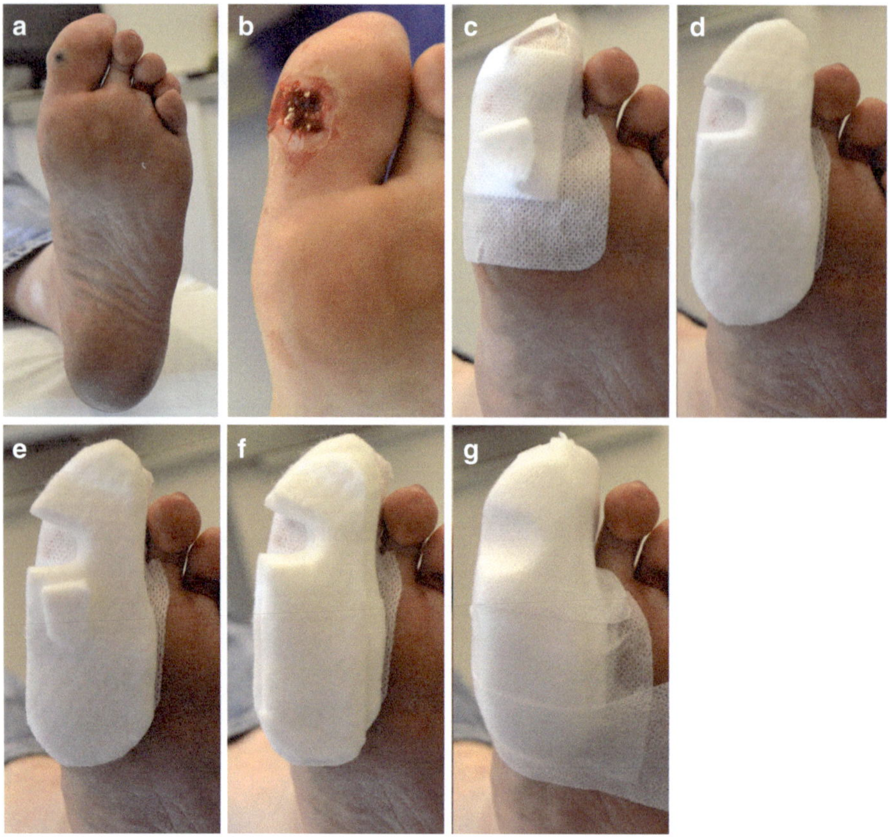

Fig. 7.9 (**a**–**g**) Distant padding of the IP joint of the hallux. The inner pressure point usually is the medial condyle which is offloaded by 2–4 layers of felt

1. Offloading the pressure point by measures in its vicinity
   - **Lowering and softening** the insole below the overstressed region. In the case of using felt to offload wounds, a recess 3 mm beyond the wounds margin is prepared. Recesses must not be circular and should not be used as a singular measure but always in combination with a support (see details in Chap. 19, Sects. 19.2.2 and 19.2.3).
   - **Adding support to the distal part of the hallux.** This can be omitted if the distal phalanx is not plantarflexed during gait, e.g., after a tenotomy of the respective flexor tendon.
2. **Raising the first MTH**. A support of the first MTH adds space beneath the hallux. A disadvantage of this pad is the enhanced distortion of the forefoot with respect to the hind- and midfoot. This distortion already exists, as hindfoot and midfoot are everted during gait, but the medial parts of the forefoot are pressed

against the ground and cannot follow this movement. Enhanced supination of the forefoot with respect to the hind- and midfoot might boost pressure in correspondence to the first MTH as well as the 5th MTH and may promote the development of a Charcot foot.

3. Reducing excessive preload of tendons or muscles by:
   - **Lowering the tip of the shoe**
   - **Elevating the heel** in case of a pes equinus ('shortening of the Achilles tendon'). This must be done with caution because it will lower the forefoot and might enhance pressure at the toes. Using a rocker bottom sole might allow integrating both elements.
4. **Raising the medial arch.** A moderate support of the medial arch might shift pressure to the lateral margin of the foot but must take into account the risk borne by the additional pressure on both areas. The medial arch is not designed anatomically to bear weight. New ulcers may occur, especially at the navicular. Therefore, the insole may be designed with softer material in the exposed area beneath the navicular.
5. Reducing pressure over time on the overstressed region using a **rocker bottom sole** with its peak beneath the MTP joint. The more distal the peak is, the better the hallux is offloaded but the more difficult it becomes to walk. Therefore, it is necessary to find a compromise. In the case of an abducted foot, the orientation of the axis of the rocker bottom sole is placed according to the direction of movement (see Fig. 19.27).
6. Avoiding flexion of the sole in terminal stance by applying a rocker bottom sole and maybe by additionally **stiffening the sole** to prevent dorsal extension of the MTP joint. This is an effective measure for many entities, but challenging for the patient because the patient has to gradually grow accustomed to walking with stiff soles.

7.5 Principles of Internal Offloading

It is necessary to conduct a careful examination while the patient is standing or walking in order to detect exactly which mechanism generates overload.

The **removal of the internal pressure points** in the medial part of the IP joint may eliminate the problem permanently. This can be done by a medial condylectomy of the head of the proximal phalanx (Fig. 7.10). As this is an intervention on the articulation and the bone, there is a higher risk of infection than with surgery on the tendons (see Chap. 20, Sect. 20.5.1.4 and Fig. 20.19).

A **tenotomy of the long flexor tendon of the hallux (FHL)** can prevent plantarisation by reducing rotation (see details in Chap. 20, Sect. 20.4.1). It can be useful to plan both interventions in a *step-by-step-strategy*. At first, derotation is made possible by a tenotomy of the FHL tendon, which is, in general, quickly done and at relatively low risk. If this is sufficient to relieve the affected region, a second

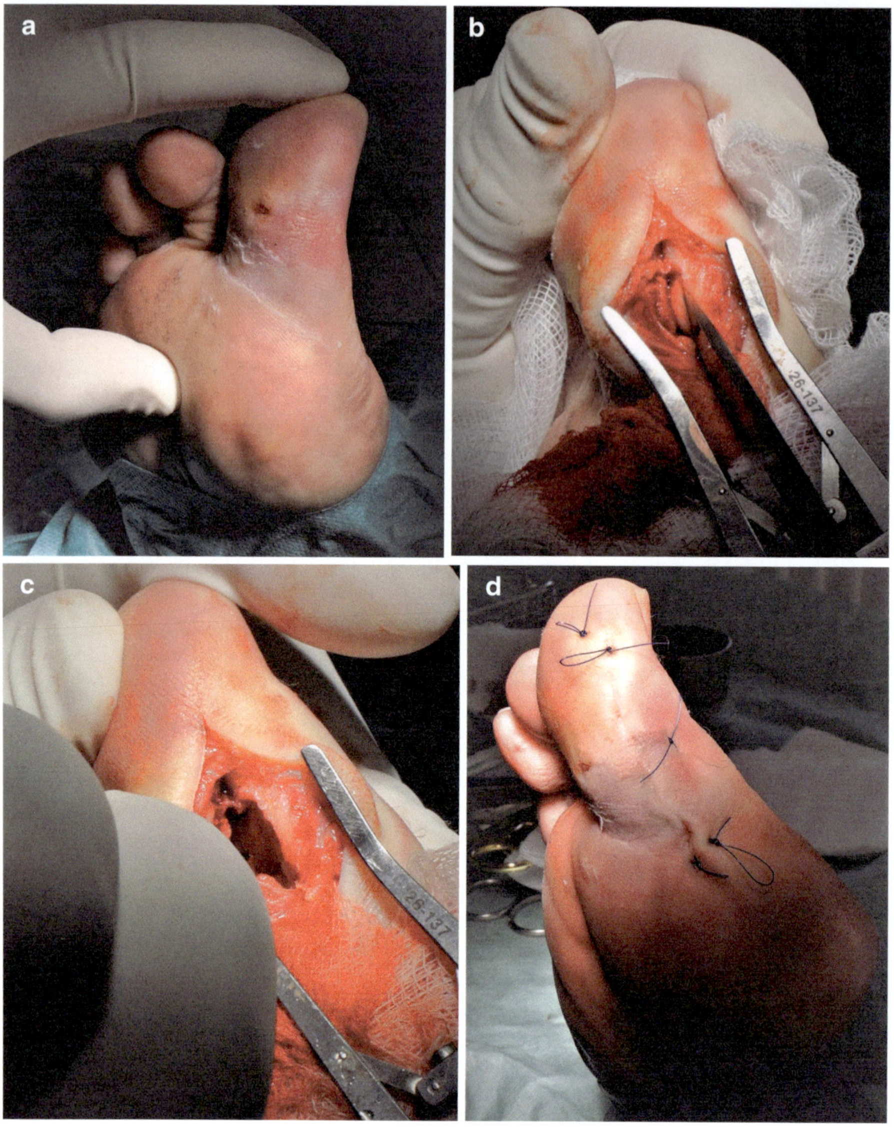

Fig. 7.10 (**a**–**d**) Condylectomy of the head of the proximal phalanx, before, during and after surgery

intervention is no longer necessary. If it is not sufficient, the inner pressure point can be removed. In the case of a *hallux valgus, an operative correction* of the deformity after wound closure might be indicated. This may sometimes be the only way to achieve a long-lasting offloading.

7.6 Summary

- **Lesions of the medial part of the hallux are due to a torsion of the hallux. In order not to miss the real cause of the ulcer, the exam has to include provocative tests.**
- **Therapy of PAD is less frequently necessary. It is a more predominantly neuropathic entity.**
- **These lesions are long-lasting and tend to reoccur. Therefore, early surgical correction should be considered.**
- **A detailed examination is necessary prior to internal offloading. The tenotomy of the long flexor tendon, removal of bony prominences and measures to correct a hallux valgus deformity, might be useful.**

Hallux Valgus (First MTH Medially, 4)

8

The medial side of the head of the first metatarsal bone is an intensely exposed prominence, which can induce the development of pressure ulcers (Fig. 8.1). It is particularly prominent and vulnerable in the case of a hallux valgus deformity.

8.1 Pathobiomechanics and Pressure Points

In the case of a hallux valgus, the first metatarsal bone generally deviates simultaneously in varus position and its head forms a significant protrusion on the medial side of the forefoot (see Chap. 2, Sect. 2.5.5). In other situations, an arthritic and thus enlarged joint may require additional space. The prominent MTH may lead to enhanced pressure and to ulcers.

Often such an ulcer is deep without exposing the bone, and it seems as if a bursa has been opened. Usually, this is a pseudobursa without contact to the MTP joint. A real bursa may also exist but generally without connection to an articulation [1].

The internal pressure point is generally the head of the first metatarsal bone in varus position. The external pressure point is almost always the shoe.

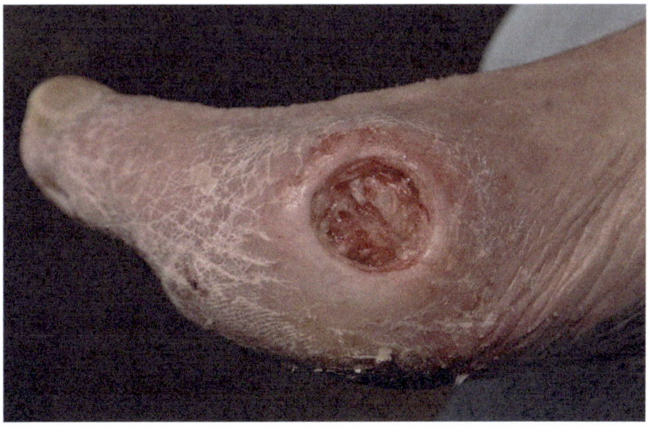

Fig. 8.1 Ulcer above the first MTH

D. Hochlenert et al., *Diabetic Foot Syndrome*,
https://doi.org/10.1007/978-3-319-92055-9_8

		Hallux valgus MTK 1 medial
Frequency		3.1%
Bone involvement		14.3%
PAD		38.2%
Revascularisation		11.4%
Amputation below ankle		7.9%
Amputation above ankle		2.8%
Days until remission		86
Duration > 180 days		30%
Reactivation following year		33.2%

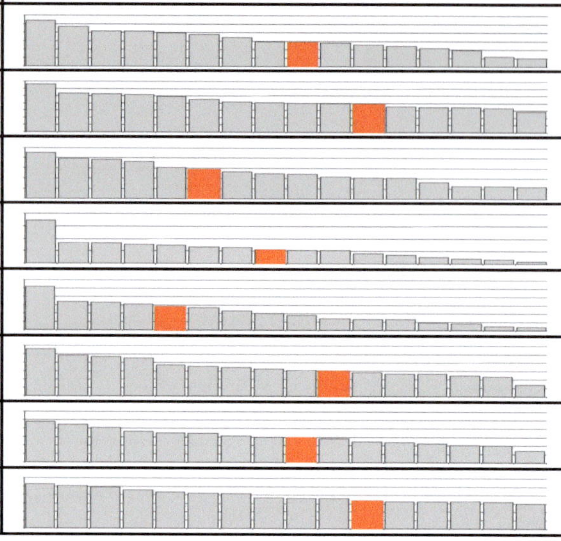

Fig. 8.2 Benchmark figures of lesions at the medial side of the first MTH (orange) in a rank of all entities in decreasing height

8.2 Statistics

The numbers presented in Fig. 8.2 do not express tendencies to extreme values.

8.3 Principles of External Offloading

Spacer pads together with sufficiently wide shoes are best suited to relieve the load on this lesion (Fig. 8.3).

After wound closure, sufficiently wide shoes are necessary to prevent reoccurrence.

8.4 Principles of Internal Offloading

Numerous operative strategies for surgical correction of the hallux valgus have been established. These procedures have common features:

1. Their aim is to re-establish the position of the sesamoid complex beneath the MTP joint. This eliminates the bowstring effect, which otherwise would contribute to maintaining the deformity.

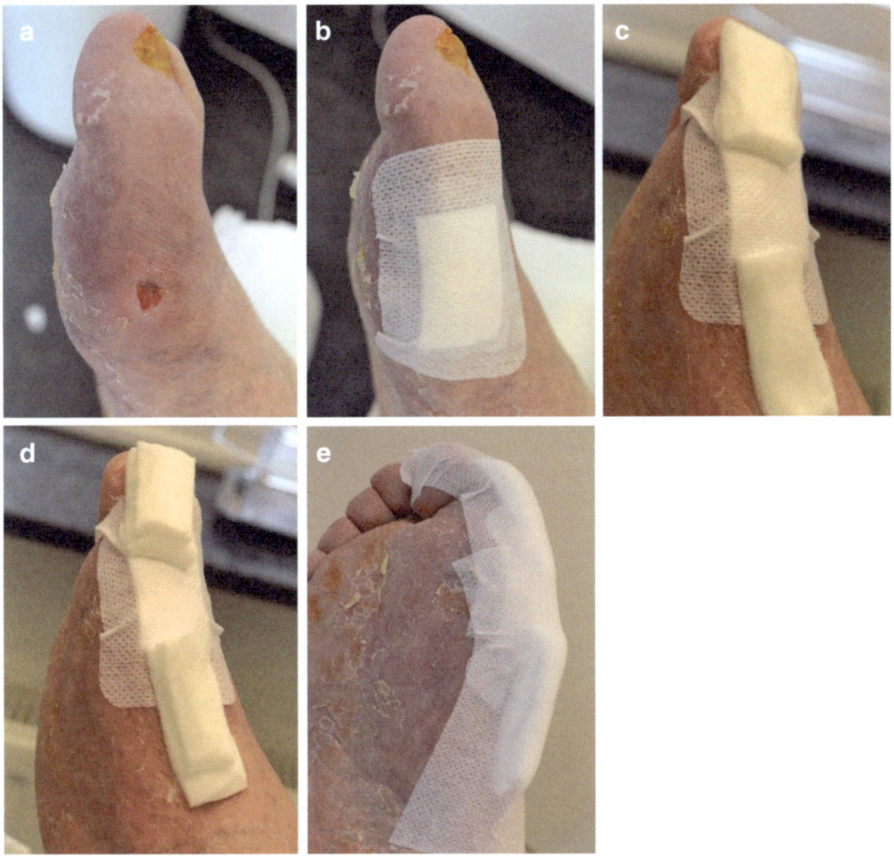

Fig. 8.3 Spacer pads relieve an ulcer at the first MTH (**a**, **b**) debridement and covering of the ulcer (**c**, **d**) two layers of felt proximately and distally to the ulcer form the spacers (**e**) the spacers are fixed

2. These complex operations involve bones, tendons and the implantation of foreign material.
3. Total immobilisation of the operated toe in the postoperative phase is essential in most cases. In order to offload the feet of people with neuropathic disorders effectively, any possible exposure to stress must be excluded.
4. Intense physiotherapeutic aftercare is essential.
5. As these corrections require the implantation of foreign material, the ulcer should be closed before surgery.

To reduce the high risk of re-ulceration, an operative correction after wound closure should be considered. Sometimes, wound closure is impossible to achieve without an operation due to a marked deformity. In this case, a '*lateral release*' may be performed [2]. This intervention is part of more complex operative strategies to correct a hallux valgus but can also be performed separately. The tendon of

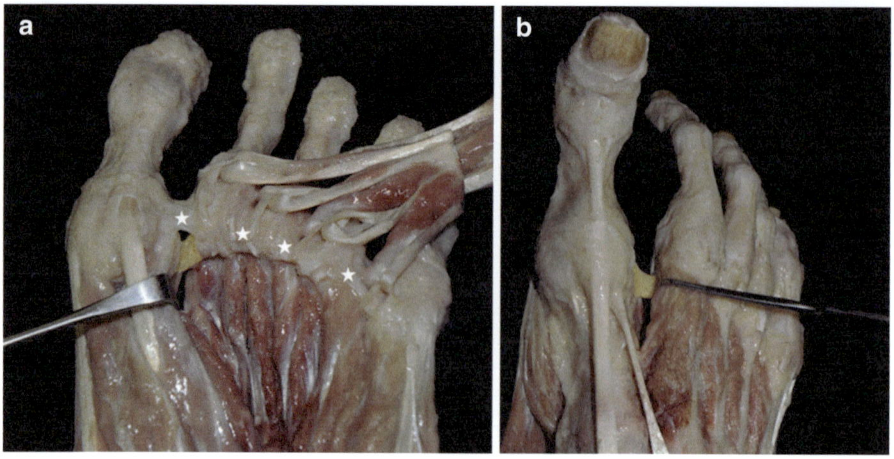

Fig. 8.4 Insertion of the transverse head of the adductor hallucis muscle (*yellow*) (**a**) plantar view with deep transverse metatarsal ligament (*stars*) (**b**) dorsal view, deep transverse metatarsal ligament removed

the transverse head of the adductor hallucis muscle is severed near its insertion at the lateral sesamoid of the first MTP joint (Fig. 8.4) (see Chap. 20 Sect. 20.4.3). In addition, the medial part of the protruding metatarsal bone and a pseudobursa might be removed. To keep this partially repositioned bone in place for several weeks, a Kirschner wire or a rigid tape dressing might be used temporarily. After wound closure, it can be assessed whether a second operation is required to further correct the malalignment. This is not one of the more established procedures in the surgery of hallux valgus, but a strategy to treat ulcers in people with neuropathy.

The best procedure to adopt depends mainly on the biological age and the amount of exercise the patient is willing and able to perform. In many cases of surgery on the hallux valgus, as in other operations on the diabetic foot, less is more.

8.5 Summary

- **Often a pseudobursa is opened without affecting joints or bones.**
- **Treatment of ulcers by external offloading is often successful.**
- **Recurrences are a common problem. During remission, the possibility of a surgical correction of the hallux valgus deformity should be discussed with the patient.**

References

1. Schweitzer ME, Maheshwari S, Shabshin N. Hallux valgus and hallux rigidus: MRI findings. Clin Imaging. 1999;23(6):397–402.
2. Hromadka R, Bartak V, Bek J, Popelka S Jr, Bednarova J, Popelka S. Lateral release in hallux valgus deformity: from anatomic study to surgical tip. J Foot Ankle Surg. 2013;52(3):298–302. https://doi.org/10.1053/j.jfas.2013.01.003.

Hallux: Plantar IP Joint (5)

9

The flexion fold of the interphalangeal joint (IP joint) of the hallux, is only rarely subject to pressure in the physiological situation of a healthy foot (e.g., in barefoot climbing). Therefore it is not equipped to withstand pressure and ulcers may emerge easily if this region is put under stress (Fig. 9.1).

9.1 Pathobiomechanics and Pressure Points

The pathobiomechanical alterations at the base of this entity are:

1. Pathological hyperextension of the IP joint secondary to inflexibility of the first MTP joint (*Hallux limitus or rigidus*). The rigidity of the MTP joint may be caused by arthrosis or by a functional limit to motion due to a metatarsus primus elevates (see Chap. 2, Sect. 2.7.4.3 and Fig. 2.55) (Fig. 9.2).

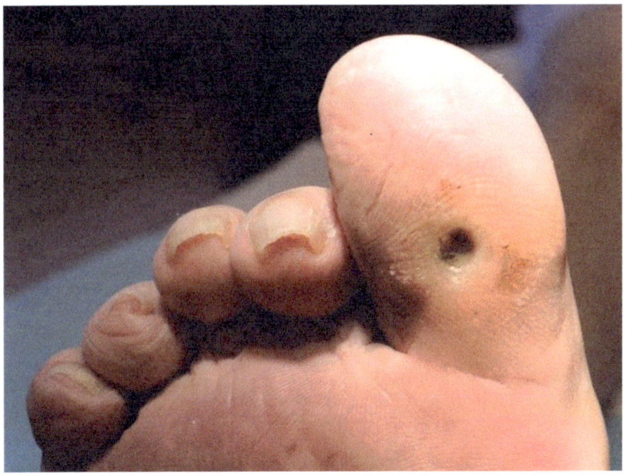

Fig. 9.1 Lesion plantar at the IP joint

D. Hochlenert et al., *Diabetic Foot Syndrome*,
https://doi.org/10.1007/978-3-319-92055-9_9

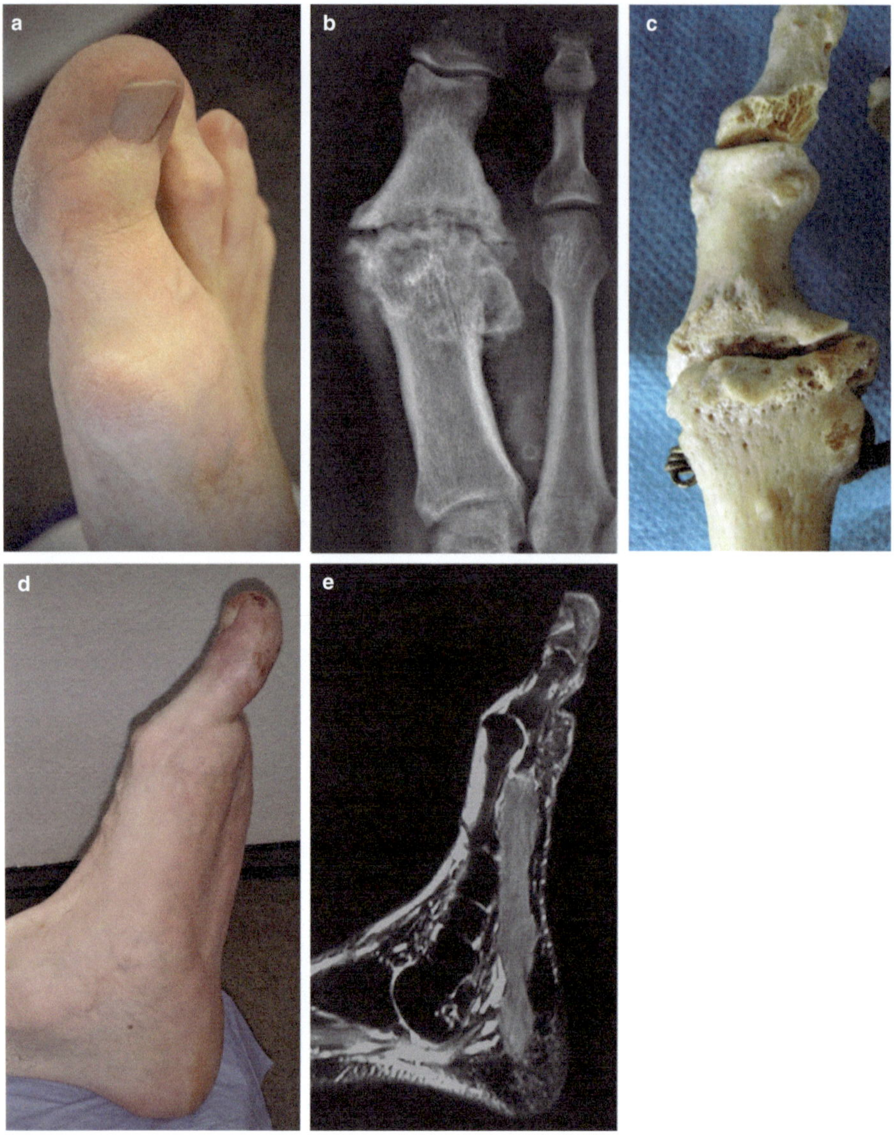

Fig. 9.2 (**a**–**c**) Hallux rigidus caused by arthrosis as seen clinically, radiologically and as an anatomical skeletal preparation. By kind permission of Prof. Dr. rer. nat. Jürgen Koebke, Centre for Anatomy, University of Cologne, (**d**, **e**) caused by functional impairment due to a metatarsus primus elevatus

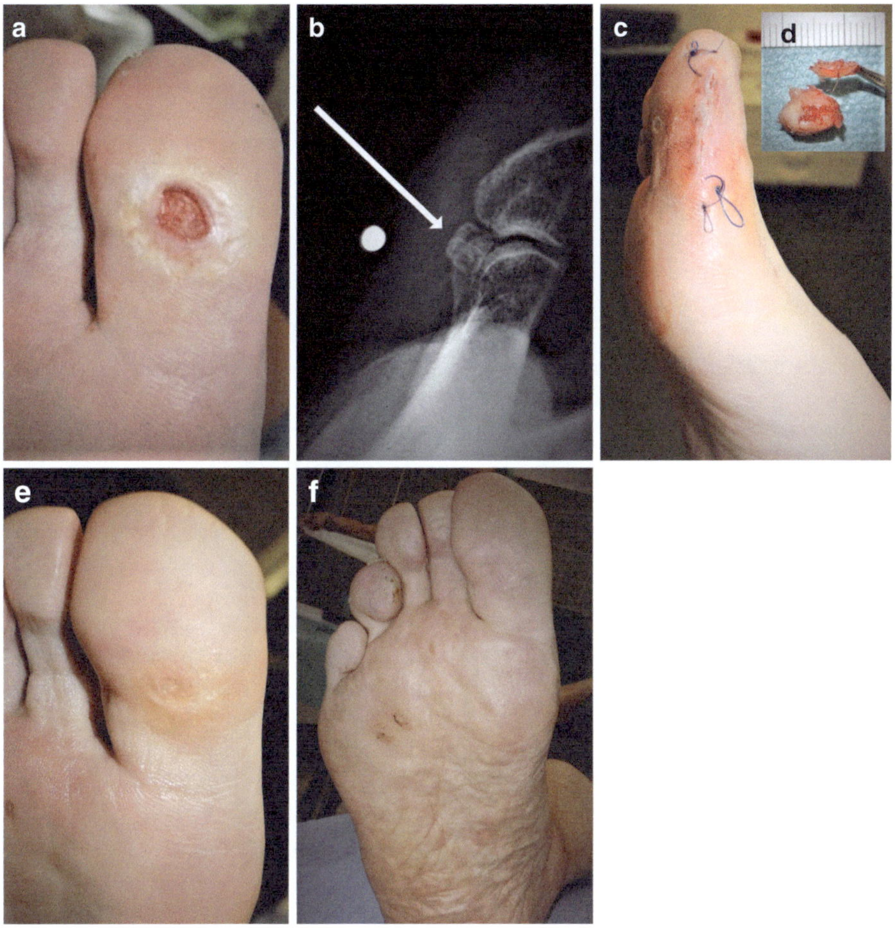

Fig. 9.3 Accessory sesamoid bone (**a**) initial picture (**b**) radiography, the lesion is marked by a pellet, the accessory bone by an arrow (**c**) postoperative picture (**d**) the removed accessory sesamoid bone (**e**) 6 weeks after the intervention (**f**) 2 years after the intervention in occasion of a tenotomy of the FDL tendon of the fourth and fifth toe

2. A possible pressure point is an *accessory sesamoid bone* in the course of the long flexor tendon (Fig. 9.3).

In the case of limited mobility of the MTP joint (hallux limitus or rigidus), the hallux is not able to dorsiflex (passive, dorsal extension) as much as is needed to perform the sequence of motions when walking. The IP joint adopts this movement because at the end of terminal stance dorsiflexion of the hallux, at least at its distal part, is mandatory. Physiologically, this joint is not built to perform any dorsiflexion beyond the neutral position. Its hyperextension exposes plantar parts of the IP joint. The bony prominences are physiologically hidden by the protective protrusion of the fat pad situated below the distal phalanx. These parts of the joint become weight-bearing and form an internal pressure point causing hyperkeratosis, preulcerative lesions or an ulcer. Ulcers occur mainly at the medial condyle of the head of the proximal phalanx (see also Fig. 2.57), but may affect also other parts of the joint. It is only necessary to search for an accessory sesamoid bone when the rigid hallux is not plausible as the sole cause of the ulcer.

Internal pressure point:

1. At the head of the proximal phalanx, which acts as an extension of the metatarsal bone, the medial condyle is particularly prominent.
2. An accessory sesamoid bone in the course of the long flexor tendon may become a pressure point.

9.2 Tests to Perform

Fixed deformities are usually easy to detect. The arthritic MTP joint often exposes osteophytes, that can be seen during inspection as humps under the skin in the area of the joint. If a functional impairment is suspected, it can be confirmed by a *functional test* which is to move the joint passively.

The only challenge arises if an arthrosis is not the cause of the limitation in movement, but the flexor tendons. This is also known as *'functional hallux limitus'* and is detected by performing a *push-up test* and *a functional test* (see Chap. 3, Sect. 3.4.1.3 and Fig. 3.7d), trying to dorsiflex the hallux with the foot in plantigrade position (approximately 90° angle to the lower limb).

It is useful to *observe the patient while walking* and to look for a rotational movement in terminal stance, when the rigid hallux becomes particularly obstructive. At that time, the joint and the distal phalanx are on the ground and under maximum pressure. If the only way to allow further evolvement of the gait cycle is to rotate the foot widening the angle of the foot and bringing the heel inwards, the sheer force on the skin will be particularly destructive.

In addition, a test should be performed to reveal a dysfunction of the Achilles tendon leading to further worsening of the overload on the forefoot (see Chap. 3, Sect. 3.4.1.3). The result of this test is important to estimate the minimum heel spring (Chap. 19, Sect. 19.7 'Elements of protective footwear'). A flat heel helps in external offloading of forefoot problems but leads to even higher pressure on the forefoot in the case of a pes equinus.

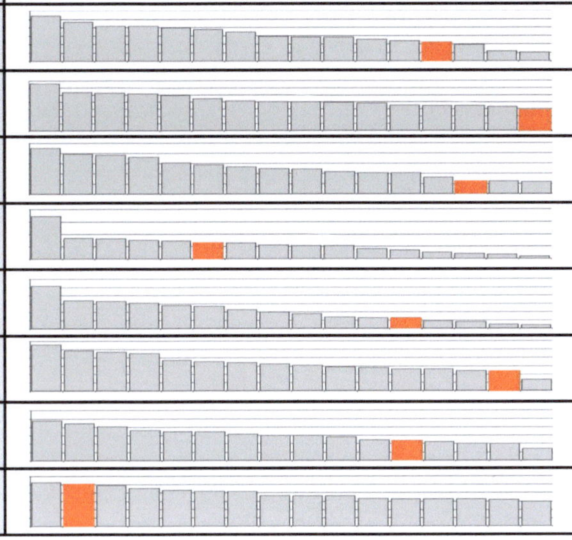

	Hallux rigidus IP plantar
Frequency	2.9%
Bone involvement	10.9%
PAD	28.4%
Revascularisation	5.1%
Amputation below ankle	9.2%
Amputation above ankle	1.3%
Days until remission	70
Duration > 180 days	32.5%
Reactivation following year	50.5%

Fig. 9.4 Benchmark figures of lesions at the plantar side of the first IP joint (orange) in a rank of all entities in decreasing height

9.3 Statistics

The data is shown in Fig. 9.4. Bone or PAD involvement is rarer than in other entities. The median duration until wound closure is amongst the lowest for all entities, which may imply that the severity of this type of lesion is seldom very high. By contrast, the rate of reactivation is very high, probably because conservative prophylactic treatment is often very difficult and surgical procedures are not considered. The high proportion of amputations below the ankle is in line with the assumption that there is significant potential for improvement at least in this cohort.

9.4 Principles of External Offloading

The most important modifications of the shoe consist in the use of sole stiffeners and a contoured outsole. These measures are considered to be helpful:

1. **Offloading the pressure** point by measures in its vicinity
    - **Lowering and softening** the material beneath the overloaded area. In the case of ulcers, a recess beneath the ulcer and about 3 mm beyond its edge offloads the prominence, which can be most accurately achieved when felt is fixed directly onto the skin.

- Adding **support to the distal part of the hallux** in the case of ulcers of the IP joint. This can be done by using self-adhesive felt placed beneath the hallux.

2. Reduction of the pressure and its time of action in the region may be achieved by using a **rocker bottom sole**. The maximum offloading is achieved when the apex of the rocker is placed slightly proximal to the joint which is to be relieved, e.g., approximately below the first MTH in this case. Inconveniently, this makes walking much more difficult. A peak placed proximal to the MTHs is much more comfortable but provides less offloading. The rocker also partially prevents dorsiflexion (=extension) of the MTP joint because it converts bending forces into a torque moment. The position of the roller also has to reflect the angle of abduction of the foot and other criteria (see Chap. 19).
3. The effect of the contoured outsole in terminal stance may be enhanced by completely eliminating the flexion of the sole adding a **stiffener**. This makes the passive dorsal extension of the MTP and IP joints unnecessary. Bear in mind that the patient has to become gradually accustomed to walking with stiff soles. In more extreme cases, the stiffener should be rigid enough to prevent any bending whatsoever.
4. Avoiding even the slightest **slipping** of the heel out of the heel cap as this will counteract the benefits of any modification the shoe might have at the forefoot. By acting as a lever, even slight slipping of the heel may lower the hallux and exert great pressure beneath the IP joint. This can be avoided by using an optimised rocker and an upper that reaches above the ankle.
5. Allowing the hallux to remain in the least possible dorsiflexion. This is achieved by reducing the elevation of the tip of the shoes (toe spring).
6. A **flat longitudinal axis** of the foot. The heel might be designed to be extremely flat only if there is no limit in the dorsal extension of the ankle. As this is rarely the case, a compromise must be found.
7. Moderate **supination** of the forefoot may be achieved by raising the ball region (support beneath the first metatarsal head and support of the medial arch).

The use of felt for offloading is similar to its use for the medial condyle with medial ulcers. In the case of a precisely centred ulcer, the recess may also be centred (Fig. 9.5).

9.5 Principles of Internal Offloading

Surgical therapy may try to eliminate the internal pressure point or to mobilise the rigid MTP joint.

- If the joint is still sufficiently mobile and the medial condyle has been identified as the inner pressure point, a *medial condylectomy* of the head of the proximal phalanx might be sufficient (see Chap. 20, Sect. 20.5.1.4 and Fig. 7.11a–d).

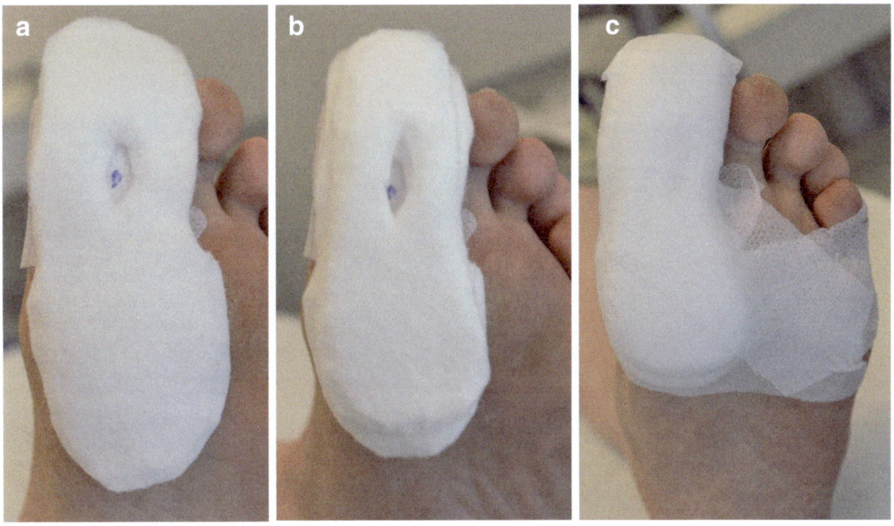

Fig. 9.5 (**a**–**c**) Cushioning to offload an ulcer in the plantar area of the IP joint of the hallux

- In some cases, it is useful to *remove the accessory sesamoid bone* within the flexor hallucis longus tendon (FHL). The accessory sesamoid bone does not need to be removed necessarily if another option can be found and the sesamoid bone is not infected.
- The operative therapy of a hallux rigidus follows a specific classification according to Vanore. Its four stages are determined considering the remaining walking capacity and the level of pain [1]. **In people with neuropathy, this is of no use** and the indication should consider the expected long-term ability to walk and the need in terms of offloading. A frequently used option is a *Valenti's operation* (see Chap. 20, Sect. 20.5.2.3). This is a modified Resection Arthroplasty that in people without neuropathy is used in stage 2 and 3 according to Vanore (initial or advanced destruction of the joint accompanied by pain). A wedge is removed, including the destroyed surface of the joint and a part of both adjacent bones, to leave a space with an angle of around 45°, which is open towards the dorsum of the foot. The plantar surface of the joint is preserved as well as the sesamoid complex, which is mobilised (Fig. 9.6).
- In case of delayed closure or frequent recurrence of ulcers, it might be useful to explore the site surgically because some sturdy fibrous tissues might exert pressure like a sesamoid bone, even if not ossified and therefore not visible in the radiological exam.

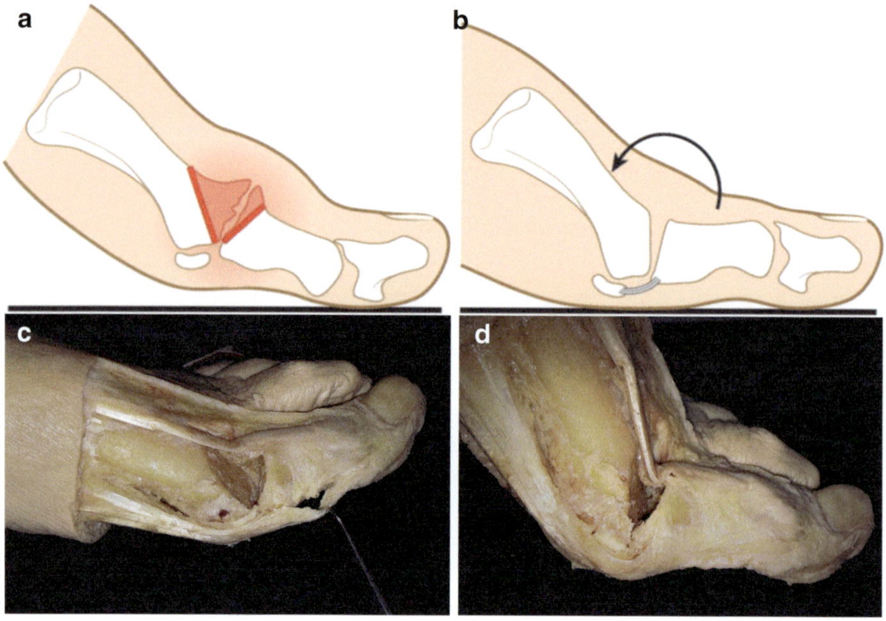

Fig. 9.6 (**a**, **b**) Principal concept of the operation according to Valenti represented schematically (**c**) seen in an anatomical preparation (**d**) the same as (**c**) but in dorsiflexed position

9.6 Summary

- **A general clinical examination will easily identify the main triggers, a hallux limitus or rigidus. In uncertain situations, the assessment should include a conventional radiological exam to look for an accessory sesamoid bone.**
- **Contoured outsole (rocker bottom sole) and sole stiffeners are most important for offloading therapy.**
- **Surgical offloading is possible. The best approach must be assessed individually.**

Reference

1. Wolfring A. Operative Verfahren beim Hallux rigidus. Implantationsarthroplastik im metaanalytischen Vergleich zur Resektionsarthroplastik und Arthrodese; 2006.

Nail Bed Lesions (6)

10

Pressure is the main factor inducing damage to the nail and its bed. Underestimated, insidious and repeated trauma facilitates deformities of the nail and infection by bacteria or fungi (Onychomycosis). Skin compensates for pressure by a thickening of its superficial layers. The nail bed can do so only to a limited extent, as each thickening of the nail (Onychogryphosis) increases the pressure exerted within a shoe or facilitates levering. As a consequence, the nail bed is less able to react and protect itself than the surrounding tissue and therefore might provide an early sign of excessive pressure and indicate the need for the introduction of protective measures.

10.1 Overview

The main categories of damage to the nail bed are:

- Ingrown toenails (Unguis incarnates). Sometimes, chronic pressure to the nail derives from plantarisation and the picture is similar, but there is no ingrowing part of the nail. The nail can be pushed into the margin of the nail bed or vice versa (see Fig. 10.4).
- Hypertrophic nails with structural changes, for example, in the case of onychomycosis or psoriasis with ulcers beneath the nail. In this context, a pathological keratosis of the nail bed takes place in areas of the nail that detach from the nail bed (see Fig. 10.8). This chronic trauma can be induced by hyperflexion of the distal phalanx.
- Trauma of the nail leading to injuries of the nail bed (Fig. 10.1). The acute trauma typically affects the nail from the front, sometimes damaging the entire nail bed and sometimes only its root.

D. Hochlenert et al., *Diabetic Foot Syndrome*,
https://doi.org/10.1007/978-3-319-92055-9_10

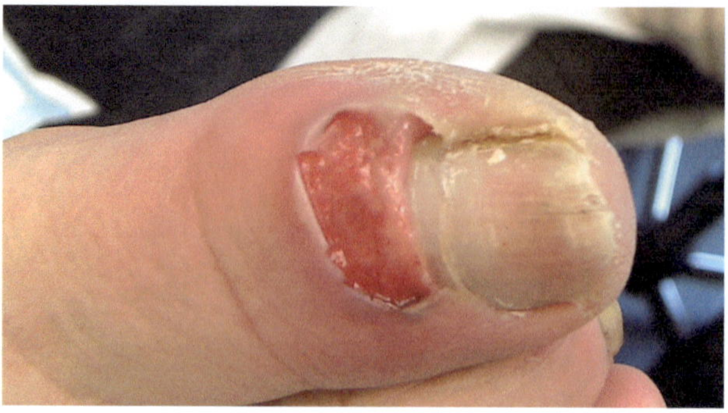

Fig. 10.1 Traumatised nail

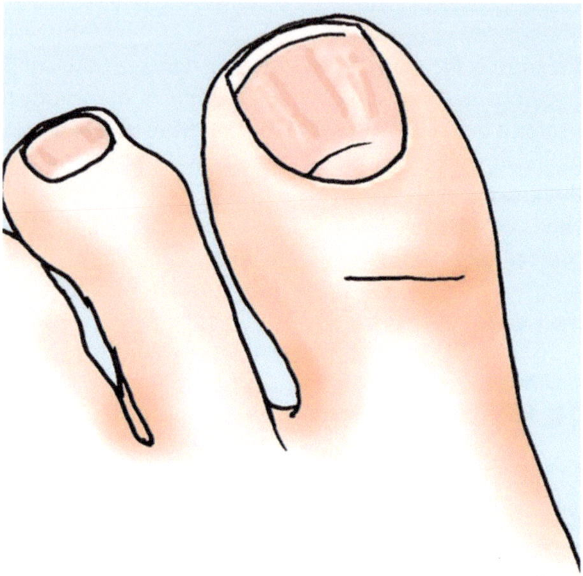

Fig. 10.2 The correct cut

10.2 Director's Cut: The Correct Cut of Toenails

The correct cut follows the tip of the toe in a way that the nail afterwards is a little shorter than the toe itself (ca. 1 mm) (Fig. 10.2). It does not matter whether this cut is straight or round as long as it follows the shape of the tip of the toe. Under no circumstances should the edges be so short that the nail fold (sulcus unguis) is no longer occupied by the edge of the nail and closes in such a way that the growing nail grows in.

10.3 Ingrown Toenail

The toenail grows in if the nail fold does no longer exist up to its distal end. With pressure from the side, the nail fold becomes deeper. It then becomes progressively more difficult to cut the nail in the deepest part of the fold and a spur may easily stay in place (Spicula). This ingrowing spur provokes an inflammatory reaction, swelling and further laceration, possible infection, hypergranulation and sometimes pain (Fig. 10.3). Swelling and pain additionally limit access and further restrict the possibilities of care until the person seeks help.

The medial nail fold of the hallux can be damaged by pressure of shoes or compression stockings or by hyperflexion and rotation of the distal phalanx. The thickened nail can also become an abutment if soft tissue at the tip of the misaligned toe is pressed against the nail.

But also the lateral nail fold can be compromised, as the entire nail plate of the hallux can be displaced laterally by pressure exerted medially. The lateral nail fold is limited by the adjacent second toe, so that pressure is generated between the displaced nail and the 2nd toe. The lateral nail fold can be squeezed even more forcefully if the 2nd toe is not positioned parallel to the hallux, but the toes take a crossed position to each other (Fig. 10.4). These situations also appear clinically as ingrown toenails, but they are caused by movements independent of nail growth. This is important because a tenotomy of the FHL-tendon is a useful measure to provide immediate relief and avoid recurrence. This may be performed in addition to nail surgery or on its own.

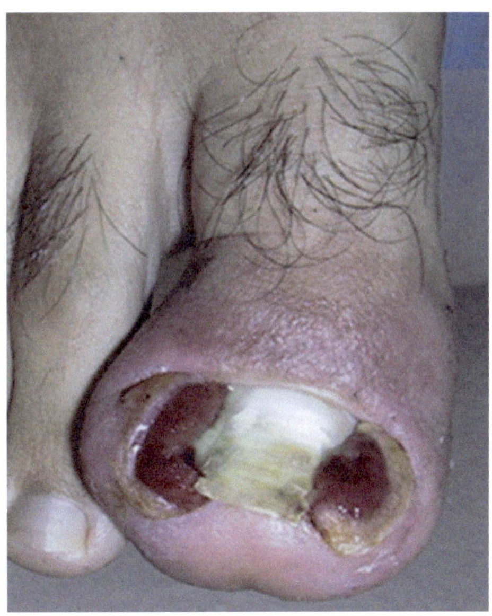

Fig. 10.3 Ingrown toenail at the hallux medial and lateral

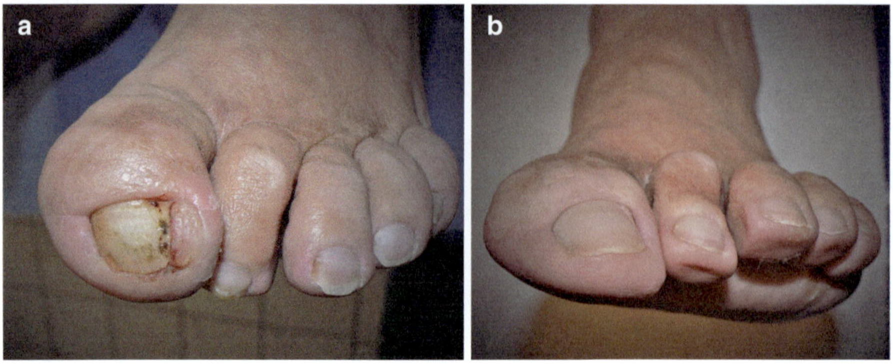

Fig. 10.4 (**a**) The nail on the misaligned hallux (hyperflexion and rotation of the distal phalanx) is pressed against the transversely positioned 2nd toe and the lateral nail fold of the hallux is therefore traumatized (**b**) 2 years after tenotomy of the FHL tendon

10.4 Statistics

The figures presented in the Fig. 10.5 show the sequent peculiarities:

- Ninety percent of all nail bed lesions are located at the hallux.
- Bone involvement, PAD, revascularisation, amputations and reactivation are relatively rare.
- The median time until resolution is half the one observed in other entities.

10.5 Principles of External Offloading

- Sufficiently large and long shoes (see also Fig. 19.26, Chap. 19) are the most important aspect of prevention. They should have a straight medial margin and no stiffened toe caps. Even apparently insignificant stiffening or pressure from the medial or lateral side may contribute to a deeper nail fold over time.

Remember: The nail and nail bed are always weaker than even the softest part of a shoe.

- The nail needs care to limit trauma:
  - Do not allow nails to grow too long.
  - Do not hesitate to grind down thickened nails.
  - Use podiatry care.

		Nail total	Nail D1 ingrown	Nail D1 trauma	Nail D1 struct.	**Nail D2-D4**
Frequency		12.1%	5.5%	1.7%	3.8%	1%
Bone involvement	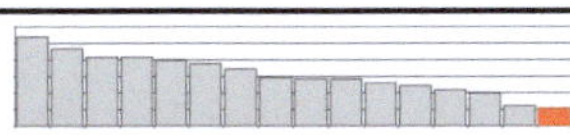	5.2%	3.2%	6.3%	7.5%	5.6%
PAD	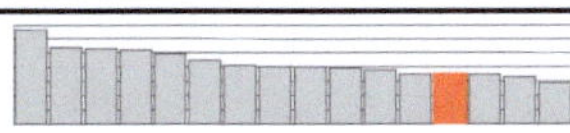	34.9%	29.2%	37.5%	39.8%	42.4%
Revascularisation	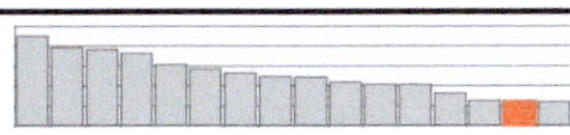	5%	4.4%	4.6%	4.6%	10.3%
Amputation below ankle	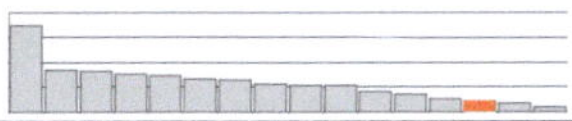	2.8%	1.7%	3.4%	3.8%	3.7%
Amputation above ankle	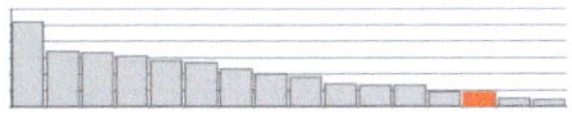	0.8%	0.3%	0%	1.8%	1.8%
Days until remission	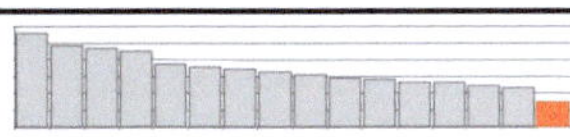	42	41	39	43	54
Duration > 180 days	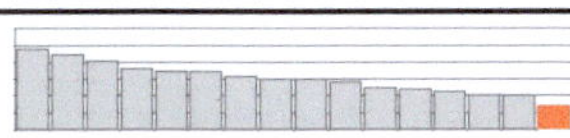	13.7%	10.6%	16.2%	16.2%	17.1%
Reactivation following year	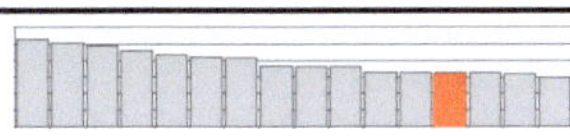	32.7%	29%	37.6%	35.7%	34%

Fig. 10.5 Benchmark figures of lesions at the onychostroma (orange) in a rank of all entities with decreasing height

10.6 Principles of Internal Offloading

- **Do not extract nails!** This is a frequent but unnecessary intervention that traumatises the nail bed and, in the best cases, leads to a healing of the injury with scar formation. The problem is not addressed and not solved. The nail often grows back with more deformities, causing the same problems that had led to the initial extraction. In case of a concurrent PAD, the consequences are particularly serious and could in extreme cases even cause amputation of the whole leg. A PAD is not always safely excluded in everyday care, even if it is considered to be self-evident.
- **Tamponade** in case of ingrown toenail: The nail is bevelled in the distal part of the fold in such a way that no edge or spur presses into the tissue. Material is placed under the border of the nail in order to spread the physiological pressure to a larger surface in the fold. Due to this tamponade, the nail is prevented from traumatising the skin in the fold (Fig. 10.6a).
- **Orthonyxia clasp**: There are several models of clasps and the correct preparation forms part of the podiatrist's professional training in many countries. The basic principle is to lift the borders using the clasp, which is in turn supported by the nail at its centre (Fig. 10.6b).

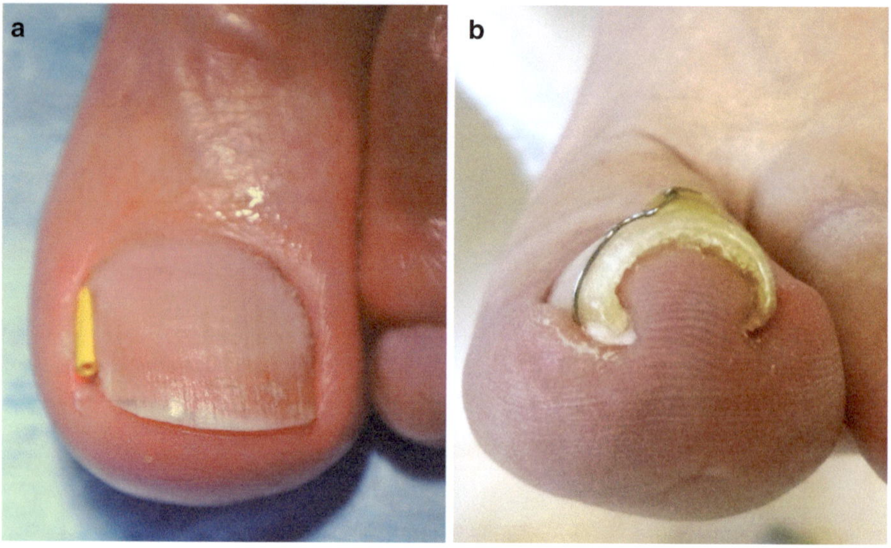

Fig. 10.6 Pressure reduction by podiatric treatment: (**a**) Protection of the nails fold (sulci protector) (**b**) Orthonyxia clasp

Fig. 10.7 Pathological growth of a nail after partial resection of its root

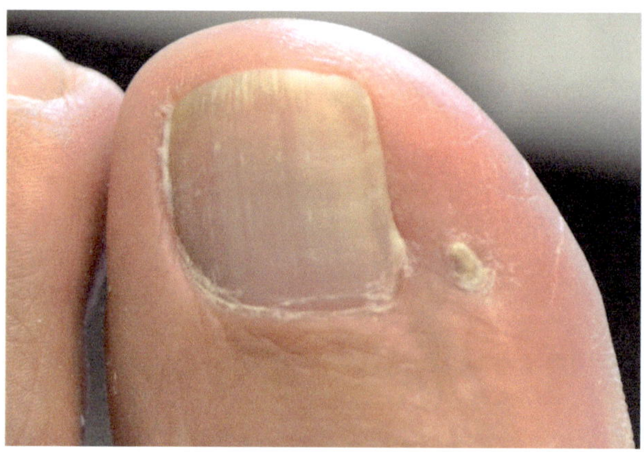

- **Partial removal of a wedge of the nail:** A section of the nail which is as short as possible including the spur is removed. This immediately relieves the irritated nail bed. Other measures of podiatry care must be taken in order to prevent traumatism by the nail, which is highly probable as it grows back.
- **Partial removal of the root of the nail**: This concerns a wedge excision of the nail fold, nail edge, and corresponding matrix. This procedure is popular in some countries and also known as 'Emmert plasty', developed by Baudens (1804–1857) [1]. Regrowth of this part of the nail should be avoided by removal of all remaining rests of the root. If this fails, it will lead to reactivation (Fig. 10.7).

- **Phenolisation**: In this procedure, the margin of the nail is removed including the root and then a swab soaked in a solution of phenol is placed for a short, defined time into the defect where parts of the root might have remained. The tissue which is reached by the solution becomes necrotic and is rejected by the vital adjacent tissue. In comparison with surgical removal alone, reactivation is rare, pain disappears earlier and patients are able to return to work sooner [2]. All interventions should be performed in a bloodless field and with regional block anaesthesia.
- **Tenotomy of the FDL-tendon** of a transversally positioned neighbouring toe might be considered.
- **Tenotomy of the FHL-tendon** of the hallux in case of a lesion of the distal medial fold caused by plantarisation due to hyperflexion and torsion can relieve the compromised nail fold (see Fig. 10.4).

10.7 Treatment of Onychomycosis

A significant number of people with DFS also suffer from onychomycosis (Fig. 10.8) [3]. It is characteristic for the fungal infection that at least one nail is spared, even if most of the nails of a person are affected. In the case of a systemic disease, such as psoriasis, by contrast, nail involvement typically affects all nails without exception.

The indication for treatment is controversial. On one hand, it is possible to eliminate the mycosis completely and therefore to reduce the reservoir of fungi and spores. On the other hand, the rate of reactivation is high, and as a consequence, the measures must be maintained for a long time in order to be successful. In the case

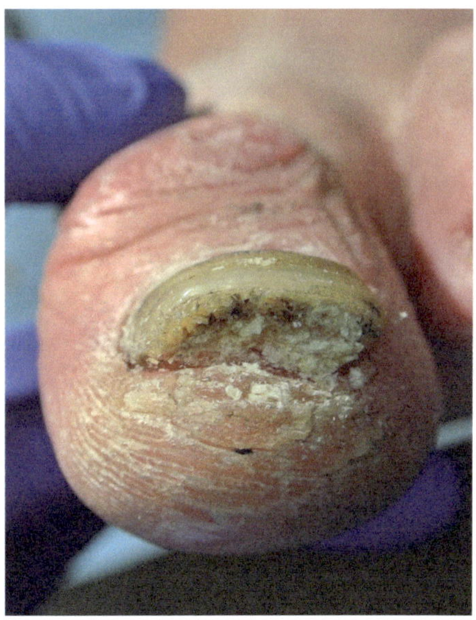

Fig. 10.8 Onychomycosis and gryphosis of the left hallux

of people affected by a DFS, this is often unrealistic. Some of the antimycotic substances in use are hepatotoxic and, as a result, the benefit is often not regarded as sufficient to justify their use [4].

In the case of younger patients suffering from an unsightly appearance or other consequences of the infection, an attempt should be made to eradicate the fungi. The following instructions [5] may be useful.

10.7.1 General Considerations

- Written information for the patient. The patient must understand that any treatment takes at least several months and that the infection often returns after treatment. To be successful in spite of this, patience, stamina and consistency are needed.
- Microbial detection and an investigation of the resistance of the fungi is needed if systemic therapy is planned or in case of reactivation. Part of an affected nail is sent to the laboratory. In general, no specific transport material is needed.
- Systemic therapy can be used if more than two nails or the matrix (root) of one of them are affected.

10.7.2 First Phase (Approximately 2 Weeks)

During the first phase, the affected nail matrix is removed. Applying an antifungal ointment, also containing 40% urea, on the affected nail each day for 2 weeks will soften the diseased nail, which can then be easily abraded. To keep the ointment in place the nail should be covered with an impervious plaster. Unaffected parts of the nail remain firm and stay in place, often with a clear edge. The nail bed remains covered by skin and normally no wound occurs.

10.7.3 2nd Phase (up to 1 Year)

During the 2nd phase, reinfection of the nail as it grows back is avoided.

- Local treatment with antifungal cream, varnish or spray.
- Disinfection of shoes and other textiles, such as compression socks, with a disinfectant which is effective on spores.
- Use disinfectant detergents to wash all the laundry of the household that has been in contact with fungi or their spores (towels, linen, socks, etc) for several weeks. A temperature of 60 °C should be sufficient to disinfect fungi and spores.
- If necessary, systemic antimycotic therapy.

10.7.4 3rd Phase (Lifelong)

During the 3rd phase, the aim is to avoid reinfection. Spores are everywhere. It is not possible to avoid contact with them altogether. The aim is to prevent them from getting established again.

- Avoid pressure on the nails by shoes and possibly by certain socks.
- Dry the feet carefully, especially between the toes.
- Wear shoes in hotel rooms or public showers or baths.

10.8 Summary

- **Ninety percent of nail lesions relate to the hallux.**
- **Nail lesions are in general less serious or dangerous than other entities of lesions.**
- **Extraction of nails in people with neuropathy rarely resolve the problem. They can be extremely harmful with severe consequences including major amputations, particularly in case of PAD. There are many alternatives which have a lower risk of complications.**
- **Pressure exerted by shoes is the main factor for the initiation and development of nail pathologies. In prevention and treatment, footwear that does not exert any pressure on the toes (except the sole) is mandatory.**
- **In addition to nail surgery, tenotomies can be used to correct the misaligned toes and prevent pressure on the nail bed.**

References

1. Waldeck M. Unguis incarnatus: Die Emmert-Plastik und ihre Alternativen. ChirurgenMagazin. 2012;10(4):42–6.
2. Scholz N. Konservative Behandlung eingewachsener Zehennägel mit Nagel-Korrekturspangen. Dtsch Arztebl. 2000;97(22):A1532.
3. Papini M, Cicoletti M, Fabrizi V, Landucci P. Skin and nail mycoses in patients with diabetic foot. G Ital Dermatol Venereol. 2013;148(6):603–8.
4. Borgers M, Degreef H, Cauwenbergh G. Fungal infections of the skin: infection process and antimycotic therapy. Curr Drug Targets. 2005;6(8):849–62.
5. Tietz HJ. Nagelpilz ist heilbar. Der Hausarzt. 2012;(16).

11 Dorsum of the IP Joints (7–8)

Lesions on the dorsum of the IP joints generally relate to deformed toes. The corresponding lesions of the 5th toe are considered together with the toe's other lesions as entity 10 due to their connected biomechanical background.

Lesions on the hallux (7) have a different background to those on the 2nd to 4th toe (8) and are therefore dealt with separately.

The possible negative impact of a rigid toe cap and the usefulness of minimally invasive surgical alternatives to amputation are particularly evident in this entity.

11.1 Pathobiomechanics and Pressure Points

At the 2nd to 4th toe generally the PIP joint is affected (Fig. 11.1). The **dorsal parts of the head of the proximal phalanx** form the dorsum of the toe at the level of the proximal interphalangeal (PIP) joint. The rarer lesions situated above the distal interphalangeal (DIP) joint generally involve excessively long toes or toes with mallet deformity.

On the dorsum of the hallux the inner pressure point is formed by the **dorsal parts of the medial condyle of the proximal phalanx** (Fig. 11.2). In toes displaying this entity, the joint is often permanently flexed causing a deformity of the toe. In this position, the perfusion of the skin at the inner pressure point is compromised even without external pressure. Only after extension is the perfusion restored.

In the case of simultaneous hallux valgus, the bones are not even in one sagittal plane. The traction at the FHL tendon, inserted at the distal phalanx of the hallux, has further consequences:

D. Hochlenert et al., *Diabetic Foot Syndrome*,
https://doi.org/10.1007/978-3-319-92055-9_11

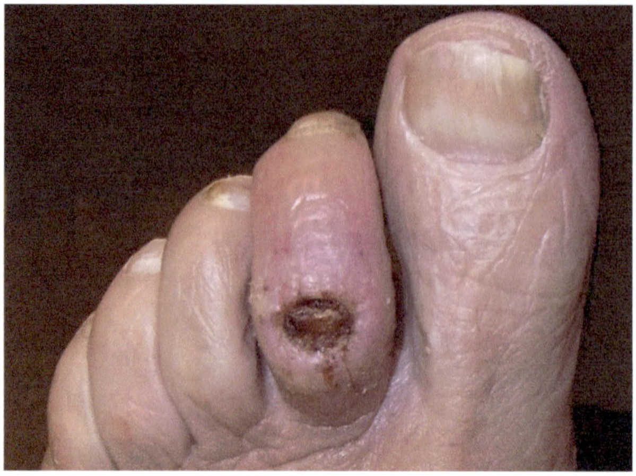

Fig. 11.1 Lesion at the PIP joint of the clawed 2nd toe

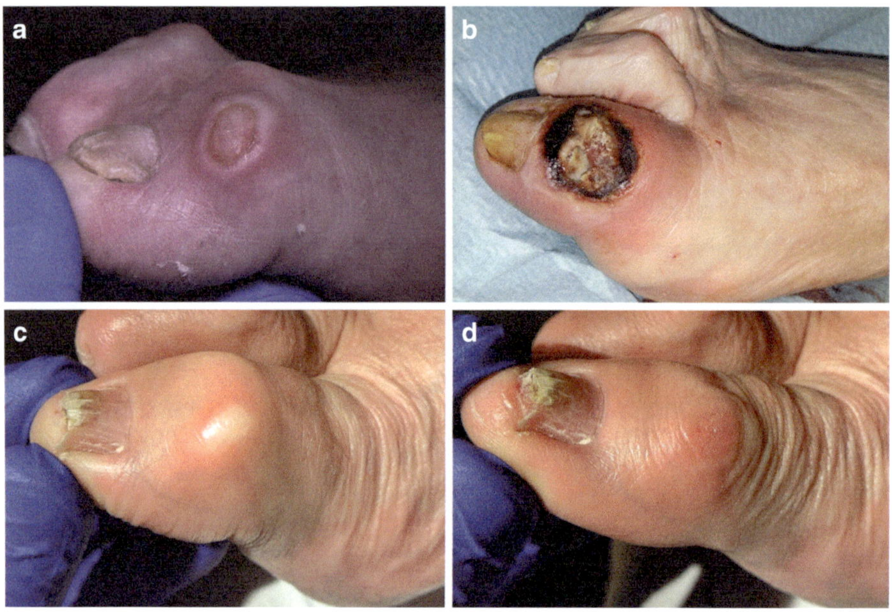

Fig. 11.2 (**a**) Superficial ulcer (**b**) if effective measures are delayed, massive tissue loss may occur (**c**) skin in ischemia due to the flexion at the dorsal hallux (**d**) reperfusion in extension

- Increased clawing (zig-zag deformity)
- Rotation of the hallux with its dorsum rotated to the medial site to form the distal-medial margin of the foot.

External pressure point:

The external pressure point is always the upper of a shoe in its distal part. Any stiffening of the toe box enhances the risk of injury.

		IPJ 1st-4th toe dorsal	IPJ 2nd-4th toe dorsal	IPJ hallux dorsal
Frequency		7.6%	6.5%	1%
Bone involvement	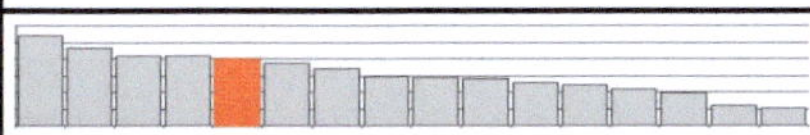	**19.8**	**20.6%**	14.5%
PAD	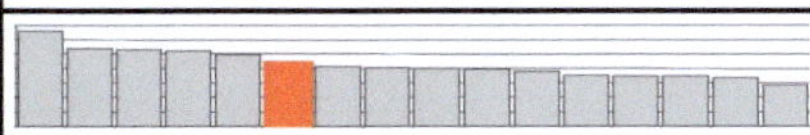	44.8	44.5%	46.6%
Revascularisation	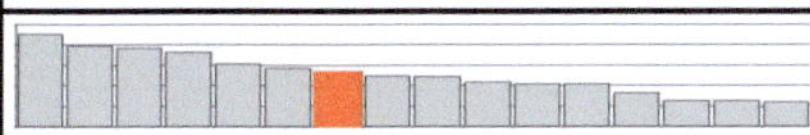	10.6	10.5%	10.6%
Amputation below ankle	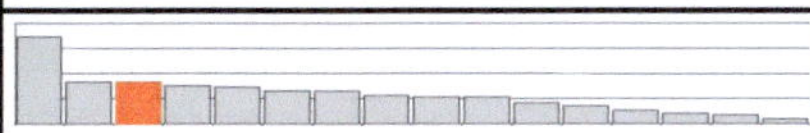	**11.5**	**12.3%**	5.8%
Amputation above ankle	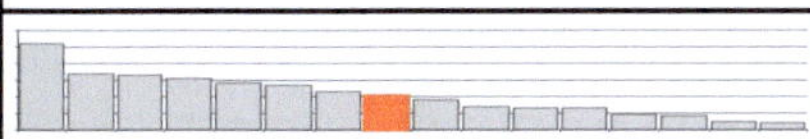	2	2.1%	1.9%
Days until remission	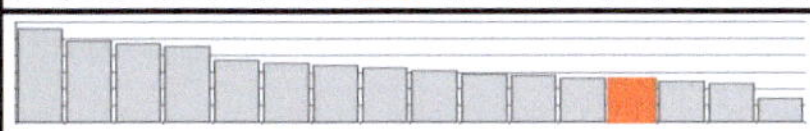	79	77	84
Duration > 180 days	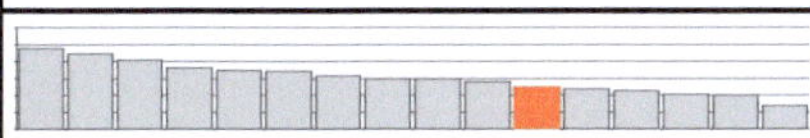	24.4%	23.5%	30.6%
Reactivation following year	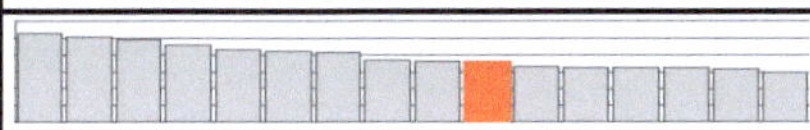	36.5	36.7%	35.3%

Fig. 11.3 Benchmark figures of lesions above the IP joints (orange) in a rank of all entities in decreasing height

11.2 Statistics

The figures are presented in the Fig. 11.3 show some remarkable characteristics:

- The lesion is 6 times more frequent on toes 2nd to 4th than on the hallux.
- Bone contact is more frequent on the lesser toes than the hallux.
- On the lesser toes remission is more rapid (on the hallux the time to remission is about average).
- Minor amputation of the hallux is rare, but twice as frequent when the smaller toes are affected.
- Despite a good prognosis and alternative therapeutic options (see below), the lesser toes are frequently amputated.

11.3 Principles of External Offloading

Details of external offloading are described in Chap. 19. The following elements might be used to offload the dorsal aspect of a hyperflexed PIP joint in a clawed toe:

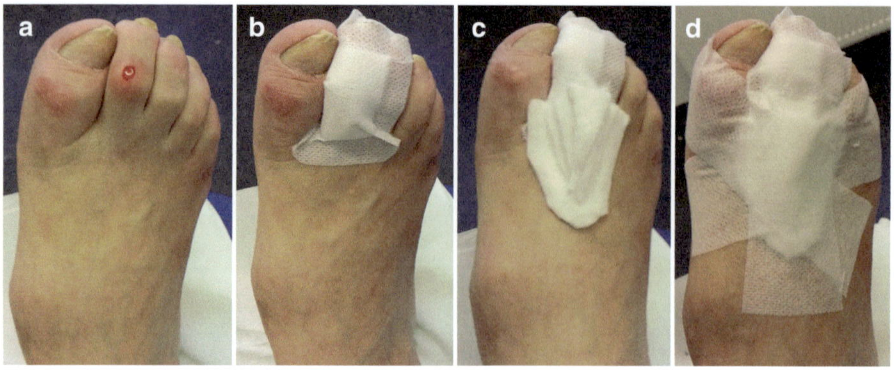

Fig. 11.4 (**a–d**) Distant cushion to protect skin above the PIP joint of the 2nd toe

- Remote padding on the adjacent parts of the dorsum of the foot using 15–20 mm of felt (Fig. 11.4).
- Remote padding at the hallux using the skin of the adjacent parts of the dorsum of the hallux.
- Shoes sufficiently spacious at the distal part with no stiffeners in the upper near the toes.

11.4 Principles of Internal Offloading of the 2nd to the 4th Toe

A detailed description of the operation techniques can be found in Chap. 19 'External Offloading'.

- A **Tenotomy** of the long flexor tendons if the DIP joint is flexible is the less invasive option. This has no direct effect on the PIP joint but may lower the toe slightly.
- **Downsizing of the wound**: A combination of tenotomy of the long and short flexor tendons with a lengthening of the extensor tendons reduces the clawing, thus extending the toe (see Chap. 20, Sect. 20.4.3). As the traction on the skin diminishes, the area of the wound is immediately reduced. The operative access for this measure is very small and the whole intervention is limited to areas of soft tissue. Compared to the defect after an amputation, these ulcers usually close more quickly and with fewer complications. This might even be suitable for people with PAD after careful consideration of all the risks and benefits as a less risky alternative to an amputation.
- In the case of fixation due to a shrinking of the capsule but without bony fixation proven by a radiological exam, a **plantar capsulotomy of the PIP Joint** through the same percutaneous access, using a lancet, is possible.
- In the case of a bony fixed deformity (anchylosis), more invasive interventions, such as **resection of the PIP joint** in combination with soft tissue surgery (see Chap. 20, Sect. 20.5.1.2), might be suitable.

- If, after all, an amputation is unavoidable, the *line of the amputation* should pass through one of the phalanges, thus preserving the MTP joint with its ligaments, which are important for the adjacent toes (deep transverse metatarsal ligament, Fig. 2.8c 'Right foot at propulsion' and Fig. 2.51 'Claw toe'). If a part of the toe can be preserved, this might be helpful to work as a spacer to avoid further deviation of the adjacent toes.

11.5 Principles of Internal Offloading of the Hallux

The decision regarding which operation is most suitable depends on the flexibility of the MTP and the IP joints.

- In the case of flexible joints, a **tenotomy of the long flexor tendon of the hallux in combination with a lengthening of the extensors** is possible. By this method, a straightening of the toe in both articulations may be achieved. The traction at the edges of the wound is immediately discontinued, the wound surface shrinks and a closure of the wound usually occurs (see Chap. 20, Sect. 20.4.3).
- In the case of a fixed deformity of the IP joint, a **resection with arthroplasty of the fixed joint together with lengthening of the extensor** might be necessary (see Chap. 20, Sect. 20.5.1.2 and combinations that are also discussed there).
- In the case of an exposed joint or bone with osteitis, a **limited resection of the infected bone** and conservation of soft tissue should be considered before the distal phalanx is amputated (see Chap. 20, Sects. 20.5.1 and 20.5.1.2). After this limited resection, wound closure might take more time than after an amputation and the toe may appear a little shorter than it was before the ulcer occurred, but it is usually seen as less mutilating than an amputation and the toe can still maintain residual function.

11.6 Summary

- **Bone involvement is frequent, which should not be confused with an indication for amputation!**
- **Intervention on tendons and remote cushioning using adjacent parts of the foot or toe as support are easy to use and particularly promising.**
- **As an alternative to an amputation of the distal phalanx, a resection of the infected bone while preserving soft tissue should be considered.**
- **In both prevention and treatment of wounds, special attention has to be paid to the toe box. Contact of the skin covering the joint with any rigid material has to be excluded.**

12 Interdigital Lesions (9)

The interphalangeal joints (IP joints) represent a physiological enlargement of the toes. When the toes are pressed against each other, the adjacent toe can exert pressure on the joint and vice versa. Hyperkeratosis and ulcers may affect the joint by exerting pressure on itself (Fig. 12.1) or the adjacent toe. If both are affected, the term 'kissing ulcers' may be used.

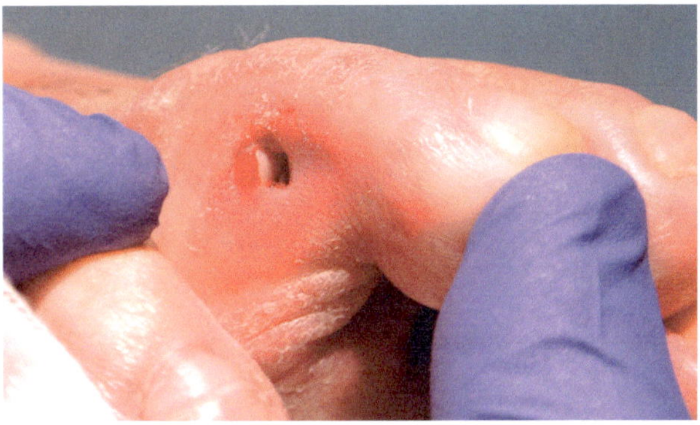

Fig. 12.1 Interdigital lesion of the PIP joint of the 2nd toe medially

D. Hochlenert et al., *Diabetic Foot Syndrome*,
https://doi.org/10.1007/978-3-319-92055-9_12

12.1 Pathobiomechanics and Pressure Points

The pathway to ulcers at this site is marked particularly by limited joint mobility due to glycosylation of soft tissue in these joints. An excessive pressure between the toes can thus arise even without external pressure due to ill-fitting shoes [1]. However, tight shoes play an important role and can increase pressure and thereby trigger ulcers.

Internal pressure points are the IP joints. The PIP joints are more frequently involved than the DIP joints.

12.2 Statistics

The figures in Fig. 12.2 do not show any marked characteristic with respect to the other entities in general besides one: In the year after wound closure reactivation is rarer.

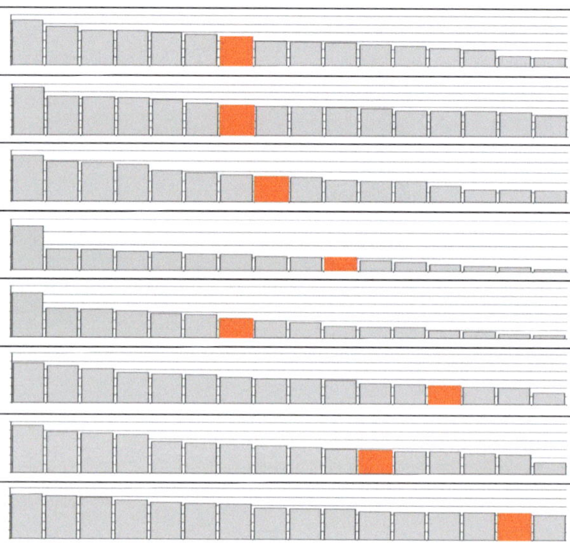

	Interdigital
Frequency	5.5%
Bone involvement	17.2%
PAD	41.2%
Revascularisation	10%
Amputation below ankle	7.5%
Amputation above ankle	2.3%
Days until remission	79
Duration > 180 days	22.4%
Reactivation following year	31.7%

Fig. 12.2 Benchmark figures of interdigital lesions (orange) in a rank of all entities in decreasing height

12.3 Principles of External Offloading

- Anything that could restrict the forefoot should be avoided. Shoes that are held in the forefoot area are a common cause of compression. These include light shoes that are used at home such as slippers or sandals or 'ballerinas'. Sandals often have a transversal strap to hold them firmly to the foot in the region of the MTP joints. Patients appreciate the light design and underestimate the pressure they might exert. 'Flip-Flops', which have a strap passing between the hallux and the 2nd toe, are particularly dangerous (Fig. 12.3).
- Spacers should be used only distally, if at all (Fig. 12.4).
- A support integrated into the insole underneath both IP joints of the toes under consideration may help to increase the space between them slightly.

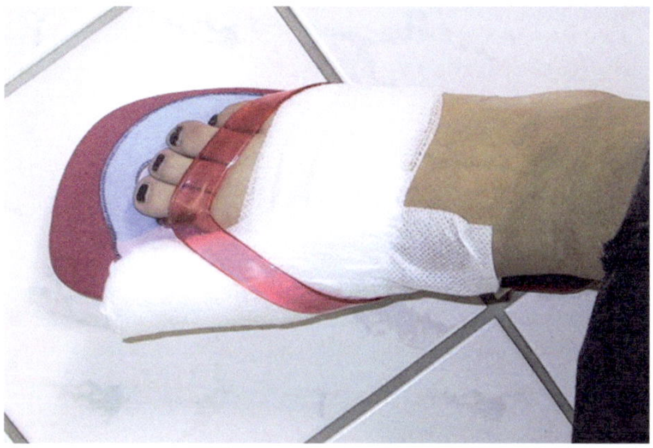

Fig. 12.3 Footwear which exerts an underestimated risk

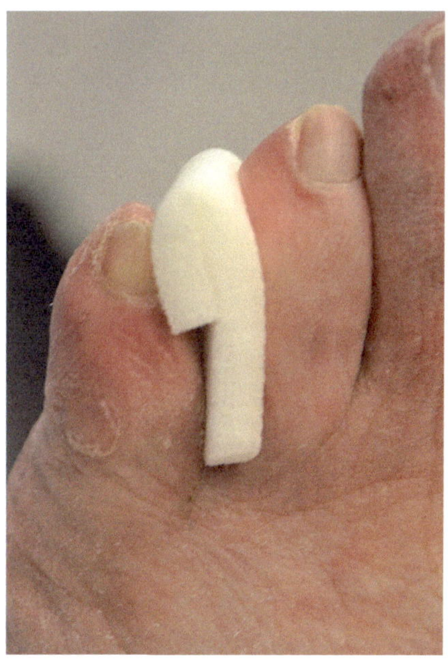

Fig. 12.4 Dressings which preserve distance

12.4 Principles of Internal Offloading

- *Resection of the IP joint*: This is particularly useful when the joint is open and blood circulation is sufficient. At the lesser toes, this is easy to perform with the help of a small Luer forceps. The intervention can be done on an outpatient basis. The dressing may afterwards fix the toe (see also Chap. 20, Sect. 20.5.1.2) and stabilise the wound region.

12.5 Summary

- **Lesions between the toes are less prone to reactivation than other entities.**
- **In the case of an open joint, it is often possible to remove the joint through the existing wound. Not every amputation performed in this case is actually necessary.**

Reference

1. Zimny S, Schatz H, Pfohl M. The role of limited joint mobility in diabetic patients with an at-risk foot. Diabetes Care. 2004;27(4):942–6.

The Lateral Side of the Foot (10–12)

13

There are five bony prominences on the lateral aspect of the forefoot and midfoot. Three of them are very close to each other on the 5th toe. Lesions on the 5th toe do not show any significant differences in pathobiomechanics, risk or therapy. For this reason, they are considered as one entity (10).

On the lateral side of the 5th metatarsal bone lesions may arise at the MTP joint (11) or at the base of the 5th metatarsal bone (12). Aspects of therapy differ largely between the two.

13.1 Pathobiomechanics and Pressure Points

1. The **lateral contour of the 5th toe** (Fig. 13.1) shows three natural prominences, the tip and the two IP joints.

   They are subjected to pressure because of two mechanisms:

   (a) *Clawing* with hyperflexion in particular in the PIP joint and excessive dorsiflexion in the MTP joint is part of a multi joint-deformity similar to those in other minor toes.

   (b) *Rotation* of the lateral contour to the plantar side is a typical plantarisation. This rotation might be due to two hypermobile joints: (1) A hypermobility in the 5th ray, which is attached in a flexible manner in its tarsometatarsal joint by a small joint surface. This flexibility in the tarsometatarsal joint might also give way to a Tailor's bunion (Bunionette). (2) An excessive laxity of the 5th MTP joint allows a larger range of movement and allows to rotate the 5th toe. This rotation can be induced by the long flexor tendon, that pulls obliquely and thus turns the toe, if not corrected by the quadratus plantae muscle. The latter might be weakened by an insufficiency of the intrinsic muscles (see more in Chap. 2).

D. Hochlenert et al., *Diabetic Foot Syndrome*,
https://doi.org/10.1007/978-3-319-92055-9_13

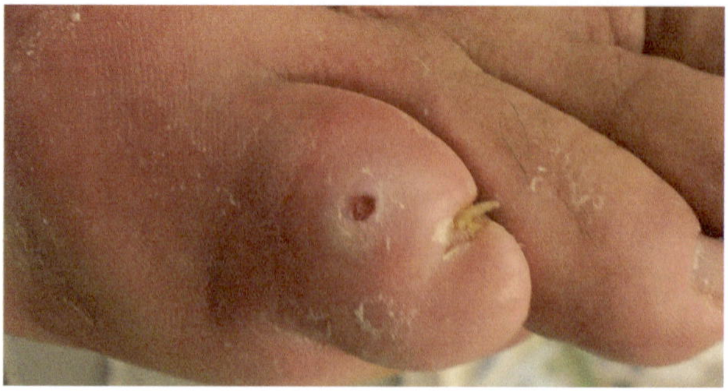

Fig. 13.1 Lesions at the outer surface of the minor toe have a good prognosis

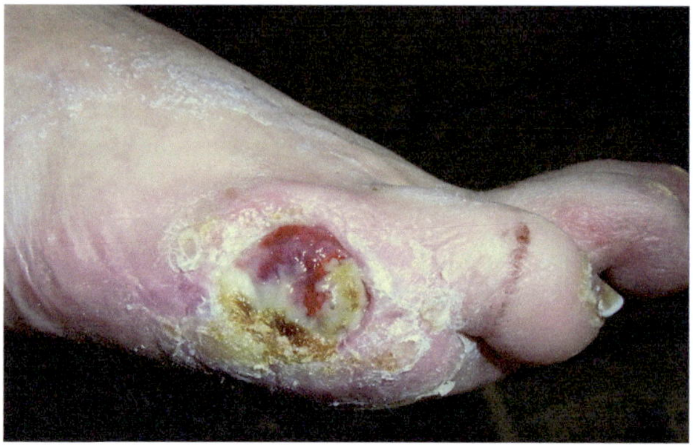

Fig. 13.2 In people with relevant PAD, wounds above the 5th MTH can easily reach structural parts of the joint

2. The MTP joint of the 5th toe represents a lateral prominence formed mainly by the **head of the 5th metatarsal bone** (Fig. 13.2).
3. At the base of the 5th metatarsal bone, a pronounced bony prominence is present, the **tuberosity of the 5th metatarsal,** where the important tendon of the fibularis brevis muscle (peroneus brevis muscle, short fibular muscle) inserts (Figs. 13.3 and 13.4). This tuberosity protrudes well beyond the surrounding area, especially in patients with reduced soft tissue due to neuropathy or other conditions. It is frequently subject to pressure. In this area parts of the shoe, such as the seams of the upper and the end of the heel stiffener, may represent an effective abutment and an external pressure point. The fibularis brevis tendon is essential for the stability of the entire foot and its balance, as it counteracts supination of the foot. A loss of function of the fibularis brevis tendon leads to a permanent drop of the outer margin of the foot and thus to an extreme exposure to pressure of the whole lateral part of the foot. This is the reason why the tuberosity must not be removed.

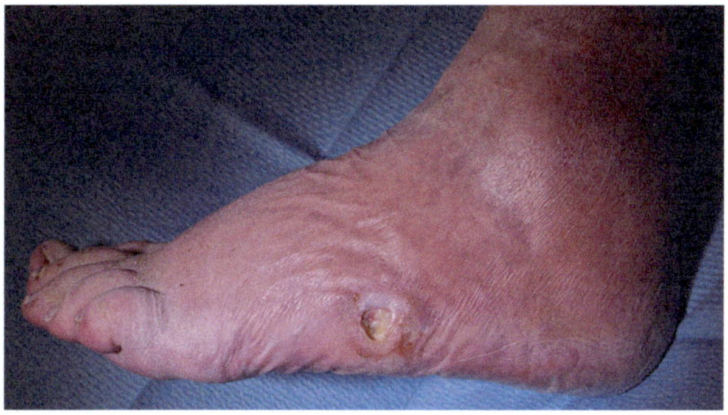

Fig. 13.3 Lesion in the area of insertion of the fibularis brevis muscle at the tuberosity of the base of the 5th metatarsal bone

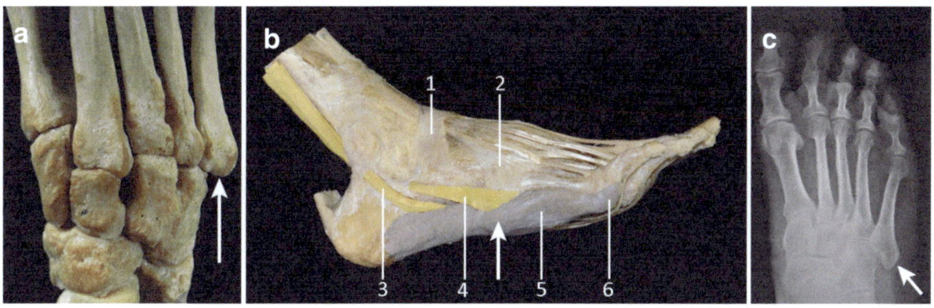

Fig. 13.4 Illustration of the prominence at the base of the 5th metatarsal in (**a**) the skeleton (**b**) the anatomical preparation (**c**) the radiological exam; 1: Retinaculum musculorum extensorum inferius; 2: tendon of the M. fibularis (peronaeus) brevis; 3: tendon of the M. peronaeus tertius; 4: tendon of the M. fibularis (peronaeus) longus; 5: Basis ossis metatarsale V; 6: M. abductor digiti minimi; arrow: Caput ossis metatarsale V

13.2 Statistics

The numbers represented in Fig. 13.5 show some specific features:

- Involvement of adjacent osseous structures is disproportionately high.
- Ulcers at the minor toe close relatively quickly. In contrast to this indicator of lower severity, amputations below the ankle are nevertheless performed in 10.5% of cases (average of all sites 7.9%). In the opinion of the authors, this discrepancy indicates potential for improvement.
- In the case of absent PAD, pressure on the lateral side of the foot tends to produce ulcers at the minor toe.
- In the case of angioneuropathy, the lateral part of the metatarsal bone is more likely to be affected than the minor toe. These lesions require revascularisation twice as frequently as the lesions of the minor toe and take much more time to pass on to inactivity. This is in contrast to the expectation that the

		5th toe	5th MTB head	5th MTB base
Frequency		3.5%	2%	0.9%
Bone involvement	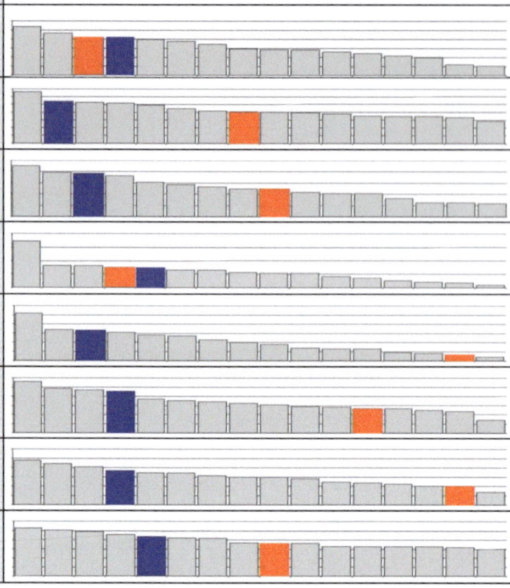	**20.9%**	**25.6%**	10.5%
PAD		40.3%	**60.5%**	40%
Revascularisation		9.8%	**17.7%**	10.5%
Amputation below ankle		**10.5%**	**12.3%**	5.2%
Amputation above ankle		**0.5%**	**2.9%**	**4.2%**
Days until remission		79	**140**	**119**
Duration > 180 days		**20.1%**	**37%**	**35.2%**
Reactivation following year		36.5%	40.6%	48.2%

Fig. 13.5 Benchmark figures of lesions on the outer surface of the foot. In the bar charts, lesions of the 5th toe are represented in orange, the two lesions of the 5th metatarsal are represented together in blue, the other entities in grey in a rank of all entities in decreasing height

more peripheral the tissue is, the more severe the circulatory problems are. The cause might be the circulation in the skin above the large joint and the large tuberosity at the base of the 5th metatarsal bone, which can be more easily compromised by external pressure than above the smaller pressure points in the minor toe.

- Lesions at the outer surface of the 5th metatarsal bone are associated with a major amputation rate that is well above average, especially those at the base of the 5th metatarsal. They also tend to need more time to close than other lesions.

13.3 Principles of External Offloading

The aim is to limit the shoe's proximity to the lateral margin of the foot. Consider using:

- Remote cushioning by the use of **spacers** in the surrounding areas in case a wound is present.
- Sufficient shoe width.

13.4 Principles of Internal Offloading

- If the surface of the joint is exposed, the **removal of the IP joints** of the 5th toe through the opening by the use of a small Luer's forceps might be indicated. This eliminates osteomyelitis and the pressure point at the same time (see Chap. 20, Sect. 20.5.1.2).
- In the case of more superficial wounds above the PIP joint of the 5th toe, a **tenotomy of the FDL tendon** might be sufficient to reduce rotation and relieve pressure at the lateral side of the toe (see Chap. 20, Sect. 20.4.1).
- The **resection of the MTP joint** (Fig. 13.6) might be indicated if the inner surface of the joint is exposed in order to remove the necrotic bone (see Chap. 20, Sect. 20.5.1.3).
- **Primary closure** can be attempted after correction of the internal pressure point as well as resection of the lesion and the affected soft tissues, possibly by using a redon drain. For this purpose, perfusion has to be sufficient, antibiotic therapy targeted and close follow-up assured.
- Regarding the tuberosity of the **base of the 5th** metatarsal, a thin layer of tissue should be removed at most. The short fibular tendon inserts here and has an important function without which the foot is inverted and even more exposed to pressure at its lateral margin.
- In the case of a **Tailor's bunion,** similar to a hallux valgus, the probability of a reactivation of wounds is high and may justify a surgical correction after wound closure.
- In the case of plantar or latero-plantar lesions at the head of the 5th metatarsal, other operations are useful that are described in Chap. 14. In rare cases, also a

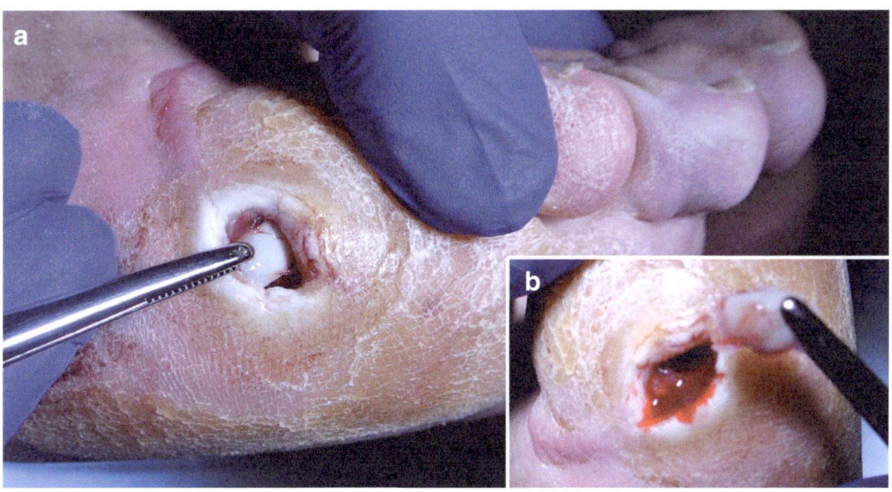

Fig. 13.6 (**a**, **b**) Removal of the cartilage of the 5th MTP joint

strictly lateral lesion in the presence of a contracted foot and a dysfunction of the Achilles tendon might profit from a lengthening of the Achilles tendon (see also Chap. 3, Sect. 3.4.1.5 and Chap. 20, Sect. 20.4.5).
- The loss of the function of the fibularis brevis tendon causes a permanent supination/inversion. If a passive correction is still possible, a transfer or split of the tibialis anterior tendon to the fibularis tertius tendon can correct the problem (see also Chap. 20, Sect. 20.4.6).

13.5 Summary

- **In the case of a marked angiopathy, lesions of the lateral aspect of the MTP joint are more likely to develop than lesions of the minor toe. If only a neuropathy exists, the minor toe is the most probable target.**
- **Lesions on the tuberosity at the base of the 5th metatarsal bone are particularly frequent in people with reduced soft tissue padding of the foot. They are associated with PAD and have a high rate of major amputations.**
- **Treatment focuses on external offloading.**
- **An intervention on tendons might be useful at the 5th toe.**
- **At the 5th metatarsal bone, surgical measures are aimed more often at the removal of affected bone and debridement than at internal offloading.**
- **Experienced surgeons can often correct flexible malalignments through a tendon transfer or extension.**

Plantar MTHs (13–14) 14

Plantar lesions at the first (13) and those at the 2nd to 5th (14) metatarsal head (MTH) are discussed in this chapter. These lesions are for many the epitome of a neuropathic diabetic foot (Fig. 14.1). They do indeed show characteristic core aspects of the diabetic foot:

1. The atrophy of the plantar subcutaneous fat pad.
2. The dysbalance in muscle function causes toe deformities and increasing plantar pressure while walking.
3. The usefulness of pressure-reducing footwear with optimised insoles and rocker bottom outsoles.
4. The presence of a typical pattern of calluses with subcutaneous haemorrhage before ulcers develop.

From a biomechanical point of view, stress under the medial (first) MTH, the median (2nd to 4th) MTHs and the lateral (5th) MTH have many similarities, but also differences. In this chapter, biomechanical phenomena and the resulting therapies of the first MTH are presented completely. For the other MTHs, only the additional aspects are described.

14.1 Pressure Points

The inner pressure point:

- In the case of stress below the first MTH, the pressure point is usually the medial sesamoid bone, rarely the lateral one.
- In the case of stress below the 2nd to 5th MTH, usually the lateral and less frequently the medial condyle of the respective MTH becomes the pressure point.

D. Hochlenert et al., *Diabetic Foot Syndrome*,
https://doi.org/10.1007/978-3-319-92055-9_14

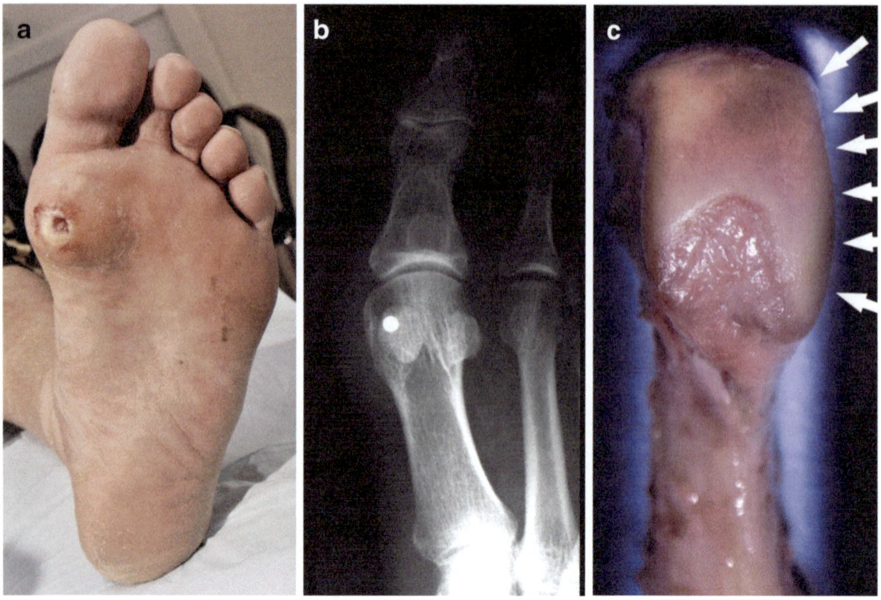

Fig. 14.1 (**a**) Ulceration below the medial sesamoid bone. (**b**) Conventional radiography with a pellet at the site of a plantar lesion in proximity to the medial sesamoid bone. (**c**) asymmetrical plantar configuration of 2nd to 5th MTH. The lateral condyle is marked by arrows

First MTH: Medial and lateral sesamoid bones frame the tendon of the flexor hallucis longus muscle in healthy people. The two heads of the flexor hallucis brevis muscle are attached to the sesamoid bones and the base of the first proximal phalanx by the plantar plate of the first MTP joint. All plantar plates are firmly connected to each other by a transverse fibre strand (deep transverse metatarsal ligament). As the foot becomes wider due to age and especially in case of a hallux valgus, the first MTH shifts medially and the sesamoid bones remain at the same place within the foot. The plantar plate remains firmly attached to the neighbouring plantar plates by the pull of the deep transverse metatarsal ligament (Fig. 14.1b, see also Fig. 2.8c and 2.22a and d). They dislocate out of the grooved facets in the metatarsal bones to which they should be attached. As a result, the medial sesamoid bone may be located centrally below the first MTH to form a marked prominence. The frequent rotation of the first ray turns the medial side downwards, which may contribute to this exposure of the medial sesamoid bone. The lesions therefore might also be situated not exactly centrally below the head, but slightly medial in position.

2nd to 5th MTH: One of the two condyles of each MTH, usually the lateral one, ends with a distinct bony cusp. This points in the direction of the plantar surface and protects the flexor tendons, which run centrally next to this cusp and reach the toe (Fig. 14.1c). These extensions of the condyle form a spiky point. At the beginning of terminal stance, this spiky point of the condyle represents the internal pressure point. Pressure is enhanced at this moment if the Achilles tendon is impaired by a shortening of the muscles soleus or gastrocnemius. Immediately after, the heel is raised by a few centimetres, the MTP joints are dorsiflexed and the surface of the lateral condyle becomes the closest part to the ground (Fig. 20.21 in Chap. 20 on internal offloading).

14.2 Tests to Perform

The deformities such as claw toes, that are important in the development of high pressure below the MTHs, are present at rest and generally don't need provocative tests to be unmasked. Nevertheless, some tests are useful to complete the picture and add aspects that are necessary to determine the most appropriate therapy. They are described in detail in Chap. 3, Sect. 3.4.1.2 and Fig. 3.7d.

Testing the *power of plantarflexion of the hallux* and the *integrity of the FHL tendon*: The power of plantarflexion of the hallux is tested (Fig. 14.2). It is possible that the plantar plate has degenerated and the plantarflexion of the proximal phalanx is weakened (see below). Furthermore, it is possible that an ulcer at the first MTH has eroded the long flexor tendon (FHL), that runs exactly between the two sesamoid bones. In this case, the distal phalanx cannot be flexed. If the power of plantarflexion of the hallux is reduced, it is not possible to offload the MTH by shifting the load onto the toes, for example, using a 'toe balcony'.

Achilles tendon dysfunction should be ruled out (see Chap. 3, Sect. 3.4.1.2 'palpation'). The *Silfverskjöld Test* can be used for this purpose or to differentiate between causes of such a dysfunction. Excessive tension on the Achilles tendon may lead to:

- an overload of the forefoot that is put under stress earlier and longer or
- an aggravation of a flat foot or
- an inversion of the heel, supinating the forefoot and overloading the 5th MTH. This aggravates a pes cavus.

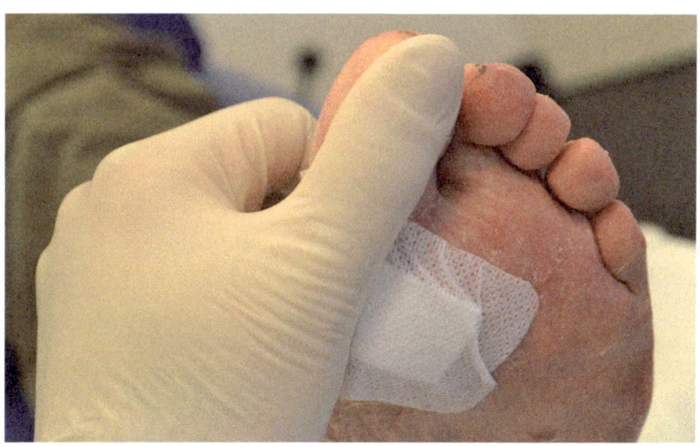

Fig. 14.2 Test of the plantarflexion strength of the hallux

Coleman Block Test (see Chap. 3, Sect. 3.4.1.5 'Coleman block test') is performed in case of a lesion at the 5th MTH and some sign of pressure at the first MTH or vice versa. If the heel is inverted and this inversion can be corrected during the test, a diagonal support of the lateral side of the foot's sole might reduce pressure.

It is necessary to *observe the patient while walking* to assess the width of the foot's angle and a possible functional impairment caused by a flat foot.

14.3 Statistics

The figures represented in Fig. 14.3 show some peculiarities:

- Reactivations in the year after wound closure occur even more frequently than with other entities. It is the highest reactivation rate of all entities.
- These lesions tend to be purely neuropathic.
- They rarely result in amputations above the ankles.
- The toes nevertheless are frequently amputated.

		Hallux MTH	2nd-4th MTH	5th MTH
Frequency		6.7%	5.6%	3.1%
Bone involvement		10.5%	15%	13.7%
PAD		31.4%	33.8%	36.5%
Revascularisation		5.9%	8%	5.1%
Amputations below the ankle		5.9%	9.8%	6.7%
Amputations above the ankle		1%	0.8%	0.9%
Days until remission		91	104	101
Duration > 180 days		33%	30.1%	30.5%
Reactivation following year		54.5%	52.2%	49.8%

Fig. 14.3 Benchmark figures of lesions beneath the MTHs. In the bar charts, ulcers beneath the MTHs are depicted in orange and the other entities in grey. All together are presented in a rank in decreasing height

14.4 Common Biomechanical Patterns

1. Due to the *thinning of the fat pad* in case of polyneuropathy, the bony spurs and the lateral condyles at the MTHs become relevant as pressure points [1]. The exact link between polyneuropathy and the atrophy of the fat pad is not yet fully understood.
2. A **claw toe** contributes to the overload beneath the MTHs in various ways:
   (a) A marked permanent clawing usually is associated with a weakening of the plantar part of the joint's capsule. This thicker part termed plantar plate is first weakened and then may even rupture. The **padding structures dislocate distally**, the MTHs lose their cushioning protection during propulsion and become palpable immediately under the skin (see more in Chap. 2, Sect. 2.5.4.2 'Plantar Plates and Interossei', Figs. 2.22 and 2.43).
   (b) Clawed toes additionally **lower the MTHs** and fix them, because they are positioned above the MTHs. The MTP joint is overstretched and the insertions of the interossei are shifted dorsally over the transverse axis by the misaligned toe. Now the interossei will act as dorsiflexors and pull the proximal phalanx further onto the dorsum of the MTH. The MTH is therefore positioned in a more plantar position. Due to the low-lying MTH, the tendons of the FDL and FDB are extremely taut under load. In combination with the overstretched MTP joint, the toe will be hyperflexed in the IP-joints. The result is a zig-zag deformity or 'claw toe'. Due to this position of the toe, the EDL and EDB tendons are now "too long" and shrink over time. This fixes the toe in its clawed position (see more in Chap. 2, Sect. 2.7.3.1 'Key Position of the MTP joint', Figs. 2.51 and 2.52).
   (c) Clawed toes don't contribute to bearing weight and the MTHs become the most distal **weight-bearing** area of the foot.
3. In the case of a **'short Achilles tendon'**, pressure on the MTHs is exerted in an earlier moment of the gait cycle when the tapered extensions of the condyle of the MTHs represent the inner pressure point. Thus the load is carried by a very small area. The maximum pressure is effective for a longer period. The time in which all MTHs and parts of the lateral side of the sole carry load decreases and the time when only some MTHs are loaded gets longer.
4. Abscesses are sometimes milled distally during gait and expand in this direction. Ulcers then might extend into the space between two MTHs or between the toes. They might also extend medially (Fig. 14.4). These secondary lesions usually are not exposed to pressure and close more rapidly when the source of secretion is eliminated.
5. Medially to the first MTH a fold may develop due to shear forces arising between skin and shoe during gate (Fig. 14.5). This fold is not prone to spread in depth and may be controlled by optimising footwear and podiatry.

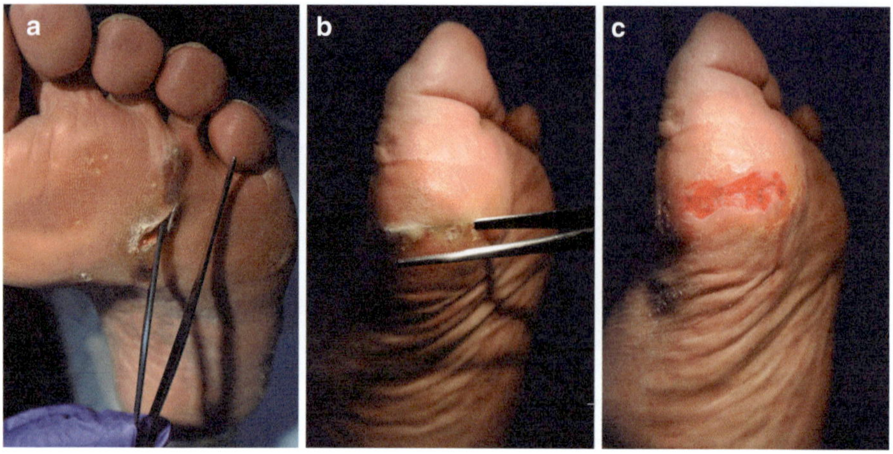

Fig. 14.4 (**a**) An Ulcer with fluids milled distally. (**b**, **c**) Secretions might also be milled medially

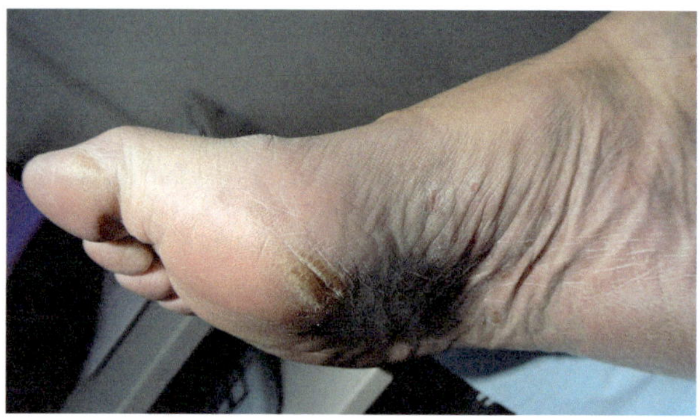

Fig. 14.5 Skin lesion with hyperkeratosis and punctate bleeding within a fold at the medial MTH caused by shear forces

14.5 First Metatarsal Head

14.5.1 Special Biomechanical Patterns

- The **long flexor tendon of the hallux** (flexor hallucis longus, FHL) passes in an area adjacent to the typical site of an ulcer below the medial sesamoid bone. Such an ulcer can nevertheless reach the tendon in the immediate vicinity, perhaps also during an earlier ulcer episode. This may cause the damaged tendon to rupture (Fig. 14.6). A *degeneration of the plantar plate*, which is common in marked clawing, may prevent plantarflexion of the proximal phalanx. In the case of a weakened plantarflexion of the toe, the pattern of callus formation shows the absence of pressure exerted there. In these cases, from a functional point of view, the first ray ends at the first MTH. This is important to know when planning measures to offload the overstressed parts.
- The first MTH in the case of a **pes cavus** (high-arched foot) is positioned lower than the adjoining 2nd MTH and the 3rd MTH. This may cause increased pressure on the low first MTH as the neighbouring metatarsals cannot contribute

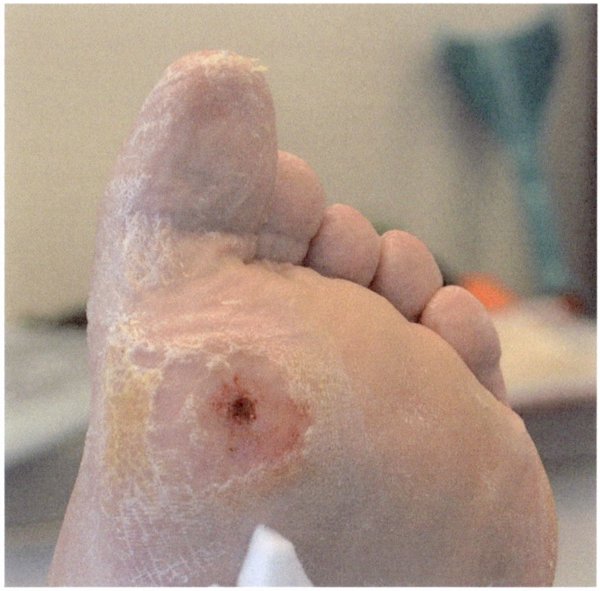

Fig. 14.6 Retracted hallux without physiological callosities as a sign of missing plantar flexion

to carrying the load. Since in midstance, the foot is lowered gradually to the ground, this low MTH forces the foot in supination and as a result, the 5th MTH might be very heavily loaded. Lesions might be located at the 5th MTH or at the first MTH or both. The first MTH has a longer lever and a larger surface of the head. Therefore, lesions here may be less profound than on the 5th MTH.

14.5.2 Principles of External Offloading of the First MTH

The techniques are depicted in detail in Chap. 19 'External Offloading and Immobilisation'.

1. The absence of the natural cushioning might be compensated by **local offload**:
   (a) Soft padding may shift load from the overloaded skin at the prominent bone to the immediate vicinity. If no ulcer is present, the surrounding tissue will resist some stress and soft padding is used frequently and successfully.
   (b) In the presence of an ulcer, even the slightest load on the wound or its margin should be avoided. A cavity ensures offloading only if supporting measures are taken simultaneously (see below).
2. **Shift load** to more proximal parts of the first ray:
   (a) A retrocapital support in form of a pad or a bar shifts load proximally. If it's built using felt and attached to the plantar surface of the foot, the distance to the margin of the wound should be 3–5 mm to allow for support, but without exerting pressure on the margin of the ulceration.
   (b) A support of the medial arch shifts load proximally and to the lateral side (see below).
3. Convert pressure in a rotating movement by adding a contoured outsole. This **rocker** has to be adequate in height, axis (positioned proximal to the MTHs),

orientation (width of the angle of the foot) and shape (integrating a flat part and adapt the curve to the walking habits of the patient).

4. Avoid a peek in pressure at terminal stance when MTP joints are dorsiflexed and load is supported by a minimal area. This is possible by adding a **stiffener** to the contoured outsole. The MTP joints are then immobilised. The plantar surface becomes both immobile and entirely weight-bearing. This very effectively reduces load but is thought to perhaps enhance the atrophy of intrinsic muscles inactivated by this stiffness. It should be applied only if necessary. Stiff soles have to be introduced to the patients walking habits gradually. When starting to use stiffened shoes, patients feel often awkward. Exercises in the first few days or weeks can help to overcome this initial difficulty.
5. In case of a dysfunction of the Achilles tendon ('short Achilles tendon') a position of the foot with elevation of the heel (**heel spring**) of about 10–20 mm may cause a reduction of the excessive load on the forefoot.
6. In the case of a positive Coleman block test, **a diagonal support of the lateral margin** might bring about relieve. In the case of a simultaneously present 'short Achilles tendon', an additional increase in the heel height helps to reduce the deformity caused by the low first MTH.
7. **Shift load** to the 2nd MTH by applying supporting pads below this MTH.
8. Shift load distally in late terminal stance by enhancing the participation of the hallux. This might be achieved by applying a *support below the hallux*. To evaluate the strength and therefore usefulness of this measure in advance, the power of plantarflexion should be tested (see also Fig. 3.9b).
9. In general, the foot has to be accommodated rather than corrected, as any type of correction exerts pressure. Nevertheless, a slight **supination** by a moderately more pronounced support of the medial arch might effectively offload the first MTH.

In the active phase, these elements might be produced in felt and fixed beneath the sole of the foot. They can also be integrated in an insole of therapeutic footwear, which features a stiffened sole, a rocker and allow the insole to be added. In the TCC they perfectly exert their effects as the ankle is also immobilised and peaks in pressure are avoided most effectively.

These elements are typically combined. To offload the first MTH by applying felt on the plantar surface of the foot, the sequent elements are used: elevation of the medial arch, retrocapital support, redistribution of the load to 2nd MTH, 3rd MTH and the hallux by placing supports there (Fig. 14.7).

14.5.3 Principles of Internal Offloading of the First MTH

The techniques are described in detail in Chap. 20 'Internal Offloading'.

- Lengthening of the extensors of the hallux (common tendon of the extensor hallucis longus and brevis, EHL and EHB) together with **tenotomy** of the long flexor tendon (flexor hallucis longus, FHL, see Sect. 20.4.1).

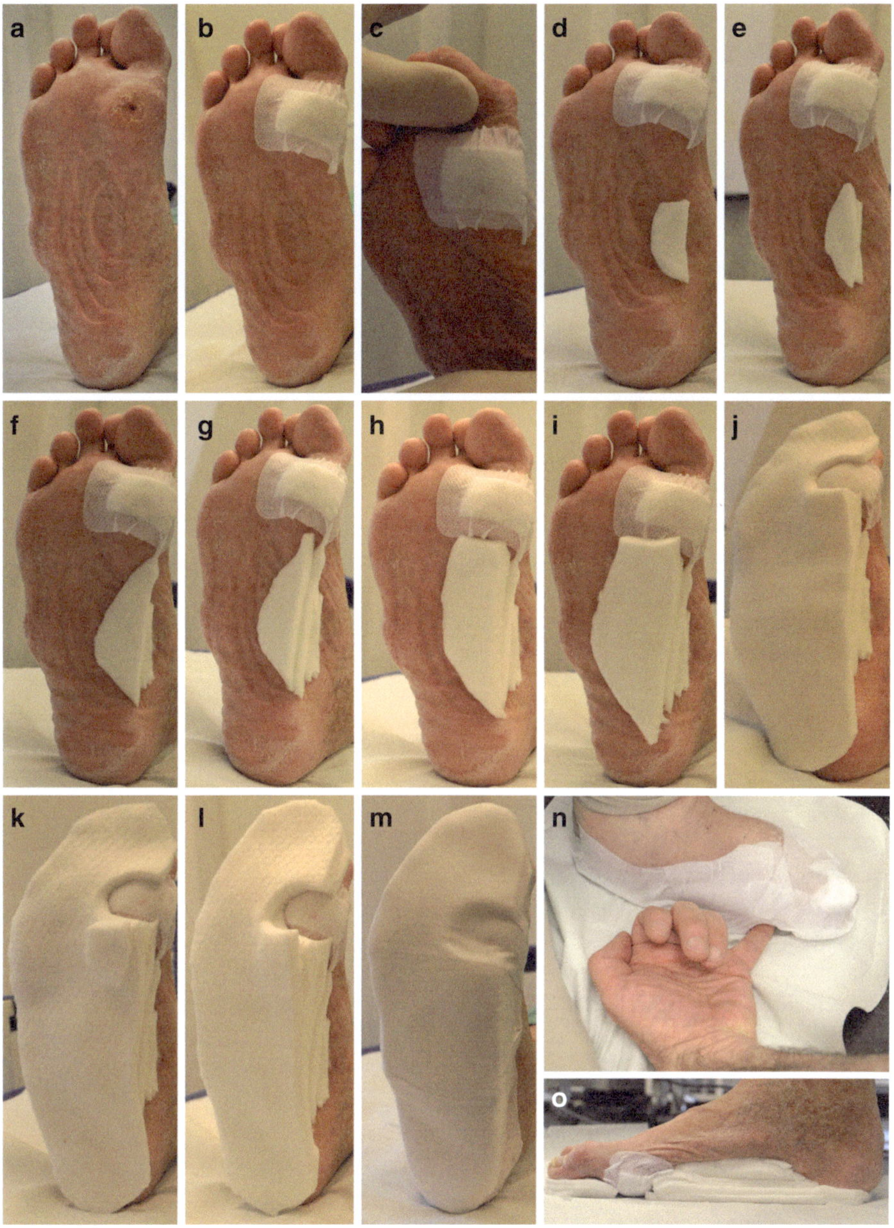

Fig. 14.7 (**a**–**o**) Offloading the first MTH: The ulcer is dressed; the strength of the hallux tested and then the offloading is built. (**n, o**) The result may be tested under load

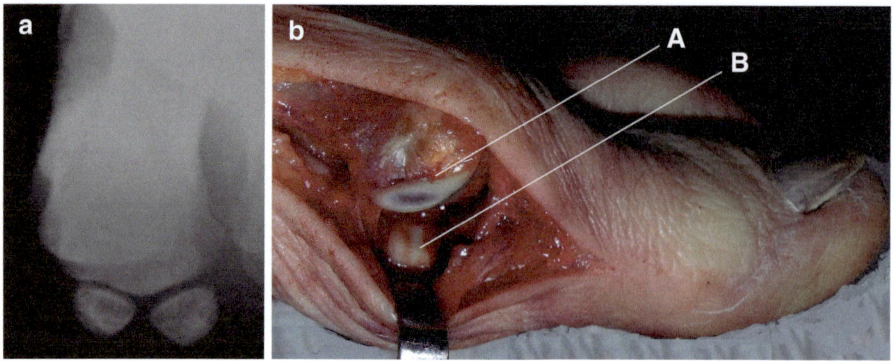

Fig. 14.8 (**a**) Axial view radiograph of the first MTP joint (**b**) surgical situation (cadaver), first MTH (*A*), medial sesamoid bone (*B*)

- **Removal of the medial sesamoid bone**. The sesamoid bone is located within the capsule of the joint, which forms the plantar plate at this point. The joint has to be opened to remove it. The risk of complications is therefore higher (Figs. 14.8, 14.9, and 14.10).
- **Operation according to Jones** (also known as Jones procedure, see Chap. 20, Sect. 20.4.4 'Jones procedure') in case of flexible first ray.

14.6 2nd to 4th Metatarsal Head

14.6.1 Special Biomechanical Patterns

- The base of the 2nd metatarsal bone is mortised between the three cuneiform bones and firmly connected to them by amphiarthroses (tight joints with limited mobility). In contrast, the first metatarsal bone is firmly connected only to the medial cuneiform bone and is held in position by muscles. Its height therefore varies. If these muscles of the first metatarsal are exhausted**,** the 2nd metatarsal is the next in row and must take up the entire load. This is the major cause of the so-called metatarsalgia if sensitivity is maintained. After loss of sensitivity, this overload causes ulcers. A rocker bottom sole, if necessary together with a stiffening of the sole and retrocapital support, might help in such cases.
- With decreased muscular strength, the 5th metatarsal can also become increasingly less powerful and the 4th metatarsal is overloaded in a similar way.
- The 2nd (and sometimes the 3rd) metatarsal bone may be the longest metatarsal bone, which means that its articulation with the toe is the most distal MTP joint. Its MTH is the most prominent during terminal stance and is exposed to the highest pressure. This is also a cause of metatarsalgia in the case of preserved sensitivity and of ulcers if sensitivity is reduced. In this case, a rocker bottom sole, possibly reinforced with a stiffener, may be very useful.
- The 2nd or the 3rd MTH may each be also lower than the ones adjacent. This might enhance pressure (Fig. 14.11).

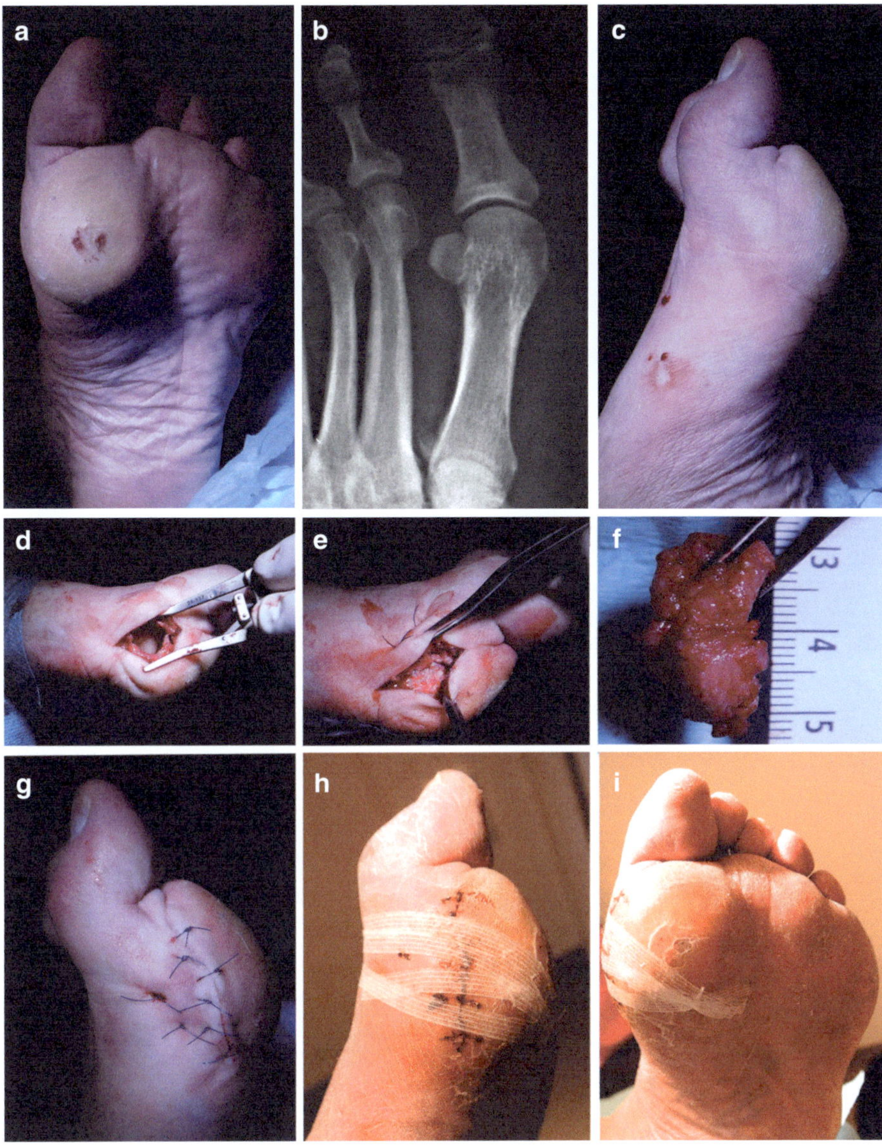

Fig. 14.9 (**a**) Radiography after removal of the medial sesamoid bone, (**b, c**) preoperative findings, (**d–g**) intraoperative development, (**h, i**) findings at the 11th postoperative day

14.6.2 Principles of External Offloading of the 2nd to the 4th MTH

The first five techniques described for the first MTH: local offloading, retrocapital support, contoured outsole, stiffened sole, elevation of the heel in the case of dysfunctional (='short') Achilles tendon may also be applied to the 2nd to 4th MTH.

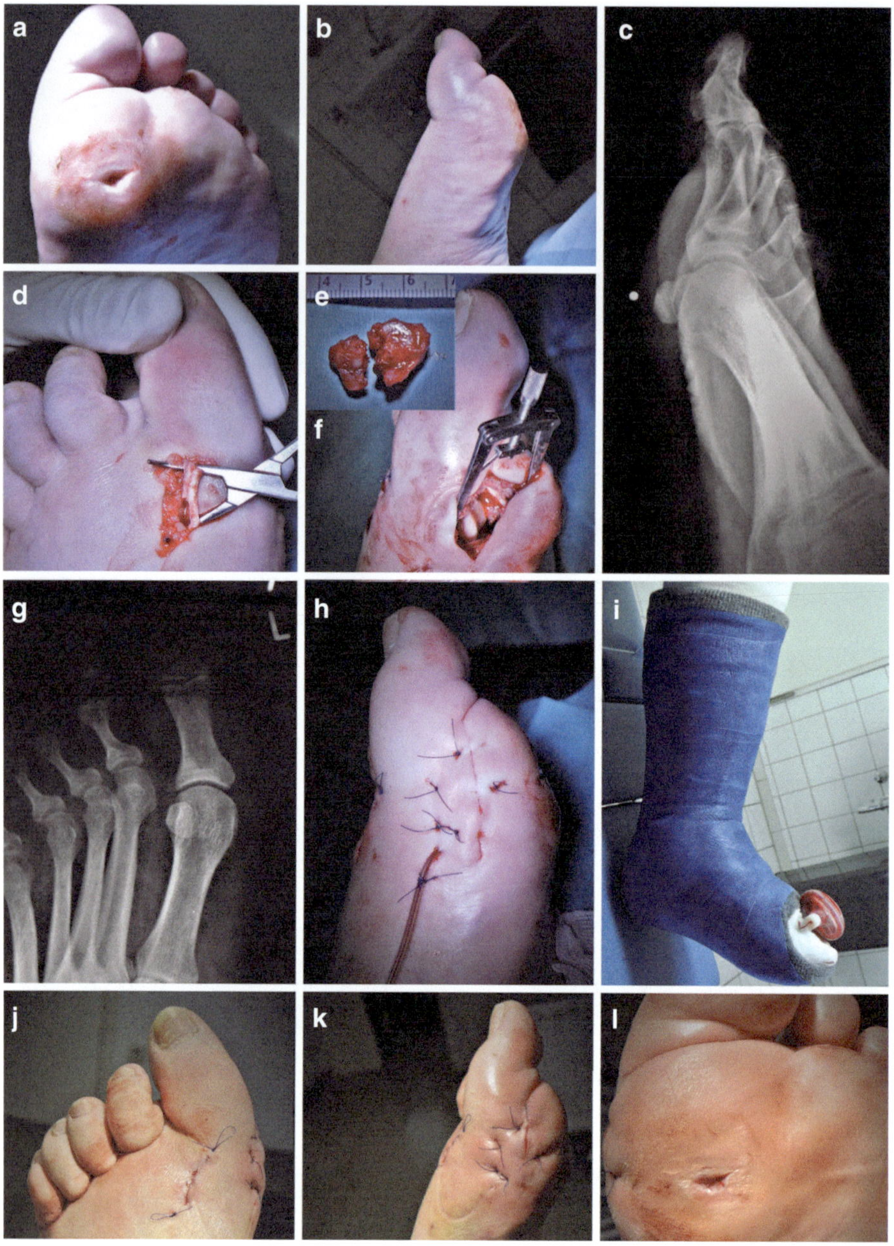

Fig. 14.10 Ulcer at the medial sesamoid bone (**a**, **b**) clinical picture (**c**) conventional x-ray, ulcer marked by a pellet (**d–f**) contemporary elongation of the EHL tendon and resection of the bone (**g**) postoperative situation (**h**) postoperative conventional x-ray (**i**) offloading in TCC (**j–l**) 2 days after surgical intervention

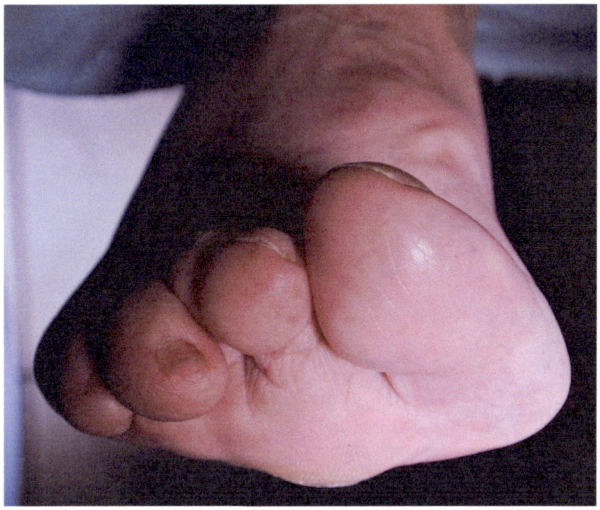

Fig. 14.11 2nd MTH lower than the adjacent rays

The techniques are depicted in detail in Chap. 19 'External Offloading and Immobilisation'. Additionally, the following measures might be useful:

- **Shift load to the adjoining** MTHs by applying supports. Often a combination is used that integrates support of the metatarsal in the retrocapital area, support of the neighbouring MTHs and lowering of the MTH of interest by a recess (Fig. 14.12).
- 2nd MTH: slight supination by a more pronounced support of the medial arch.
- 4th MTH: slight pronation by a support of the outer (lateral) margin. If a lowering of the first MTH is considered useful (Coleman bloc test positive), a diagonal support of the outer margin can be used.

The 2nd MTH is typically offloaded by a combination of: retrocapital support, shifting load on the first and the 3rd to 5th MTH as well as the 5th metatarsal and a support beneath the Hallux (Fig. 14.13).

14.6.3 Principles of Internal Offloading of the 2nd to the 4th MTH

The surgical procedures with effects on 2nd to 4th MTH use various effects that increase resistance of the MTHs and can therefore be combined:

In order to shift load from the ulcerated region distally, the sequent measures are useful.

- A **tenotomy** of the FDL tendon together with a lengthening of the long extensor of the toe (EDL) reduces the extent of the deformity of the claw toe (see Sects. 20.4.1–20.4.3). Straightening the ray, the cushioning tissue that had been displaced distally might partially return beneath the MTH. Without pressure on the MTH due to the dislocated toe, the MTH rises a few millimetres and pressure is relieved. **It is a measure with low risk and often unexpectedly marked effect.**

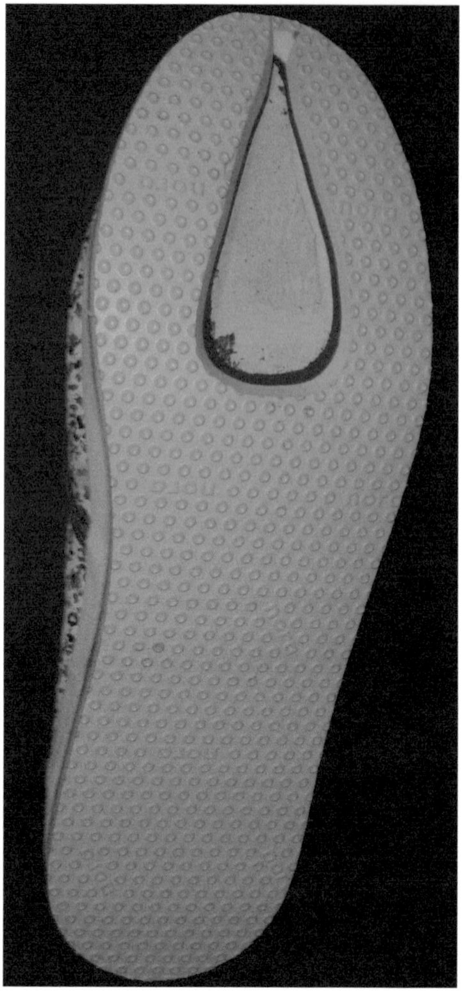

Fig. 14.12 Recess in the sole as an example of an offloading element for lowering an MTH

- A dorsalising relocation of the MTH (dorsal open **wedge osteotomy**) shifts the inner pressure point proximally for some millimetre and raises it (see Sect. 20.5.2.1).
- The **removal of the MTH** terminates the stress at this point. This procedure is biomechanically unfavourable and transfer lesions may occur on neighbouring MTHs or proximal at the edge of the resected metatarsal bone. Thus, this procedure should be avoided. An indication might be a necrosis of the MTH (see Sect. 20.5.1.3).
- **Achilles tendon lengthening** (ATL) mainly changes the time of weight-bearing. Pressure is applied later and shorter (see Sect. 20.4.5).

The techniques are described in detail in Chap. 20 'Internal Offloading'.

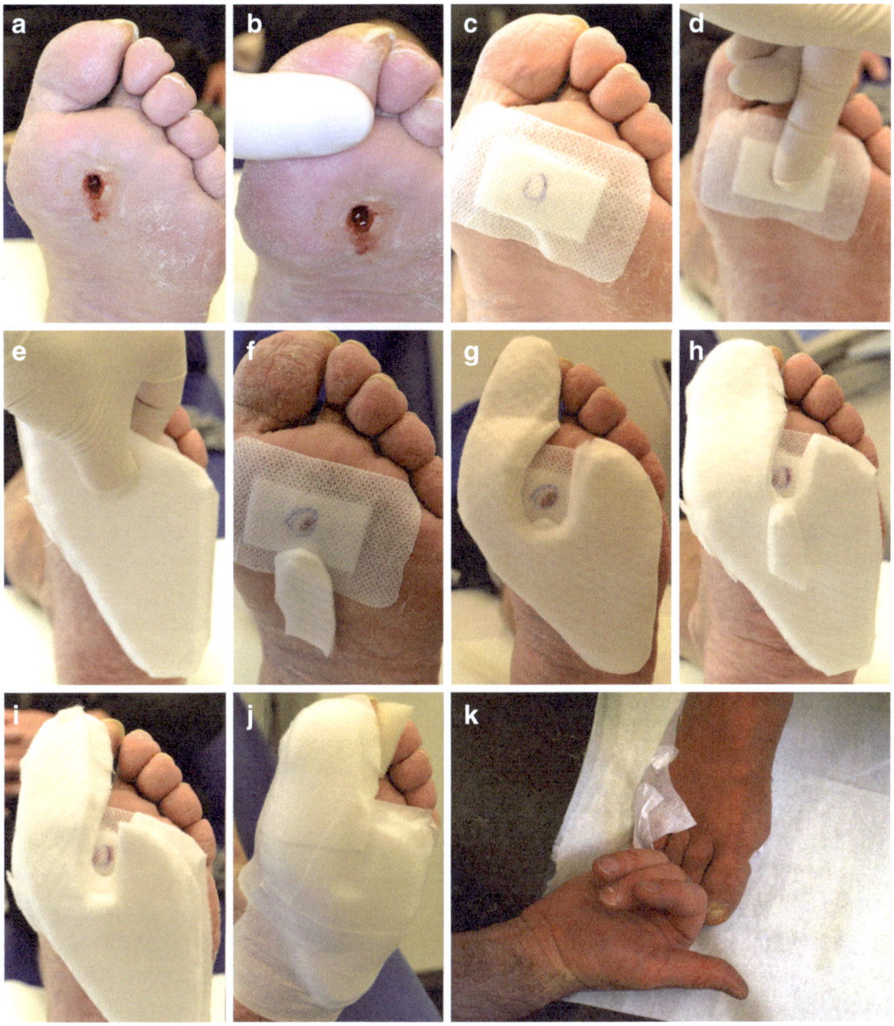

Fig. 14.13 (**a–k**) Offloading of a lesion beneath the 2nd MTH. (**b**) The resilience of areas that are planned to accept further loading is tested and the wound is dressed. (**f–i**) In the retrocapital area four layers are applied, on the others two layers, each 5 mm thick

14.7 5th Metatarsal Head

14.7.1 Special Biomechanical Patterns

A pes cavus (high arched foot) may induce supination and pressure beneath the 5th MTH (see Chap. 2, 'Pes cavus').

This might be due to a low first MTH, that supinates the forefoot under load. It has a longer lever and larger surface than the 5th and thus may induce more profound lesions at the 5th MTH. The cause for lesions at the 5th MTH in a pes cavus might also be an inverted hindfoot. Since the therapy differs, a distinction must be made between the two variants. The steps of the exam are described in detail in Chap. 3, Sect. 3.4.1.5 'Coleman Block Test'.

14.7.2 Principles of External Offloading of the 5th MTH

The first five techniques described for the first MTH (local offloading, retrocapital support, contoured outsole stiffened sole and more heel spring in the case of a 'short Achilles tendon') may be applied also to the 5th MTH.

Additionally, a slight pronation of the foot may be achieved by a **support of the outer margin.** This should be applied proximally to the 5th MTH and might elevate the 5th MTH a little.

A typical combination to offload the 5th MTH include retrocapital support, redistributing load to the 4th MTH and a support of the outer margin of the foot (Fig. 14.14).

In the case of an overload of the first and the 5th MTH due to a lowered position of the first MTH (Coleman block test positive), a combination of a diagonal support of the outer margin which entails a lowering of the first MTH might be used together with a retrocapital support of the 5th MTH and a recess beneath the 5th MTH (Fig. 14.15).

The techniques are depicted in detail in Chap. 19 'External Offloading and Immobilisation'.

14.7.3 Principles of Internal Offloading of the 5th MTH

The techniques useful for the 2nd to 4th MTH and described there (partial straightening of the toe by combined tenotomies, wedge osteotomy, removal of MTH in the case of necrosis and lengthening of the Achilles tendon) are also effective for the 5th MTH. In addition, the following are to be considered:

- **Lateral condylectomy**: The bone prominence which represents the internal pressure point at the end of midstance and at the beginning of terminal stance is removed (see Chap. 20, Sect. 20.5.2.2 'Resection of the Condyle of the 5th MTH').
- In the case of a tailor's bunion, a Chevron (Austin) osteotomy can be helpful, which brings the laterally deviating 5th metatarsal bone closer to the other metatarsals.
- At the 5th MTH in case of a 'short Achilles tendon', lengthening the Achilles tendon (ATL) might be indicated. The possibility of therapy using a diagonal elevation of the outer margin should be previously ruled out in the Coleman Block Test.

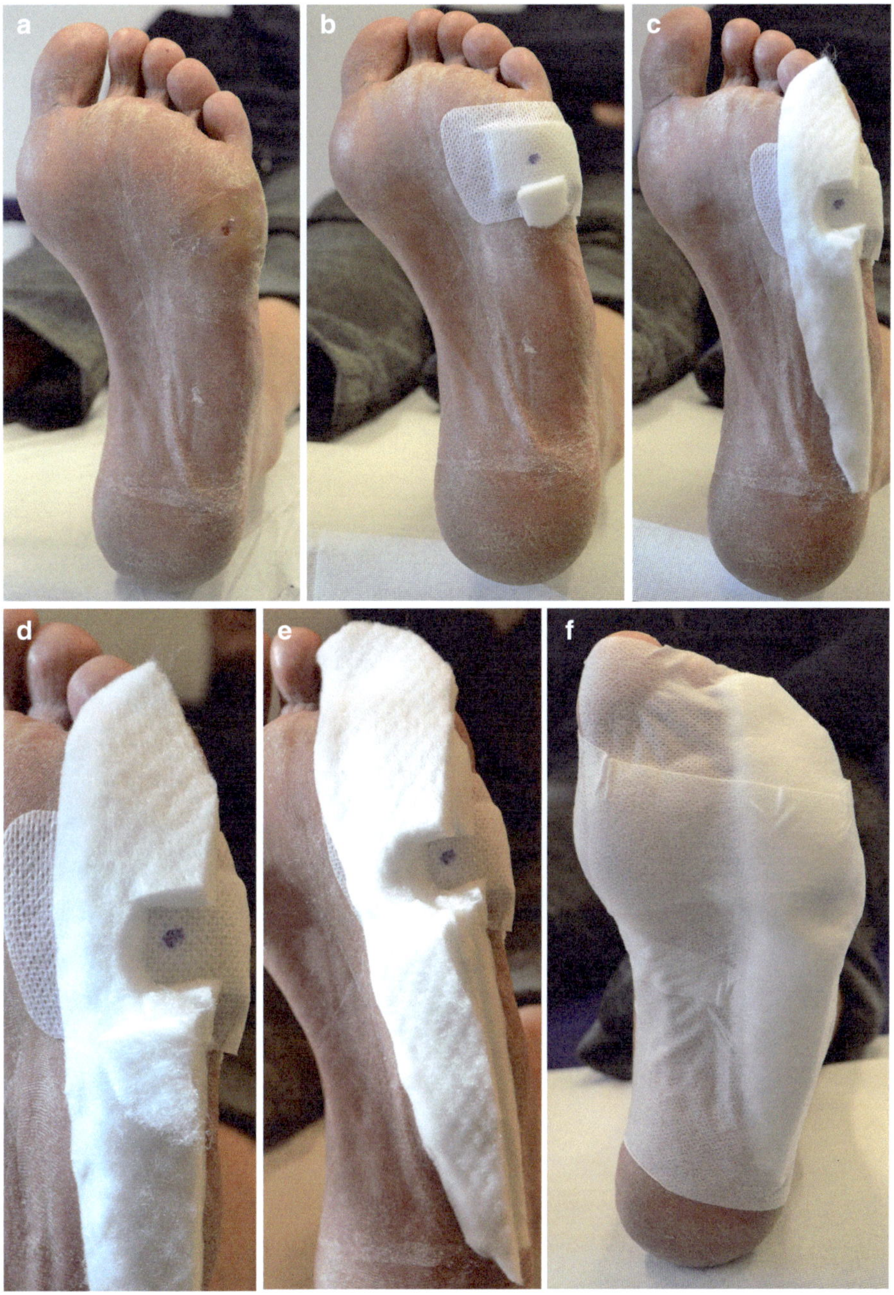

Fig. 14.14 (**a–f**) Offloading a lesion beneath the 5th MTH

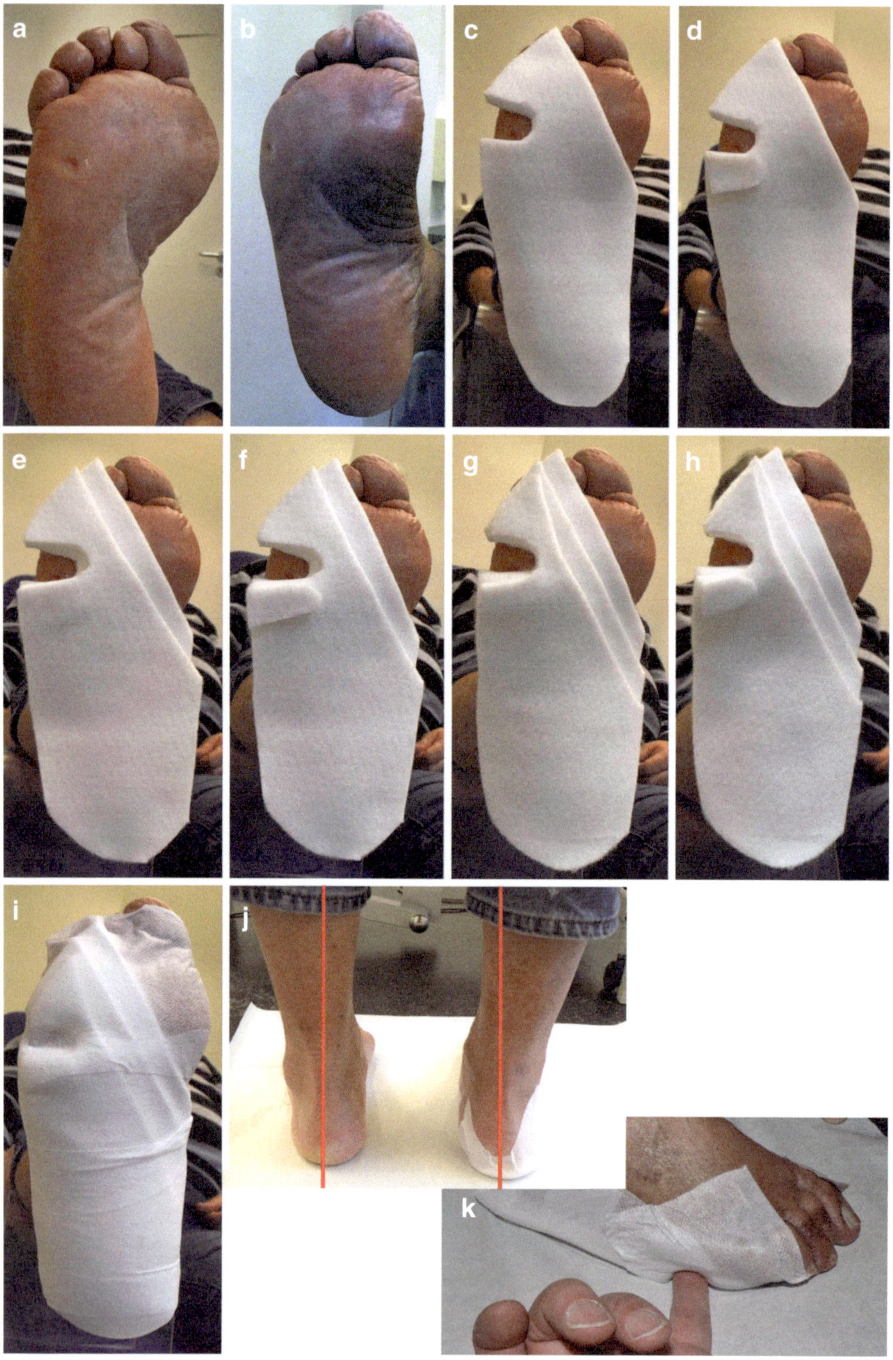
a
b
c
d
e
f
g
h
i
j
k

Fig. 14.15 (**a**) The area of a recently and superficially closed ulcer of the 5th MTH. (**b**) The first MTH shows signs of overload. (**c**) The support has recesses for the first and the 5th MTH. (**d**) The 5th MTH is additionally supported by a retrocapital support, while the first MTH is allowed to sink into the recess. (**e–h**) Other two or three layers are added together with a retrocapital support for the 5th MTH. The recess for the first MTH is wider in each layer. In doing so, also the 2nd and the 3rd MTH sink in the recess and the forefoot is pronated. (**i**) The whole support is fixed. (**j**) Eversion of the heel due to the diagonal support of the outer margin. (**k**) Test of the efficacy of the offloading

14.8 Summary

- **Plantar lesions beneath the MTHs are frequent, usually purely neuropathic, and rarely require vascular interventions.**
- **They show the highest frequency of reactivation among all entities.**
- **Numerous surgical procedures are available for the permanent improvement of resilience but are rarely used. The high risk of recurrence may indicate the need to consider surgical offloading earlier in the course of the disease, especially in physically active people.**
- **Combined tenotomies which straighten the toes may be performed transcutaneously in an outpatient clinic and are often surprisingly effective in offloading the MTHs.**

Reference

1. Brash PD, Foster J, Vennart W, Anthony P, Tooke JE. Magnetic resonance imaging techniques demonstrate soft tissue damage in the diabetic foot. Diabet Med. 1999;16(1):55–61.

15 The Malleoli (15–16)

Lesions that are primarily located centrally on top of the malleoli (15) (Fig. 15.1) show markedly different characteristics when compared to the ulcers that arise in the surrounding area (16) (Fig. 15.2). An important PAD raises the vulnerability of the prominence on top of the malleoli to such an extent that this dominates the way this kind of lesions present.

15.1 Pathobiomechanics and Pressure Points

The *prominences of the malleoli* may turn into an inner pressure point as a result of the presence of an external abutment. Examples of such abutments are the shoes, the bandages of a compression therapy or the bed of people with decubital problems. In the case of a traumatic event, it can be represented by a walking frame, a wheelchair or obstacles in the surrounding environment. The skin above the malleoli is often atrophic, sometimes due to a disturbed local perfusion.

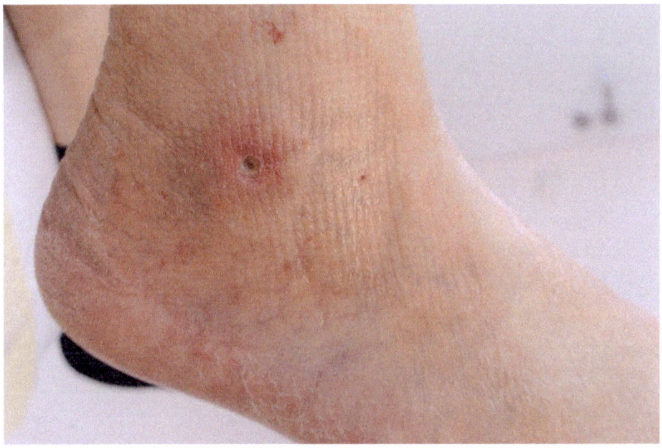

Fig. 15.1 Lesion at the lateral malleolus

D. Hochlenert et al., *Diabetic Foot Syndrome*,
https://doi.org/10.1007/978-3-319-92055-9_15

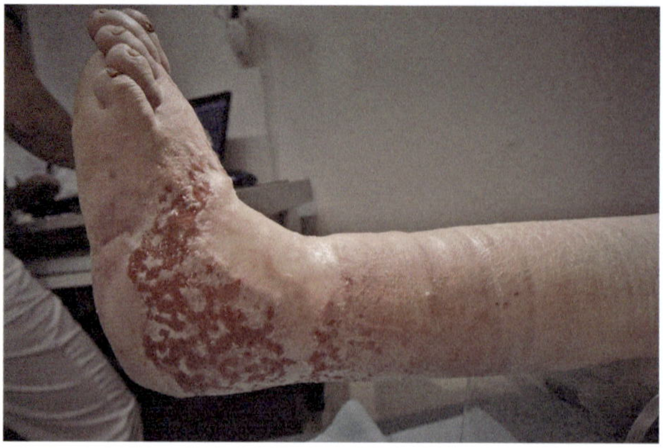

Fig. 15.2 Lesion in the region of the lateral malleolus

Ulcerations in the *area of the malleoli* that might include the malleoli without being particularly accentuated at the top of the ankles and without having started there, have the same spectrum of differential diagnoses as ulcers of the lower leg. Compression therapy is often regarded as the cornerstone of therapy in these cases. It is difficult to apply evenly distributed pressure in the area around the ankle. Compression bandages raise a 'tent' between the heel, Achilles tendon, tibialis anterior tendon and ankle. Without a further device that fills this space, the compression does not reach the skin in need, whilst the skin on the prominences receives too much of it.

15.2 Tests to Perform

A detailed anamnesis (trauma, known PAD or venous insufficiency) and exploration of the arterial and venous *perfusion* usually indicate further steps.

The gait should be carefully observed to identify ataxias and causes for trauma.

15.3 Statistics

The figures represented in Fig. 15.3 show some remarkable features:

- The lesions appearing just above the ankles show more frequent bone involvement and often require revascularisation. They are associated with a high rate of amputations above the ankle.

> **Note: Especially above the summit of the lateral ankle, there is a remarkably high risk for critical impairment of perfusion and amputations of the leg!**

- Lesions in the ankle region rarely show bone involvement and the rate of amputations is far below average.

		Mall. Centre	Mall. ext.ctr.	Mall. int.ctr.	Mall. Regio	Mall. ext.rg.	Mall. int.rg.
Frequency		1.9%	1%	0.8%	2.1%	0.6%	1.4%
Bone involvement	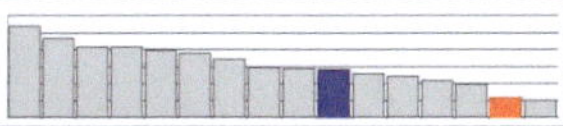	14.1%	15%	12.9%	6%	7.3%	5.4%
PAD	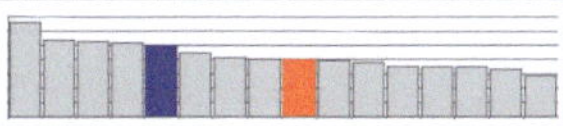	49.4%	51.4%	47%	39.8%	41.1%	39.1%
Revascularisation	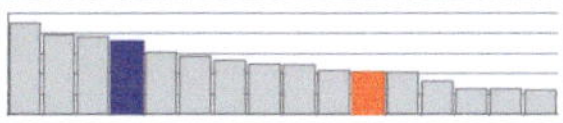	14.5%	14.9%	14.1%	8.3%	8.9%	8.1%
Minor amputation	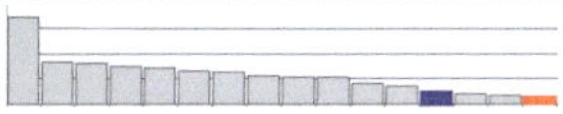	3.6%	1.8%	5.8%	1.3%	0%	2%
Amputation above ankle	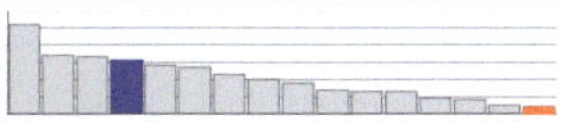	3.1%	4.7%	1.1%	0.4%	0%	0.6%
Days until remission	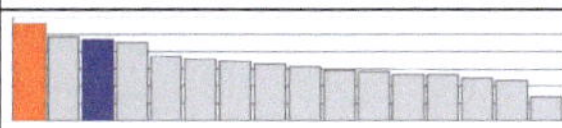	141	132	212	168	189	186
Duration > 180 days	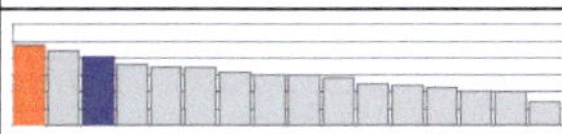	40.8%	29.2%	55.7%	47.9%	50%	46.9%
Reactivation following year	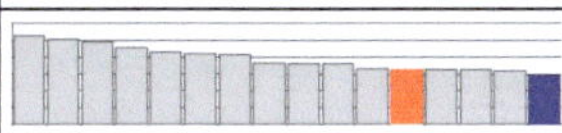	30%	31.6%	27.8%	32.7%	31.2%	33.3%

Fig. 15.3 Benchmark figures of lesions at the malleoli. In the bar charts lesions of the area surrounding the malleoli are represented in orange, the ones on top of the malleoli in blue and the other entities in grey. They are all ranked in decreasing height

- All forms tend to take a long time until the wound closes.
- All forms are less prone to reactivation than other entities.

15.4 Principles of Conservative Therapy

Compression therapy is the cornerstone in the treatment of venous insufficiency and other oedema-causing diseases but is potentially harmful in combination with a simultaneous PAD. The exact share of the different pathologies in the genesis of the lesion must be specified more precisely than with other entities. Poor decisions not only lead to an ineffective therapy but are able to cause harm themselves. Protective measures are available to allow compression therapy, at least to some extent, also in the presence of PAD.

- **Compression therapy** with relatively non-elastic bandages called '*short stretch bandages*' (SSB) is preferred in many countries. The bandages can be applied to legs that vary in volume, which is an advantage over stockings. They are supposed to be able to decongest more effectively than flexible bandages as they exert pressure discontinuously and predominantly during muscle contraction.

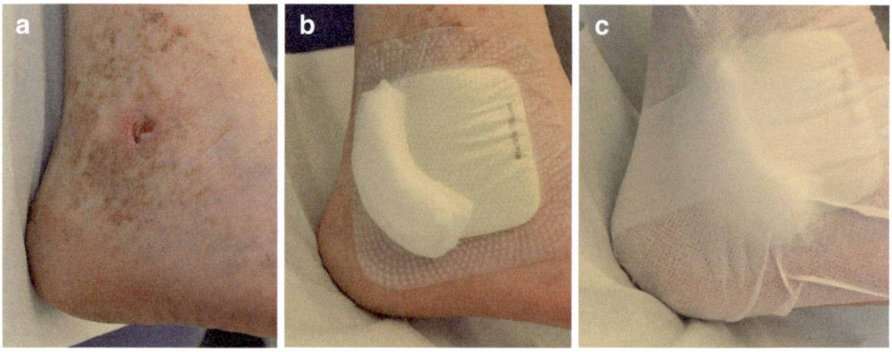

Fig. 15.4 Perimalleolar pad, two layers of 5 mm each

More flexible '*long stretch bandages*', in contrast, are easy to apply but exert pressure continuously. This is thought to be less efficient and sometimes even harmful due to the uninterrupted restriction of the blood flow. Compression stockings, instead, are often thought to be too difficult to apply at the malleolar region.

- **Perimalleolar pads** (Fig. 15.4) exert pressure to the skin in the region of the *Bisgaard's coulisse* or *Bisgaard (perimalleolar) region*, a slightly depressed area between the malleolus, the Achilles tendon and the heel. They help to distribute pressure evenly. These pads protect the tops of the malleoli as they absorb part of the pressure that would otherwise reach the tops of the malleoli unrestrictedly.
- **Protection of the tibialis anterior tendon** (see Chap. 19, Fig. 19.15) prevents damage caused by excessive compression therapy. It is used in case the tendon is particularly prominent.
- **Protection for traumatic impact** (Fig. 15.5), for example, by using two layers of felt at 5 mm each, with bevelled borders and a central recess.

15.5 Surgical Therapy

The prominences of both malleoli cannot be removed due to their multiple functions.

In the case of an important venous insufficiency, several therapies such as surgery of varicose veins, ligation of perforator veins or sclerotherapy, might be useful [1]. It should be borne in mind that these patients often need their veins during the rest of their lives for bypass surgery.

Plastic surgery, using split skin transplantation (mesh graft), is performed in the surrounding area, while flaps such as the suralis-flap or local advancement flaps are used to cover the summit of the malleoli [2, 3]. In the preoperative phase vascular imaging and maybe revascularisation are needed [4].

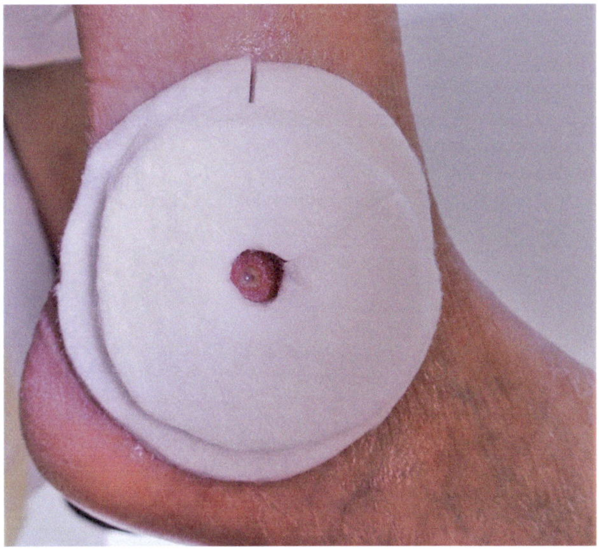

Fig. 15.5 Multilayer protection against impact

15.6 Summary

- **Venous insufficiency is often the dominant underlying disease if the ulcers are situated in the area of the malleoli. In contrast, a leading PAD is disproportionately common in lesions at the summit.**
- **When carrying out compression therapy, attention has to be paid to a simultaneous PAD and to possibly high pressure on the malleoli. A protection for the malleoli is mandatory in these cases, for example, by use of perimalleolar pads in the shape of a curved pad. These perimalleolar pads not only protect the malleoli, but also allow compression of the Bisgaard's coulisse between malleoli and Achilles tendon.**
- **Trauma or constant pressure as in the case of decubital lesions might be detected by meticulous research and then avoided by protective measures.**
- **Lesions at the malleoli need a long time to pass on to remission but are less prone to reactivation than other entities.**
- **Located at the summits and associated with a PAD they are associated with amputations above the ankle far above average.**

References

1. van Gent W, Wittens C. Influence of perforating vein surgery in patients with venous ulceration. Phlebology. 2015;30(2):127–32. https://doi.org/10.1177/0268355513517685.

2. Blume PA, Donegan R, Schmidt BM. The role of plastic surgery for soft tissue coverage of the diabetic foot and ankle. Clin Podiatr Med Surg. 2014;31(1):127–50. https://doi.org/10.1016/j.cpm.2013.09.006.
3. Schirmer S, Ritter RG, Fansa H. Vascular surgery, microsurgery and supramicrosurgery for treatment of chronic diabetic foot ulcers to prevent amputations. PLoS One. 2013;8(9):e74704. https://doi.org/10.1371/journal.pone.0074704.
4. Ignatiadis II, Tsiampa VA, Papalois AE. A systematic approach to the failed plastic surgical reconstruction of the diabetic foot. Diabet Foot Ankle. 2011;2. https://doi.org/10.3402/dfa.v2i0.6435.

The Heel (17–18) 16

Lesions can be located in different areas of the heel. These sites are:

- The calcaneal tuberosity (17)
- The sole of the heel and (18)
- The transition zone in between both (18)

There are three varying types of lesions in these areas, which are discussed separately in this chapter. The tuberosity is under pressure if the foot is upright and the skin of the tuberosity is in contact with the supporting structure (Fig. 16.1).

The lesions on the sole of the heel and in the transition between hairless and hairy skin are characterised by the fact that there is no bone prominence beneath and many statistical properties are similar. Therefore, they are grouped together as entity 18.

Heel injuries are important because they may develop based on other serious diseases and because the possibility of surgical treatment is limited.

16.1 Pathobiomechanics and Pressure Points

The heel is well equipped to withstand substantial pressures when bearing load [1–3]. The fat pad of the heel is about 2 cm thick and can meet all the demands in pressure resistance that may arise in the course of an active life. The flow of blood is ensured as all three major arteries of the lower leg supply vessels to the arterial plexus of the heel. In order to severely damage the heel's structure, it is necessary to have either significant trauma or restricted perfusion or both.

Different patterns of damage can be identified:

- The inner pressure point is the *lateral process of the calcaneal tuberosity* as a predilection site for a decubitus ulcer. The calcaneal region in the area of the insertion of the Achilles tendon shows several bony prominences. If the

D. Hochlenert et al., *Diabetic Foot Syndrome*,
https://doi.org/10.1007/978-3-319-92055-9_16

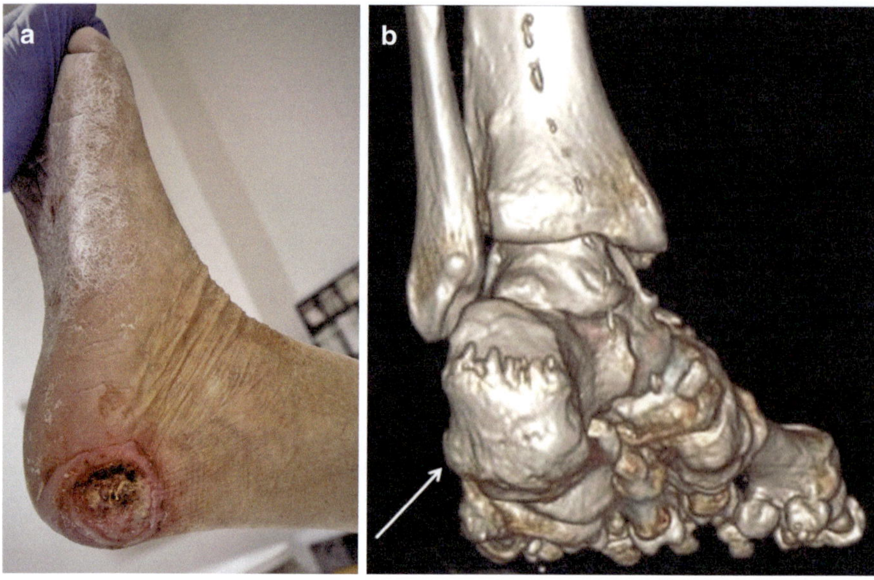

Fig. 16.1 (**a**, **b**) Clinical aspect of a lateral heel ulcer and the lateral bony prominence (arrow) of the calcaneal tuberosity in three-dimensional CT reconstruction

calcaneal tuberosity is placed on a mattress and supports the leg, the weight of the leg alone will exert enough pressure to prevent the microcirculation of the skin and to initiate necrosis [4, 5]. Patients affected are typically restricted in their spontaneous movements. Such critical situations occur especially during and after long operations and in the case of immobility due to poor general condition. The resting position of the foot of a person in a supine position is plantarflexed and slightly abducted. Decubital lesions develop on the skin covering the lateral process of the calcaneal tuberosity as a result of pressure, friction and shear force (Fig. 16.1).

- *Transition between hairless and hairy skin* as a common site for rhagades (Fig. 16.2). Rhagades on the heel are cracks at the edge of the corpus adiposum (fat pad). This zone becomes hyperkeratotic and inelastic due to repeated loading and unloading of the fat pad. This pad becomes flat and wide at every step to return to the original shape afterwards. This is neccessary because it is non-compressible and reacts to vertical pressure by widening its diameter. Once a first crack has developed, a weak spot is created and all further movements keep narrowing and widening the crack preventing it from closing.
- One particular situation is the *extreme vulnerability of the plantar fat pad* (see Chap. 2, Fig. 2.39). The heel must bear load at each step, which is made possible by the fat pad of the heel. A significant trauma, or even a minor event in the case of a PAD, may overcome this protection. Together with an infection, they may induce a serious loss of tissue in the fat pad. This loss may be facilitated by the fact that the septs are generously perfused but the fat deposits between them are not.

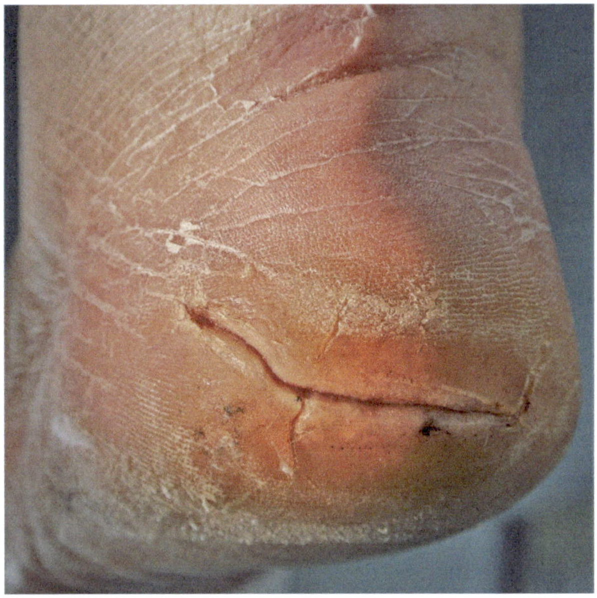

Fig. 16.2 Rhagade of the heel

- The heel is offloaded by traction on the Achilles tendon, which shifts load to the midfoot and the forefoot and thus limits the time and the amount of strain to the heel. *Loss of function of the Achilles tendon* might cause a pes calcaneus, for example after a rupture of the tendon (Fig. 16.3). The possibility of such a loss of function must be ruled out in the case of a plantar heel ulcer.

16.2 Tests to Perform

A detailed anamnesis, a precise assessment of the arterial perfusion and, if the patient is not bedridden, a biomechanical observation of the gait must be carried out in each patient with heel lesions [6].

16.3 Statistics

The figures in Fig. 16.4 show some peculiarities:

- Lesions above the tuber calcanei reach the bone frequently. This can be easily explained considering the thin layer of soft tissue covering the bone.
- Ulcers at the heel need revascularisation more frequently than the average. They are more frequently associated with major amputations and take longer to pass on to remission. The lesions above the calcaneal tuberosity display a more dramatic picture than the others, the lesions at the border, in contrast, a less dramatic one.
- Reactivation is less frequent than in most other entities.

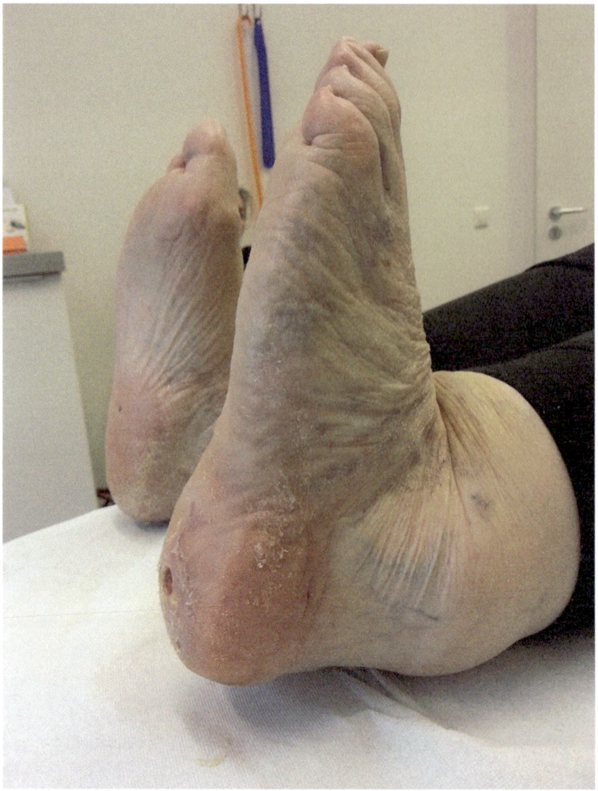

Fig. 16.3 Heel lesion after rupture of the Achilles tendon, movement in an attempt to plantar flex the foot and press the forefoot in plantar direction (!)

Note: Rhagades at the edge of the heel are less frequently associated with a PAD and have a more favourable prognosis. However, in cases of coexisting critical PAD they might become very harmful, thus surprising the professional caregivers. The danger might be expressed by an unresponsive perifocal necrotic seam [7]. **Even a single millimetre of necrotic seam becoming visible during treatment is a signal of imminent danger and should be recognised as an urgent warning sign.**

16.4 Principals of External Offloading

In the case of decubital ulcers [8–10] these measures might be useful:

- Devices to offload the heel while lying in bed or sitting in a chair.
- Splints made of slightly flexible cast material named e. g. '*Bed cast*' (Fig. 16.5) (see Chap. 19, Sect. 4.1).
- Spacers in the shape of a ring. These must be used with care as they are supported by the surrounding tissue and as a result, the tissue is compressed. Pressure might become critical and cause necrosis.
- So-called '*fur shoes*' offer insufficient protection and pressure redistribution.

		Sole of heel	Sole not heel	Rhagade not heel	Dorsum	Scars
Frequency		1.8%	1.7%	1.3%	2.2%	5.7%
Bone involvement	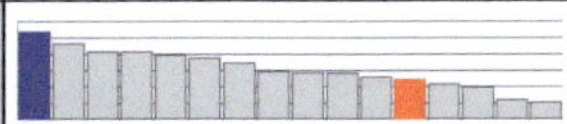	14.2%	11.6%	7.6%	14.9%	26.9%
PAD	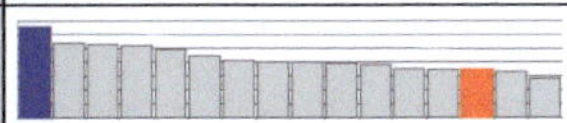	46.9%	29.8%	24.4%	44.9%	66.4%
Revascularisation	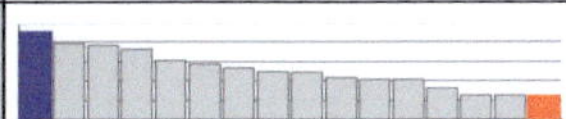	10.4%	2.9%	3.8%	6.6%	18.1%
Amputation below ankle	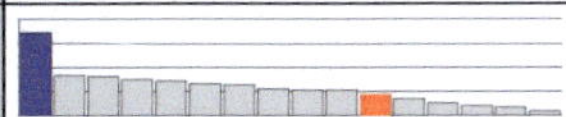	2.7%	5.2%	5.3%	6.6%	24.1%
Amputation above ankle	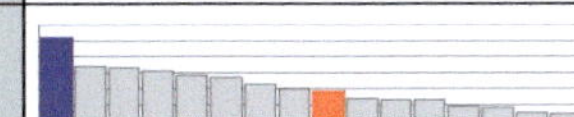	3.8%	0%	1.5%	3.5%	5.2%
Days until remission	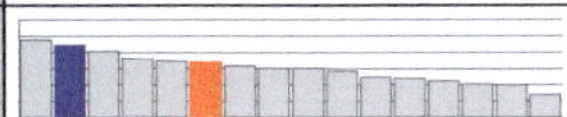	129	145	84	102	146
Duration > 180 days	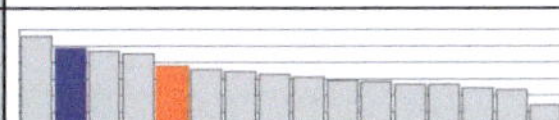	41.7%	42.4%	28%	32.2%	44.6%
Reactivation following year	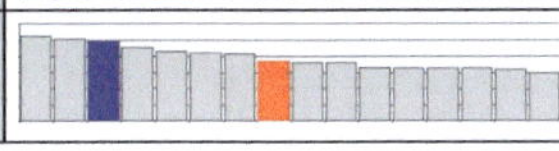	37.5%	45.3%	29%	35.2%	48.9%

Fig. 16.4 Benchmark figures of lesions of the heel (orange) in a rank of all entities (grey) in decreasing height

- Similar devices, which increase the contact surface due to their softness, might be sufficient to protect endangered bone prominences but are less effective than devices that transfer load to a distant part of the leg. They are thought to be harmful when ulcers already have developed because they transfer load to the edge of the ulcer and to adjacent skin that should provide tissue repair.

In the case of rhagades the following measures can be used:

- To maintain elasticity:
  - Remove hyperkeratosis of the border of the rhagade
  - Apply ointments or special foams
- Apply *tape dressings* at the heel
- An easy and generally successful way to deal with rhagades is to seal them by use of *acrylates*, possibly in combination with tapes (Fig. 16.6)

In the case of lesions at the plantar fat pad the following measures may help:

- The heel as a whole must be offloaded. This is possible only in complex systems as a TCC, a Walker or a custom-made orthosis involving the lower leg.
- Remote cushioning can be provided for example by applying felt or using a rear-foot offloading shoe. It should be borne in mind that the pressure at the edge of this support is high. This often results in the formation of new ulcers.

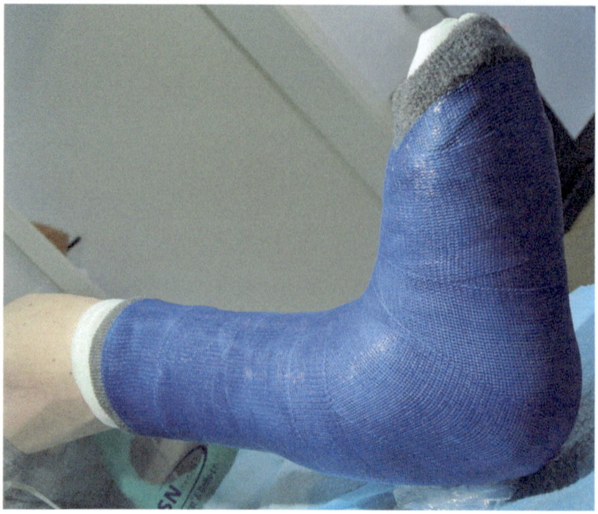

Fig. 16.5 Bed cast

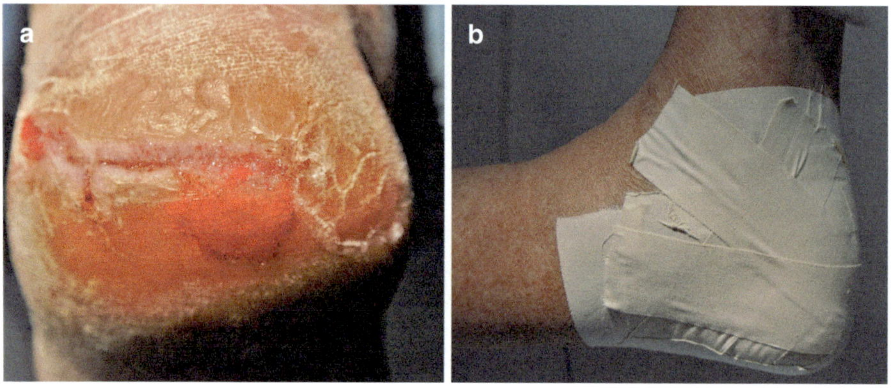

Fig. 16.6 (a) Rhagade of Fig. 16.2 treated with acrylate sealant and (b) tape dressing

- More heel spring: If the position of the heel is slightly higher, load is transferred to the mid- and forefoot.
- If a pes calcaneus is the cause of the lesion, the orthosis should support the condyles of the tibia if the patient is mobile.

16.5 Principals of Surgical Therapy

- There are no standard procedures for internal offloading that the authors are familiar with and would recommend using.
- After a trauma in the region of the fat pad of the heel meticulous exploration and assessment is needed. This is described in detail in the next chapter.

- Some ulcers fail to proceed towards closure. These are for example ulcers extending deep inside the fat pad or longstanding ulcers with borders formed by scar tissue. In these cases, an excision of the ulcer and plastic-reconstructive surgery might be helpful. It should be borne in mind that split-skin-transplants such as Mesh graft are not suitable in weight-bearing areas.

16.6 Summary

Decubital lesions at the heel...

- **... occur in immobile patients or after surgery. As a rule, they can be avoided, e. g. by using offloading devices in prevention.**
- **... are treated with external offloading. In many cases, a wound closure can be achieved despite severe initial lesions.**

Rhagades...

- **... are common.**
- **... can lead to high amputations in the presence of critical PAD.**
- **... are treated with skin care. Deep-reaching rhagades can be closed with acrylate sealants or plaster strips.**

Lesions in the area of the fat pad of the heel...

- **... can cause massive tissue loss due to infections.**
- **... often require revascularisation and lead to above-average amputation rates.**
- **... are relieved using the entire lower leg. Walkers, TCCs or a custom-made orthosis are used for this purpose.**
- **... require considering plastic-reconstructive procedures if no closure of the wound is to be expected.**

16.7 Case Report

A 62-year-old male patient with Diabetes mellitus Typ 2 for a period of 14 years presented with a rhagade at the medial border of the right heel. Critical PAD and infection led to a limb-threatening ulceration. Inpatient care with revascularisation, repeated debridement, reconstructive surgery by a plantaris medialis flap finally achieved wound closure (Fig. 16.7).

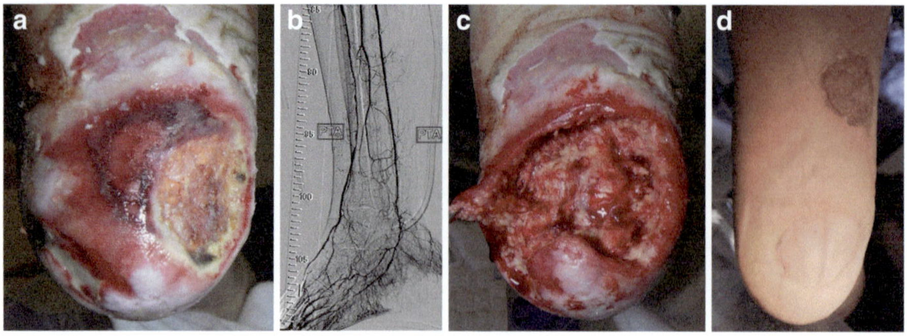

Fig. 16.7 (**a**) Plantar, infected ulcer of the heel (**b**) complete loss of local perfusion in angiography (**c**) after surgical debridement, (**d**) after plastic-reconstructive surgery (plantaris-medialis-flap)

References

1. Cichowitz A, Pan WR, Ashton M. The heel: anatomy, blood supply, and the pathophysiology of pressure ulcers. Ann Plast Surg. 2009;62(4):423–9. https://doi.org/10.1097/SAP.0b013e3181851b55.
2. Gefen A. The biomechanics of heel ulcers. J Tissue Viability. 2010;19(4):124–31. https://doi.org/10.1016/j.jtv.2010.06.003.
3. Sopher R, Nixon J, McGinnis E, Gefen A. The influence of foot posture, support stiffness, heel pad loading and tissue mechanical properties on biomechanical factors associated with a risk of heel ulceration. J Mech Behav Biomed Mater. 2011;4(4):572–82. https://doi.org/10.1016/j.jmbbm.2011.01.004.
4. Masaki N, Sugama J, Okuwa M, Inagaki M, Matsuo J, Nakatani T, Sanada H. Heel blood flow during loading and off-loading in bedridden older adults with low and normal ankle-brachial pressure index: a quasi-experimental study. Biol Res Nurs. 2013;15(3):285–91. https://doi.org/10.1177/1099800412437929.
5. Wong VK, Stotts NA, Hopf HW, Froelicher ES, Dowling GA. How heel oxygenation changes under pressure. Wound Repair Regen. 2007;15(6):786–94. https://doi.org/10.1111/j.1524-475X.2007.00309.x.
6. Treiman GS, Oderich GS, Ashrafi A, Schneider PA. Management of ischemic heel ulceration and gangrene: an evaluation of factors associated with successful healing. J Vasc Surg. 2000;31(6):1110–8.
7. Salcido R, Lee A, Ahn C. Heel pressure ulcers: purple heel and deep tissue injury. Adv Skin Wound Care. 2011;24(8):374–80.; quiz 372–381. https://doi.org/10.1097/01.ASW.0000403250.85131.b9.
8. Chipchase SY, Treece KA, Pound N, Game FL, Jeffcoate WJ. Heel ulcers don't heal in diabetes. Or do they? Diabet Med. 2005;22(9):1258–62. https://doi.org/10.1111/j.1464-5491.2005.01665.x.
9. Gilcreast DM, Warren JB, Yoder LH, Clark JJ, Wilson JA, Mays MZ. Research comparing three heel ulcer-prevention devices. J Wound Ostomy Continence Nurs. 2005;32(2):112–20.
10. Junkin J, Gray M. Are pressure redistribution surfaces or heel protection devices effective for preventing heel pressure ulcers? J Wound Ostomy Continence Nurs. 2009;36(6):602–8. https://doi.org/10.1097/WON.0b013e3181be282f.

Atypical Areas (19–22) 17

This chapter covers lesions on the sole not discussed in the preceding chapters (19), at the dorsum of the foot (20), in the transition zone between hairy and hairless skin (rhagades) on the midfoot and the forefoot (21), and recurrence of ulcers in pre-existing scars (22). None of these areas has a typical internal pressure point.

Lesions in the region of the plantar fat pad of the heel and in the border area of the heel represent a special condition. These lesions have specific characteristics and are discussed in Chap. 16 together with other lesions of the heel.

17.1 Pathobiomechanics

Plantar ulcers in localisations not featuring an underlying protruding bone as discussed in previous chapters, have two major causes: harmful external agents such as trauma or heat (see Fig. 1.1a) and acquired deformities secondary to a Charcot foot (Fig. 17.1) or an amputation. While a prominence is easy to detect, it can be difficult to identify the traumatic event or the traumatising factor. Sometimes it takes more than one discussion with the patient and his or her relatives until the cause is finally found. Diagnosis and therapy of the Charcot Foot is discussed in Chap. 21.

Lesions at the **dorsum** of the foot (Fig. 17.2) often occur above tendons that might be very prominent due to muscle atrophy secondary to motor neuropathy. Trauma and thermal damage might also play a role. Thermal damage can be recognised by the fact that lesions are not located above prominences, but rather depict the contact surface of the source of heat (see Chap. 5, Sect. 5.1).

Rhagades have been discussed as part of the lesions at the heel. They also occur at the forefoot or midfoot (Fig. 17.3) in hyperkeratotic areas in the transition from hairless skin to hairy skin or in the case of mycosis. The *transition from hairless to hairy skin* is subject to tensile, bending and shear force in such a way that hyperkeratosis of particular severity can develop. These might be capillarised and cause bleeding during treatment even before sufficient removal of hyperkeratosis has been achieved.

D. Hochlenert et al., *Diabetic Foot Syndrome*,
https://doi.org/10.1007/978-3-319-92055-9_17

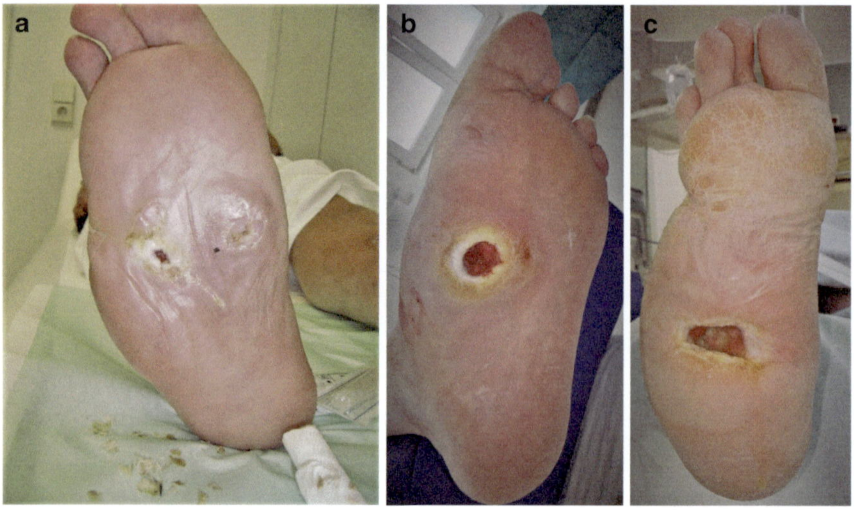

Fig. 17.1 Plantar ulcers as a consequence of a Charcot Foot (**a**) superficial (**b**) profound (**c**) invading the bone

Fig. 17.2 Lesion with exposed long extensor tendons of the toes (EDL)

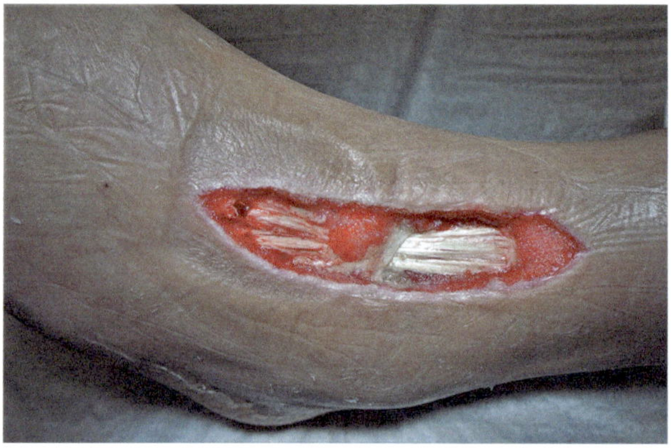

Lesions in the region of pre-existing scars encounter most arduous conditions in the hypotrophic area of the scar (Fig. 17.4) ('wound in the scar of a scar...').

17.1.1 Statistics

The figures illustrated in Fig. 17.5 show some peculiarities.

- Lesions of the sole take a long time to pass on to remission. At the heel, they often are related to PAD and need revascularisation. They often result in amputation. On other parts of the sole, the association with PAD is less frequent.

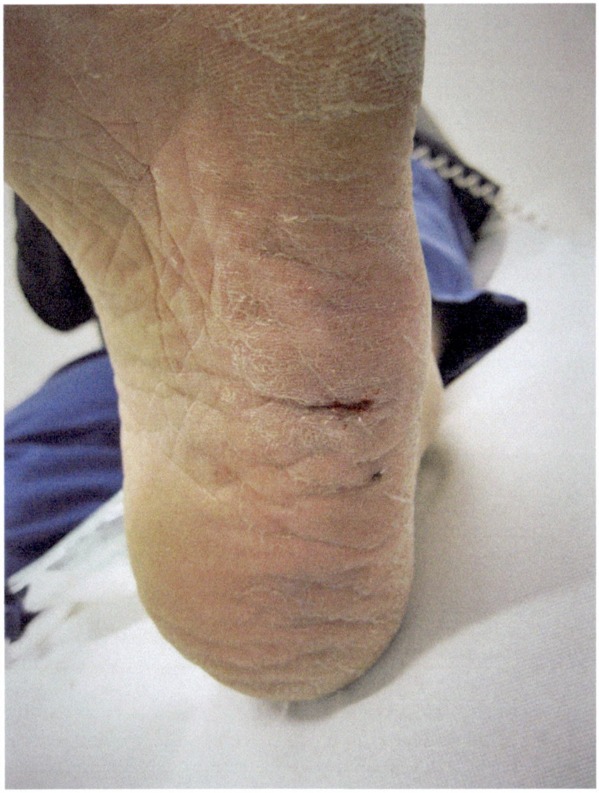

Fig. 17.3 Rhagade in the case of anhidrosis and hyperkeratosis

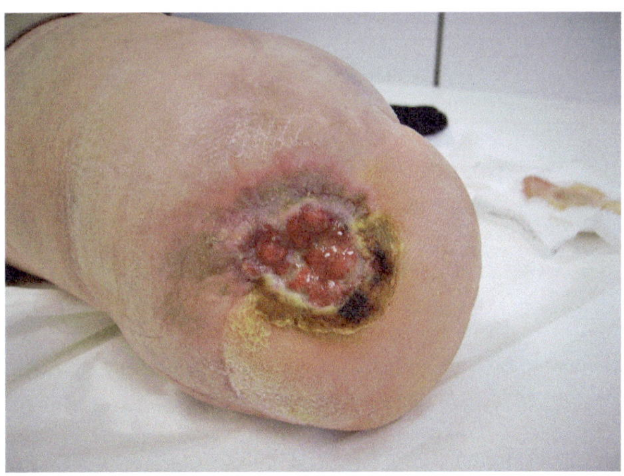

Fig. 17.4 Ulcer in the area around a scar after atypical amputation of the hindfoot

- Rhagades are generally superficial and benign.
- Re-ulceration in scar tissue is a serious event. It tends to be more profound, momentous and protracted than any other entity of the diabetic foot.

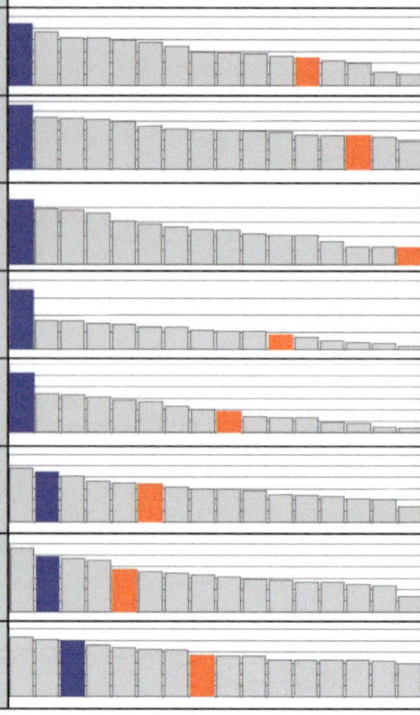

		Sole of heel	Sole not heel	Rhagade not heel	Dorsum	Scars
Frequency		1.8%	1.7%	1.3%	2.2%	5.7%
Bone involvement		14.2%	11.6%	7.6%	14.9%	26.9%
PAD		46.9%	29.8%	24.4%	44.9%	66.4%
Revascularisation		10.4%	2.9%	3.8%	6.6%	18.1%
Amputation below ankle		2.7%	5.2%	5.3%	6.6%	24.1%
Amputation above ankle		3.8%	0%	1.5%	3.5%	5.2%
Days until remission		129	145	84	102	146
Duration > 180 days		41.7%	42.4%	28%	32.2%	44.6%
Reactivation following year		37.5%	45.3%	29%	35.2%	48.9%

Fig. 17.5 The column in blue corresponds to lesions in scar tissue. The columns in orange show the other three entities of this chapter, the remaining columns in grey concern all other entities. The figures of the plantar heel lesions are added to give additional information to this adjacent area with completely different characteristics. Plantar heel lesions are discussed in Chap. 16

17.2 Principles of External Offloading

- Plantar lesions distant from the heel might be offloaded by remote padding similar to lesions at the MTHs.
- Remote padding might also be used to offload lesions of the dorsum of the foot.

17.3 Principles of Internal Offloading

- On the dorsal part of the foot, lesions often develop at prominent tendons. The tendons are easily exposed, and serious infections might spread along the tendon sheets. If tendons are involved, an immobilisation of the joint bridged by the tendon in question is essential. With the help of an adequate device, immobilisation limits movements in the tendons compartment and helps to prevent the spreading of the infection. Surgical debridement removes the destroyed fibres and sometimes the tendon is lost.

- After traumatic injuries, small and contaminated foreign bodies may remain in the wound. Therefore, it is important to explore the depth of the lesion with a thin probe. The extent of the traumatic destruction of tissue and bacterial contamination must also be estimated. If the lesion has reached deep compartments and there has been considerable contamination or trauma, surgical revision is essential. In other cases, when less tissue has been lost and arterial blood flow is adequate, it is possible to completely offload the foot, administer antibiotics and wait for 1–2 weeks.
- If the formation of granulation tissue or epithelisation in the region of a pre-existing scar is slow or stagnant, this matter of fact should be well documented and become apparent with no delay. In this case, excision of the scar and closing the defect by means of plastic-reconstructive surgery should be considered at an early stage.

17.4 Summary

- **Abscesses and deep, contaminated canals after penetration require surgical therapy.**
- **Re-ulceration in scar tissue easily becomes deep, affecting large parts of the hypotrophic tissue with serious consequences.**

Transition to the Lower Leg

18

This chapter reviews practical aspects of lesions of the lower leg in people with diabetes. The high rate of comorbidities frequently leads to a more complex course of the disease compared to people without diabetes. Many patients with diabetic foot syndrome suffer from ulcers on the lower leg and ulcers on the feet at the same time. Therefore, in many countries the treatment of ulcers at the lower leg is also part of the typical workload of a diabetic foot outpatient clinic.

18.1 Statistics

The figures illustrated in Fig. 18.1 show specific characteristics of leg ulcers. Bone involvement usually applies to concomitant foot ulcers. In summary, these figures show that:

- For each case in which an ulcer on the lower leg dominates the scenario, 13 cases with predominant ulcers on the feet have been documented.
- Bone is reached late in the course of the disease.
- Dorsal leg ulcers are more often decubitus ulcers and are frequently associated with ulcers at the heel. They tend to be profound involving the Achilles tendon and are associated with prolonged time to healing (Fig. 18.2).
- Lateral ulcers of the lower leg (and on the malleolus) are associated with the highest major amputation rates.
- The extraordinary threat posed by ulcers on the lateral leg is particularly striking in comparison to those on the medial side.

D. Hochlenert et al., *Diabetic Foot Syndrome*,
https://doi.org/10.1007/978-3-319-92055-9_18

	Lower leg all	Ventral	Medial	Lateral	Dorsal
Frequency	7.8 / 100 foot lesions	4.7%	1.3%	1.1%	0.7%
Bone involvement	4.5%	3.5%	3.7%	5.3%	10.9%
PAD	34.3%	30%	43.1%	33.9%	46.5%
Revascularisation	3.2%	1.9%	5.3%	3.5%	8.2%
Amputation below ankle	1.6%	1.6%	0.7%	1.7%	2.7%
Amputation above ankle	1.5%	0.8%	1.5%	4.4%	1.3%
Days until remission	94	76	112	142	177.5
Duration >180 days	30.8%	23%	38.8%	45%	48.1%
Reactivation following year	31.7%	31.6%	33.3%	27.7%	36.5%

Fig. 18.1 Benchmark figures of ulcers of the lower leg

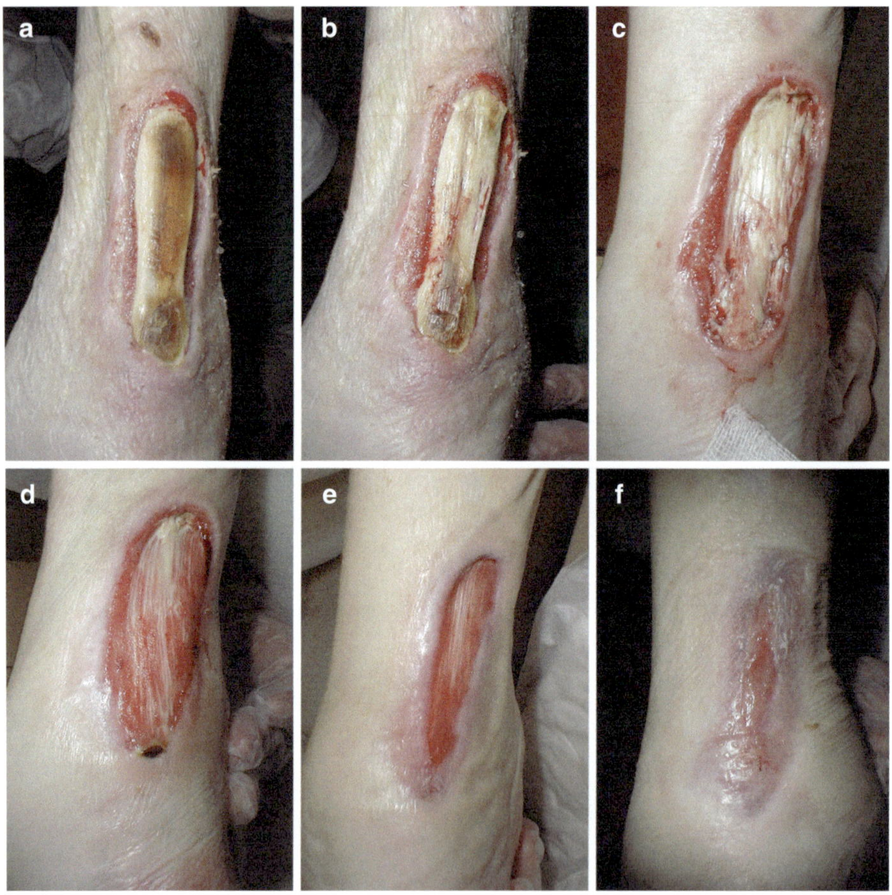

Fig. 18.2 (**a**–**f**) Decubitus lesion of the dorsal side of the lower leg involving the Achilles tendon, conservative treatment included shaving of the tendon; duration of treatment 5 months

18.2 Pathophysiology and Background

Ulcers of the lower leg require a meticulous analysis of the underlying disease:

- Oedema as a result of cardiac, renal or hepatic disease
- Chronic venous insufficiency and insufficient compression therapy either due to contraindications or because of poor application
- PAD
- Pressure (decubital) problems
- Trauma due to a collision
- Defects of the epidermis (e.g. Pruritus causing scratching)
- Rare causes
  - Autoimmunity (leukocytoclastic vasculitis of the small vessel, polyarteritis nodosa, etc.)
  - Pathological deposits in the interstitial space (amyloidosis, calciphylaxis)
  - some types of anaemia (sickle cell anaemia, thalassaemia)
  - Diseases with unknown genesis (pyoderma gangrenosum, necrobiosis lipoidica)
  - Neoplastic diseases (squamous cell carcinoma, cutaneous lymphoma, melanoma)
  - Drug-induced skin diseases (hydroxyurea, coumarin-based anticoagulants)

18.3 Communication with the Patient

Communication with the patient is particularly important as the offered treatment is often in contrast to some deep-seated convictions. Additionally, patients' attitudes and usual lifestyle will have a major influence on the success of the therapy. Topics for discussion include:

- **Walking and lying are helpful, sitting or standing may not be**. In a seated position, even with elevated legs, muscle pumps are not active and if the legs are lower than the heart, the difference in height determines the accumulation of fluids in the lower limbs. Sitting with elevated legs may even obstruct the return of venous blood and lymph at the level of the groin. Therefore, it might be useful to discuss the optimal rest position. A supine position on a sofa with the concerned limb positioned slightly higher on a pillow or similar is beneficial. Sitting in an armchair with legs elevated on a stool may not prevent oedema sufficiently.
- **Diuretics are to be taken regularly**: Each day the patient may find a number of reasons why it is inconvenient to take diuretics at precisely the time they are prescribed. A possible solution is to postpone the intake to another hour of the day, but not to omit it.
- **Limit liquid intake**: Recommendations on minimum daily liquid intake are subject to trends and have to be questioned even in the general population if not expressed

by a healthcare professional considering the whole picture of health, clinical need and medication. In people taking diuretics, it is even less sensible to replace a volume of liquid immediately after they have been removed by the diuretics.
- **Limit salt consumption**: The taste of salt is often less intense as people age and thus the amount of salt consumed may increase. This is important for the development and therapy of hypertension and oedema.
- **Pain caused by compression**: Removal of oedema in firmly filled legs by mechanical means such as compression therapy might result in severe pain, especially in the area of wounds where there may be some inflammation. Pain may be sufficiently severe to require opiate analgesia. Pain management should be performed according to guidelines such as the WHO-scheme, paying particular to any renal insufficiency. In general, it may be better to use several different methods to treat the oedema at the same time, each of which may not need to be applied with such an intensity that major problems including pain are caused. In patient's eyes, it may seem more obvious to remove the compression than to take painkillers that are perceived as loaded with side effects. This must be discussed with empathy so that compression therapy is seen as useful and will be continued unless side effects are genuinely intolerable and can't be managed.
- **Health beliefs**: Patients often have their own clear views of why and how the wound has developed. As a consequence, they sometimes adopt strange practice strategies in the belief that they will counteract these causes. It is very beneficial to know of any such beliefs and to be able to discuss them with the patient.

18.4 Special Aspects of Therapy

18.4.1 Oedema Control

Oedema almost always contributes, at least in part, to delayed closure of wounds on the lower leg. This makes decongestive measures one of the cornerstones of therapy. Measures to remove and prevent oedema are:

- Treatment of medical diseases such as heart failure
- Compression with multilayer bandages, compression stockings or zinc paste bandage
- Lymphatic drainage, manually or by means of mechanical aids
- Elevation of the limb
- Behavioural change such as altering liquid intake, salt consumption and compliance to medication

A failure to implement this fundamental part of the treatment may completely prevent wound closure. In the case of coexisting relevant PAD moderate compression only may be possible, or compression might be considered only after improving perfusion [1]. In this case, meticulous assessment of the extent of PAD and the risk brought about by compression needs discussion in an interdisciplinary consultation. Light compression, frequent review, and interdisciplinary consultations to find the best solution for an individual patient in addition to well-trained staff can lead to successful outcomes even in this difficult situation [2]. A pressure of approx. 20 mmHg can be utilised, which is the case for short-stretch bandages if they are used without special pulling. Finding a method of mild compression is also important if the border of an ulcer is oedematous. With a difference in height between the level of the surrounding skin and the granulation tissue at the base of the ulcer, epithelialisation may be difficult to achieve [3].

Hence, coexisting PAD is not an absolute contraindication to compression therapy.

18.4.2 Exudate Control

Highly absorbent dressing pads with superabsorbers accept liquids and do not release them when put under pressure. They can be used between skin and a compression bandage. The liquids contain autolytic enzymes and their absorption is an effective protection of the unharmed tissue in the wound as well as the skin surrounding the wound.

18.4.3 Control of Inflammation

Protection of the intact skin at the wound's edge: Autolytic enzymes within wound exudate are able to extend inflammatory processes and enlarge wounds. Absorbing this exudate and drawing it away from the healthy periwound skin is therefore important. Antibiotics are used too frequently. If there is only the impression that an infection cannot be excluded, they should be avoided. It should be remembered that not all inflammation is due to infection, and overuse risks the development of multidrug-resistant organisms. The use of *corticosteroids* locally is often beneficial, together with antibiotics or alone.

A sign of good control of the inflammation is substantial reduction of pain.

18.4.4 Invasive Correction of Problems in Venous Flow

To enhance wound closure and reduce the probability of recidivism, invasive measures to partially correct defects in venous blood flow should be considered [4].

18.5 Summary

Special aspects of wounds of the lower leg of people with Diabetes:

- **Lesions on the lateral side of the lower leg (as well as lesions on the lateral malleoli) are associated with high rate of major amputation.**
- **Compression therapy, even if only at low pressure due to concomitant PAD, is a cornerstone of the therapy.**
- **Consider additional invasive measures to correct venous dysfunction.**
- **Particular attention has to be paid to communication with the patient because measures such as compression therapy and adherence to prescribed medication may encounter understandable but deleterious resistance.**

18.6 Case Report

Compression therapy in the case of concomitant PAD: In a 74-year-old woman with Diabetes mellitus type 2 for 22 years treated with insulin, a cruro-pedal bypass occluded after 3 years and was opened by a PTA of the bypass. An ulcer of the affected limb laterally with clinically marked wound oedema and stagnant wound closure was present. Treatment consisted of moderate compression by several short stretch bandages in an inverted application (Fig. 18.3) for a duration of 4.5 months.

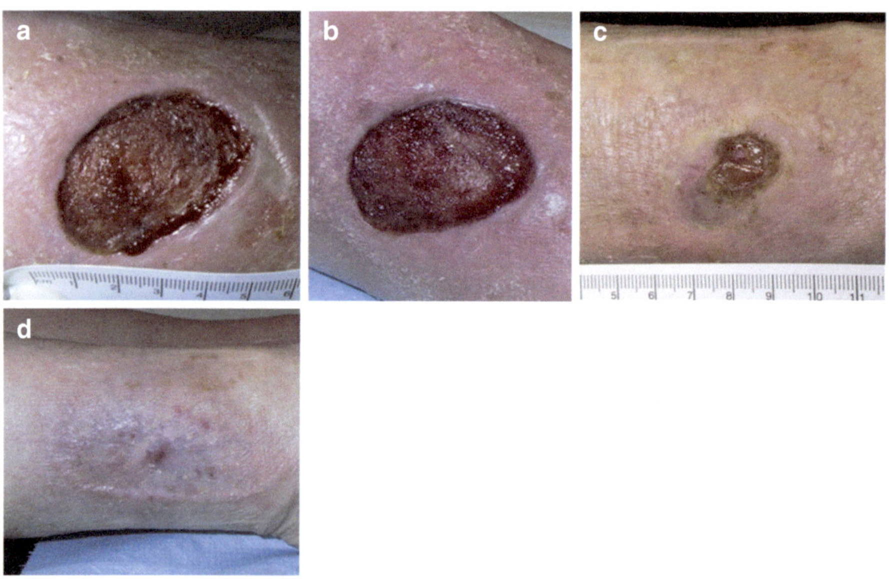

Fig. 18.3 (**a–d**) Compression therapy to reduce oedema at the edges of the wound and facilitate epithelisation despite coexisting PAD

References

1. Apelqvist J, Larsson J, Agardh CD. The importance of peripheral pulses, peripheral oedema and local pain for the outcome of diabetic foot ulcers. Diabet Med. 1990;7(7):590–4.
2. Wu SC, Crews RT, Najafi B, Slone-Rivera N, Minder JL, Andersen CA. Safety and efficacy of mild compression (18-25 mm Hg) therapy in patients with diabetes and lower extremity edema. J Diabetes Sci Technol. 2012;6(3):641–7.
3. Armstrong DG, Nguyen HC. Improvement in healing with aggressive edema reduction after debridement of foot infection in persons with diabetes. Arch Surg. 2000;135(12):1405–9.
4. Armstrong DG. Addition of surgical correction to compression therapy reduced recurrences in chronic venous leg ulceration. ACP J Club. 2007;147(3):73.

External Offloading and Immobilisation 19

Redistribution of load is the most important measure to prevent or to treat diabetic foot ulcers. Redistributing load efficiently means that it is possible to offload the region in question without the need to drastically limit the steps the patient takes. This allows the patient to maintain mobility and to continue the life she or he is used to. Remaining mobile also allows the individual to maintain control of their diabetes and an overall healthy lifestyle.

Load redistribution assigns part of the load bearing duties to areas of the foot that would normally be less load bearing. This is not usually feasible using one singular procedure, and hence a combination of measures may be necessary.

Emphasis is placed on methods that offload without immobilisation of joints. The latter may offload very efficiently but might reduce mobility of the affected person and may be interpreted as increasing frailty.

This chapter focuses on those methods that do not require surgery. Surgical solutions are definite, whilst the non-surgical solutions might be discontinued.

19.1 Overview

Mechanical stress on a certain area of the foot can be reduced either by limiting the number of steps taken or by limiting the pressure exerted on this area at each step.

The first method is easy to prescribe but difficult to apply. It appears contradictory if the main goal for the treatment of DFS is to strive for preserved mobility. Mobility is a key factor for independence and quality of life. Limiting mobility for several weeks or maybe months may compromise this overriding goal to such an extent that it may not be reached again for the remainder of the patients' life. As a consequence, **reduction of the number of steps made should not be used** for more than a short period of time.

For a person with DFS, living with as little impairment as possible means reconciling walking with preserving the integrity of the foot. To avoid overload, the mechanical stress during each step can be reduced by redistributing load to

D. Hochlenert et al., *Diabetic Foot Syndrome*,
https://doi.org/10.1007/978-3-319-92055-9_19

sufficiently resistant parts of the foot. Therefore, it is important to find, elaborate and teach techniques of load redistribution as they are the cornerstones for the prevention and treatment of the vast majority of people with DFS.

Offloading should aim to redistribute pressure as much as possible on sufficiently resistant parts of the foot, instead of preventing the patient from walking.

Immobilisation of joints of the foot helps to redistribute pressure and may be very effective. The use of immobilising devices is, however, limited by several undesirable effects. For example, measures such as rigid, debilitating footwear are less acceptable to the patient, tend to be used less and therefore may be less effective. Rigid footwear may also lead to muscle disuse. These muscles will then weaken and atrophy, which may lead to further damage. Therefore, an individualised plan for the necessary extent of offloading and immobilisation is crucial. A motto to describe this approach could be: '**As little as possible, as much as necessary**.'

This chapter focuses on techniques that do not require surgery. Techniques describing surgery are described in the next chapter. In contrast to the explanations in the chapters on the various entities, the emphasis here is on aspects that cover several entities. In the chapters concerning the entities, these techniques are described with the emphasis on the particular indication for the respective entity.

19.2 Internal and External Offloading

Using measures to reduce pressure on one part of the foot automatically means that this load is transferred to another part of the foot. Offloading without limiting the mobility of the patient is therefore equivalent to load redistribution. The drawbacks of increasing the load on other parts of the foot should be limited by the use of a combination of several different procedures.

Changing the inner pressure point is referred to as '*internal offloading*'. By contrast, '*external offloading*' optimises the transmission of pressure from the skin to the environment.

- *Internal offloading* is provided by surgery and aims to permanently reduce the impact of an internal pressure point. Its effect is independent of the behaviour of the patient.
- *External offloading* is provided by use of devices or might be applied directly to the skin. They can be customised individually or be prefabricated, sometimes with individual modification. Their efficacy depends, however, on uninterrupted use by the patient.
- During acute treatment, offloading has to be much stricter than in the subsequent phase of secondary prevention.

19.2.1 Uninterrupted Use

The uninterrupted use of a measure of external offloading is difficult to achieve. If the device can be taken off or the procedure can be interrupted it is likely that it will be. Theoretically, maximum relief is achieved by *bed rest* or *immobilisation in a wheelchair* or if the leg is *in traction*, when the foot should be without any load. But without such apparatus, the foot may be fully loaded on several occasions each day such as when visiting the toilet and other such events erroneously considered insignificant. The most efficient method is the *Total Contact Cast* (*TCC*) because it applies offloading and immobilising techniques in both, inpatient and outpatient settings, and must be worn in bed. In its irremovable version it is considered to be the gold standard of external offloading [1–3].

In the case of prevention, very few patients discard all their standard shoes after acquiring protective footwear. These shoes are usually retained because patients plan to wear them in future. **Uninterrupted use of voluntary protective measures is thus difficult to achieve** as in other areas of life. For example, measures of occupational safety are only enforced through monitoring and sanctions. Furthermore, people with DFS are asked to wear protection in every aspect of their life, even on occasion while sleeping or taking a shower. Exceedingly few people are able to consistently put this into practice.

Another difficulty for the patient's perception in dealing with the disease is the individual relatively low probability of recurrence, considering the number of occasions a patient may not wear his or her prescribed footwear. A patient presenting with three recurrences per year is thought to have an exceedingly high recurrence rate. However, no reactivation occurred in 99 out of 100 days, despite the fact that there were plenty of opportunities to develop new ulcers.

In view of these many uncertainties, there has been a call for intensified research into new interventions that target psychological and behavioural factors [4]. It may be appropriate however to consider surgical measures of internal offloading more frequently if the risk is acceptable.

19.2.2 Soft Padding

A *soft pad* between a firm prominence and a hard, supporting area offloads the immediate contact zone by involving adjacent areas. This is the way plantar soft tissue protects bony prominences. A soft insole in a shoe clings to the sole of the foot, enlarges the contact area and offloads the areas that had been originally the prominent part. Without such an insole less than 50% of the sole is in contact with the ground. This portion can be significantly extended with the insole resulting in a reduction of pressure above exposed parts.

A defect in the sole of the foot caused by pressure on a bony prominence completely changes the conditions. The bony prominence sinks into this defect. Soft padding leads to more subsidence of the prominence through the defect into the soft padding adding tensile load and pressure to the periphery of the defect. In other words, soft padding of a plantar pressure ulcer protects the prominence beneath the ulcer using the margin as support. It adds further load to the proliferation zone at the margin. As a single measure, therefore soft padding of the ulcer is not such a helpful approach.

19.2.3 Distant Padding

In contrast, measures to redistribute load to areas distant from the ulcer are very useful in the therapy of pressure ulcers. The redistribution needs a thoughtful approach and combines relatively firm material (supports) with recesses or inserts made of soft materials. A support is necessary to determine which part will carry the redistributed load and thus prevent transfer to vulnerable regions. Because weight cannot be eliminated but only redistributed, it is crucial to select sufficient resistant parts of the sole. This shift should not be left to chance, but firm material should determine precisely where the load should go.

19.2.4 No Circular Plantar Notches as a Sole Measure

Another frequently used but often unfavourable measure is a circular plantar recess as singular measure to offload plantar ulcers. In this case, the subsidence of the bony prominence causes tension at the wounds margins and may be unable to prevent its tip from touching the supporting area. Furthermore, interstitial fluids are kneaded towards the recess forming 'window oedema' (see Fig. 19.4). The third drawback of plantar circular recesses is the possibility of traumatising contacts with the distal border of the recess while sliding forward during gait. To avoid this drawback, the distal margin is sometimes tapered off, shaping the notch similar to a drop.

19.3 Immobilisation of Joints

Immobilisation of joints of the foot is a concept to consider distinct from pure offloading. Immobilisation focuses on preventing the movement of joints and thus preventing any leverage that might involve the articulating bones. For example, a soft shoe without stiffeners in combination with an insole may offload MTHs, but does not immobilise the MTP joints. Immobilisation of MTP joints using sole stiffeners, on the other hand, also provides offloading.

Immobilisation is often more invasive than mere offloading. A stiffened shoe, for example, may be perceived as heavy and as hampering movement. Furthermore, it is possible that avoiding exercise of the intrinsic muscles enhances their atrophy. **If immobilisation of joints is considered in addition to redistribution of load, a**

risk assessment must be performed for each patient. Overprotection by footwear is not only pointless and a waste of economic resources but compromises the use and therefore the efficacy of the footwear. Moreover, it causes the unused muscles to atrophy. Overprotection can therefore be harmful in many cases.

19.4 How to Build a Total Contact Cast (TCC)

The *Total Contact Cast* (*TCC*) in its irremovable version is considered to be the gold standard in immobilisation and external offloading of the diabetic foot [5]. It immobilises joints, has a stiff and moulded sole, and the wall bears a substantial part of the load [6].

Techniques in building a total contact cast vary widely. Common features of most of them are:

- Padding is applied at prominences considered vulnerable.
- The TCC ends some centimetre below the head of the fibular bone.
- Several materials are used, one of which becomes very stiff and splints the sole.
- A rocker bottom sole is strapped or foamed beneath the TCC and enables walking.

The main differences are whether the TCC:

- Can be removed and applied again by the patient *(Removable TCC*). For this purpose, slots are usually created that divide the TCC into two segments (*'bivalved TCC'*).
- Can be opened and closed only by the therapeutic team. These TCC's are often closed using a plaster bandage that has to be opened with a saw (*rendered irremovable TCC*).
- Is irremovable but allows access to the ulcer in order to change dressings (*windowed TCC*). The window may be situated in the weight-bearing area or in the non-weight-bearing part of the TCC. A TCC offering access through a ventral window but being otherwise irremovable, developed by the Cologne Network, has been named ventral windowed non-removable TCC or VW-TCC (see Fig. 19.2).
- Is planned to be used only once and is disposed afterwards. These in general can't be opened by the patient (*traditional TCC* or *standard TCC*).
- In the area of the toes only a sole is present (open) or a complete toe box (closed).

In addition to these, the so-called '*instant TCC (i-TCC)*' is described in the literature, in which prefabricated orthotics are closed with cable ties [7] or with a plaster bandage [1, 8, 9] and shouldn't be removed by the patient.

TCC's planned for multiple use are designed to be durable and can be applied for months or years, whilst the ones for single use are thin and light. In the construction of reusable models, *spacers* are placed upon the more delicate parts of the skin that are removed after opening the cast and leave a depression on the inner surface of the cast. This provides further protection against injuries.

The *toe box* is supposed to protect against the entrance of foreign bodies and against trauma. If it is omitted, the toes can be examined and warning signs of possible ischemia can be monitored. The toe box might itself exert pressure and cause ulcers. In techniques avoiding the patients access to limb, often an open toe box is preferred, and in removable versions the advantages of a toe box are often thought to prevail.

It is mandatory in many countries to obtain *informed consent* before starting treatment with a total contact cast (TCC). This cast restricts the patient's freedom. The patient must also be aware of the safety precautions to be taken when walking and driving. Risks such as injuries within the TCC and falls due to the use of a TCC must be known to the patient. The information should be given in a structured way, at best with written literature containing all the necessary elements for the patient to make a free decision.

For a specialised diabetic foot clinic it is very useful to have a cast technique at their disposal. The clinic may then use the gold standard without delay and diversify the technique in unusual circumstances, which might be anatomical conditions such as equinus deformity or deformities after amputations. Variations might also adapt to therapeutic necessities such as corrections of position or inclusion of a fixateur externe.

In the production process several skills have to be mastered:

- Cushioning: Correct cushioning and possible consequences of errors.
- Applying the cast material skilfully to create a smooth series of layers by manipulating the direction of the rolls.
- Stiffening of the ankle with special tracks in the form of a figure of eight around the heel similar to bandages supporting the ankle after sprains.
- Keeping track of the cast's thickness at every location. Shaping the cast according to the foot and the lower limb.
- Define the optimal cutting lines to open the cast.
- Handling of the saw and the scissors to open the cast.
- Masking the edges and patching flaws.

These suggestions should facilitate learning:

- If possible, visit a course to learn the technique.
- As many of these techniques as possible can be practiced beforehand using elastic bandages or applying a 'cotton wool boot' (Fig. 21.10).
- Choose a certain day to apply the first cast and purchase all the necessary material.
- Practice the technique on a 'model' some days before with a tutor for several hours intensively.

Necessary **instruments** for the majority of these techniques are:

- One pair of scissors to cut unhardened cast material (cheapest version is sufficient)
- One pair of scissors to cut cushioning material and adhesive tapes (The scissors have to be sharp. The cheapest version is sufficient)

- Small trestle to support the upper part of the leg
- Spray bottle to wet the cast
- Marker to trace the cutting lines
- Oscillating saw
- Small and large scissors for slicing the cast

The **material** used differs widely due to technique and preferences. Here is an example of the technique preferred by some of the authors:

- 5 mm thick, self-adherent felt to cushion delicate parts
- 2 cm thick open-pored foam material to cushion the toe box
- Adhesive tape to stabilise cushioning and mask uneven parts
- Towelling tubular bandage that will be the inner surface of the TCC
- Flat fiberglass casting material large 12.5 cm to stiffen the sole
- Plaster bandages made from polyester large 7.5 cm to be applied to the foot
- Plaster bandages made from polyester large 10 cm to be applied to the lower leg
- Shrink film 10 cm wide is to be used after wetting the cast to distribute the humidity, to enhance the attachment of the layers and to smooth the surface which would otherwise be relatively rough.
- Hook and loop fastener (Velcro), one of both should be self-adherent
- Rocker bottom soles in different sizes

Steps applying a TCC (Fig. 19.1):

1. Firstly, a compress is placed between the toes to ensure sufficient minimum width of the toe box.
2. Then spacers are placed at the malleoli, at the anterior tibial crest, at the tibialis anterior tendon and its transition onto the foot.
3. Two layers of spacers are placed above the area of the ulcer that shall be offloaded in a stricter manner. If the TCC is applied to treat a Charcot Foot without ulcers, this step might be omitted. (Fig. 19.1a)
4. Cotton wool is applied in one or two layers starting with the toes. At the toes five layers are applied one above the other. This measure is also meant to ensure a minimum space for the toe box. (Fig. 19.1b)
5. Now the towelling tubular bandage is pulled over the cotton wool layer. This soft terry cloth material will represent the inner lining of the TCC. Everything between the leg and the towelling tubular bandage will later be removed and is needed to ensure sufficient distance between leg and cast material.
6. On the towelling tubular bandage other cushions are applied that will provide a soft inner surface in critical parts. In the area of the toe box this is achieved by using open-pored foam 2 cm thick. In other parts such as the malleoli, the shin-bone, the calcaneus and the sole this is achieved by 5 mm of felt (Fig. 19.1c). The sole is cushioned with one layer of felt if it is intended to immobilise a Charcot Foot and with three layers containing cut-outs in two of them if ulcers need a redistribution of load. These cut-outs correspond exactly to the spacers allied beforehand on the ulcer areas.

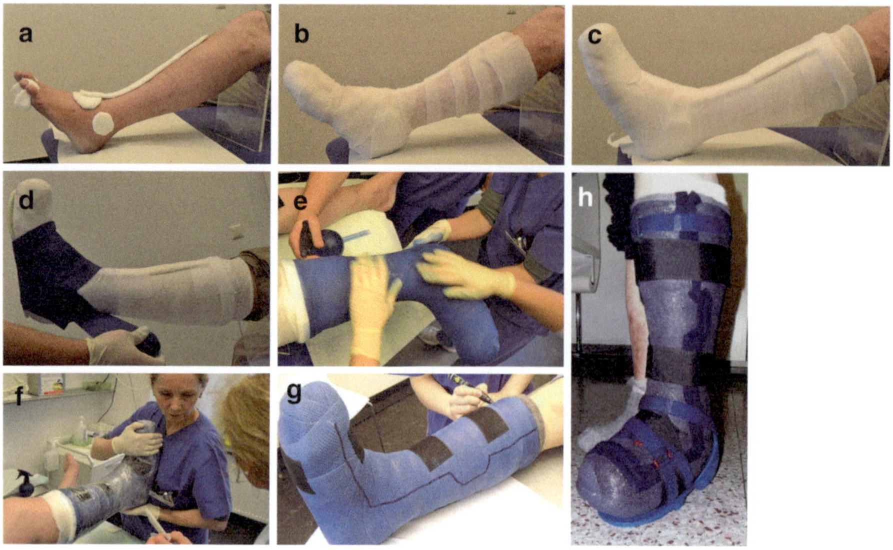

Fig. 19.1 Applying a TCC (**a**) spacers below the cotton wool, both intended as spacers removed later (**b**) apply cotton wool (**c**) cushioning on the towelling tubular bandage (**d**) the first bandage applied as a figure eight around the heel (**e**) wetting the cast (**f**) shaping the TCC (**g**) marked lines of cutting (**h**) TCC closed

7. The cushioning material is fixed by adhesive tape applied under slight tension. This is also useful to level out uneven areas. Larger gaps are filled with felt beforehand. This step is important as the inner layers of the cast material will swell and enter in these gaps. Later, this will result in lumps and bumps on the inner surface of the cast.
8. To protect the therapist, gloves and protective clothing are used. The sole is cut out of a flat fiberglass casting material and initially fixed onto the foot with the first plaster bandage large 7.5 cm. This first bandage is used for the heel that is wrapped by several layers wound in a figure of eight (Fig. 19.1d).
9. The initial part of the 2nd bandage is used to produce five layers applied one over the other to form a dome as a toe box. This bandage is intended to complete the cast at the forefoot.
10. Another 4–8 bandages are used depending on height, weight and the assumed distances the patient may walk.
11. The TCC is sprayed with water so that it is entirely soaked (Fig. 19.1e).
12. The self-adhesive Velcro straps are applied.
13. Shrink film (normally used for packaging) is wound tightly around the TCC.
14. The TCC is shaped, especially at the plantar area and between Achilles tendon and the malleoli (Fig. 19.1f).
15. After about 10 min the TCC is firm enough to maintain its shape if not compressed. After about 20 min the patient can be transported in a wheelchair.

16. To be cut by the oscillating saw, the TCC has to be inelastic and hardened. Ideally, it is only cut open on the 2nd day. Sometimes, this is not possible due to organisational issues.
17. The lines of cutting are drawn in such a way that the front shell results slightly smaller than the rear shell and the patient is able to enter or leave the rear shell easily (Fig. 19.1g). Then the rigid materials are cut with the saw, the soft parts with the scissors and the margins of the two shells are masked with special cushioning tapes (Fig. 19.1h).

The patient must not move the ankle while the plaster bandages are applied. If movement occurs, creases develop that must be milled away tediously. If the patient is unable to hold the leg firmly, an assistant must help him or her to keep the foot in its position.

Each time the TCC is opened, the inner surface must be checked for protruding edges. The cushioning materials shrink under stress, so that uneven parts previously covered can become exposed over time. During each visit, the TCC must be checked not only for new edges, but also to ensure a precise fit at the lower leg.

According to published research, patients wear walkers that can be opened and removed (RCW), only for a fraction of the steps made [10]. This is associated with delayed wound closure, so the authors of this study recommend a non-removable TCC or walker. In the opinion of the authors of this book, such behaviour is closely related to healthcare professional to patient *communication*. A statement such as: '*You should wear this TCC day and night, in bed and while taking a bath or shower*', is easy to understand and unequivocal. A statement such as *'If you are sitting in front of the TV you might take the TCC off'* gives the patient choice. It might not be erroneous from a mechanical point of view but destroys the clarity of the instruction and should be avoided. It is difficult for patients to imagine what devastating consequences a 'small mistake' could have. Therefore, individual team members should make great efforts to avoid ambiguous communication.

Guidelines call for knee-high, non-removable offloading devices [11]. For practical reasons this device must also permit wound care. One possibility is to fabricate the TCC anew each time the dressing is changed. However, if the patient cannot come to the outpatient foot clinic for every change of dressing, a community nurse must have access to the wound, but patients should not be able to take off the device themselves. One possibility is to use cable ties or similar methods for the closure. Some patients, understandably do not accept such an obviously disciplinary measure.

Windows in the loaded area have been preferred by some, but do not work particularly well in the view of the authors. The inlay can tilt and exert pressure. The edges of the window can also exert pressure and liquids can penetrate even faster than would otherwise.

An appropriate possibility is to divide the front shell into two halves to produce a **irremovable bivalved TCC** (Fig. 19.2). The distal half can be removed and the foot can be pulled out of the TCC for 10–15 cm. Dressings can be changed and the integrity of

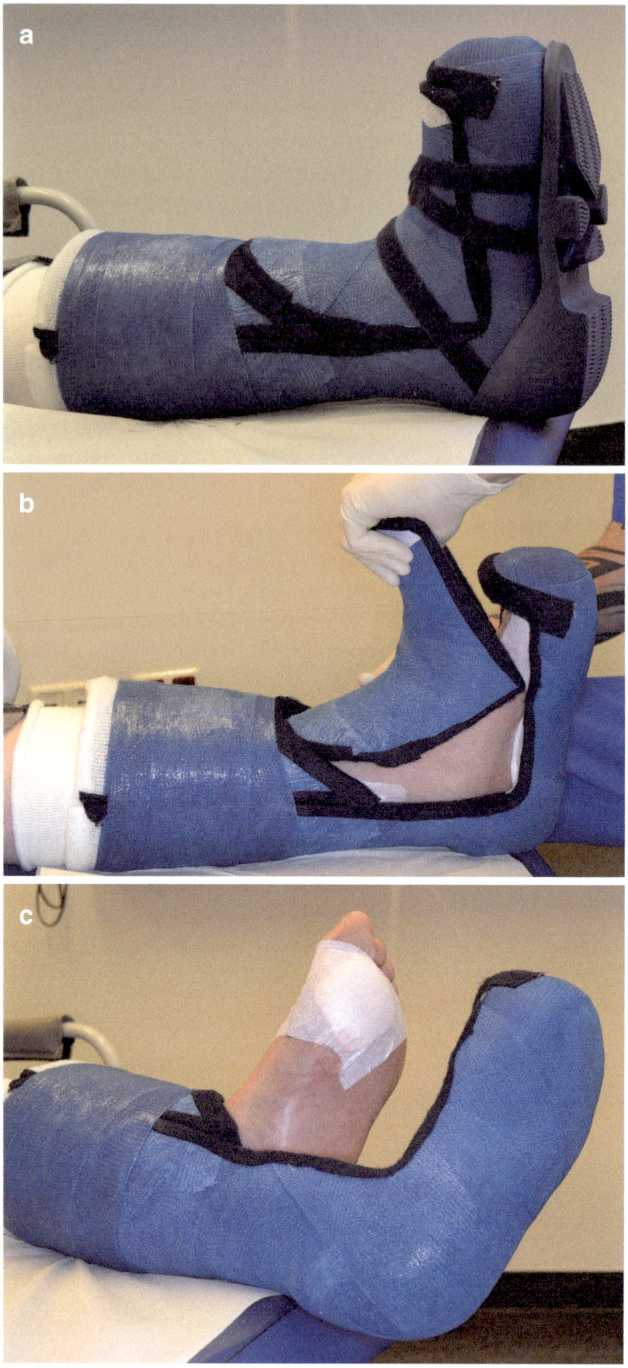

Fig. 19.2 (**a**) Ventrally windowed, non-removable TCC (VW-TCC) with (**b**) distal part of the anterior shell removable (**c**) permitting access also to plantar or heel ulcers

skin and TCC can be checked. Since the padding is regularly reworked, it does not lose its pressure redistributing properties. This technique is not feasible with a completely atrophic calf. The proximal end of the frontal cup needs more padding than usual in the area of the tibia, as it is exposed to greater pressure. If easy access to the heel is required, the incision lines run in a slightly more dorsal plane than usual. In this case, the dorsal shell becomes slimmer and must be reinforced. The technique was developed by the Cologne network and was called a 'ventrally windowed, non-removable TCC' or '**VW-TCC**'.

A TCC or walker may lengthen the leg by 3–4 cm. For this reason, it is generally necessary to **raise the sole of the contralateral shoe**. In general, **walking aids** such as crutches have to be provided even if the patient is highly reliant on them only in the initial phase.

19.4.1 Bed-Cast

Flexible cast material might be used in combination with a rigid, L-shaped splint to build a lighter version of the cast. This can be used to offload the heel in bed. Frequently used terms are '*bedcast*' and '*flexcast*'. The material can be cut with scissors so that no special saw is needed. The toe box is usually omitted. Soft pads and spacers are used to protect the region of the ulcer, the malleoli and the heel. The spacers are removed later and leave a depression in the inner surface of the cast. The cushions between the towelling tubular bandage and cast uses soft material such as felt to cover the stiff sole and to protect the malleoli (Figs. 19.3 and 19.4).

19.5 Offloading by Distant Padding within a Dressing

An individually cushioned dressing has the advantage of providing offloading that is independent from the patients' behaviour. It is attached to the foot and it remains there day and night. The added height is limited. So normally there is no needed for compensation at the contralateral foot and walking stability is preserved. Some basic rules have, however, to be considered when these pads are applied:

1. Distant padding by use of spacer pads redistributes the load to slightly more distant parts which are able to withstand it. Only the most suitable places in the area are selected to be involved in additional load-bearing with materials such as felt.
2. Adaptability: The foot is not a rigid block to step on but adapts to the contact surface. A cutout in the sole to relieve a prominence means that the prominence dips into the cutout and the edge of the cutout provides the support. This may have several adverse effects: (1) It prolongs and increases the pressure on this area during gait. (2) The soft tissue covering the prominence is stretched and thus becomes thinner and less resistant. (3) It generates pressure peaks on the margin. These damaging effects are greater the larger the recess is and the deeper the

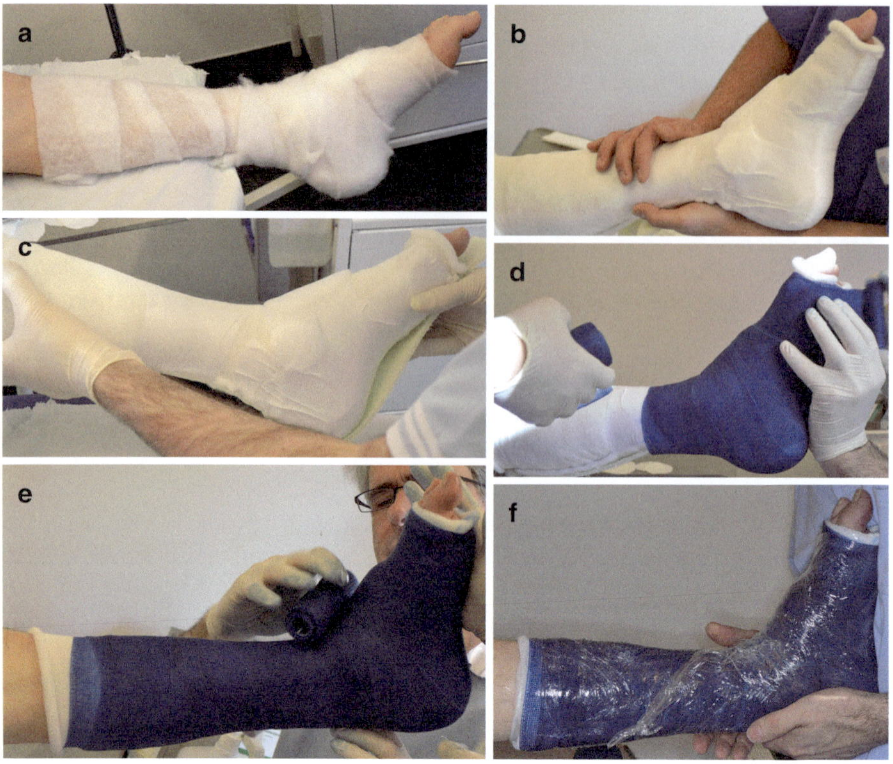

Fig. 19.3 Manufacturing a bed cast. (**a**) Spacers at the heel and the malleoli (**b**) towelling tubular bandage with protective inlays (**c**) splint made from rigid cast material (**d**, **e**) flexible material is applied (**f**) wetting and shaping

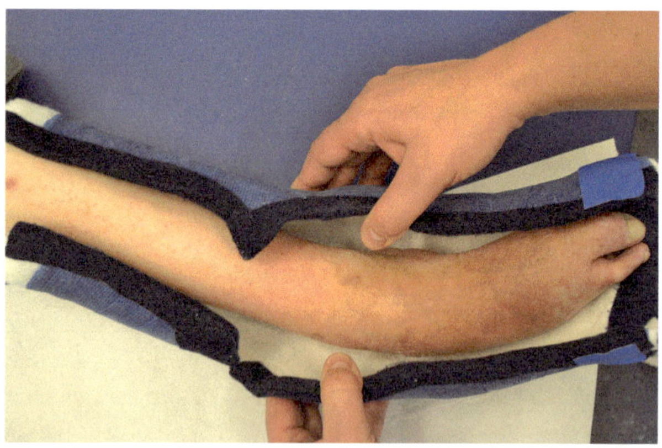

Fig. 19.4 Bed cast for a patient with repetitive ulcers at the heel and at the lateral margin of the foot

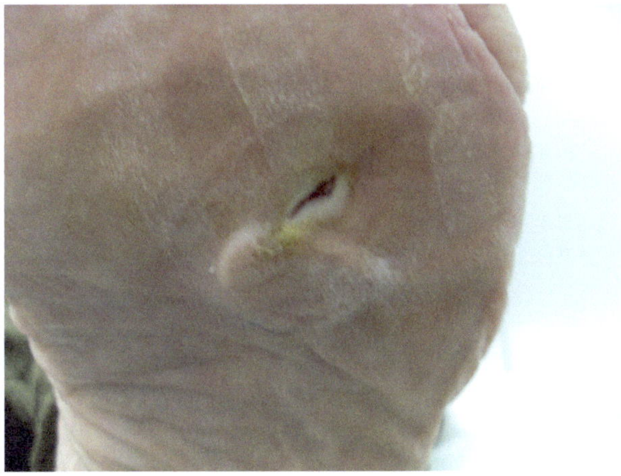

Fig. 19.5 Risks using plantar cushion: (1) window oedema in case of circular pad and (2) displacement of the pad

prominence can sink. To avoid this, **a recess should be kept small** and the edge of the recess should be reinforced at a suitable location to compensate for the loss of support within the recess. As a rule, a recess should never be the only functional principle, but **should be accompanied by adequate support** at a suitable location.

3. On the other hand, the foot's adaptability might be used for the benefit of the patient: **targeted pronation or supination** can help to reduce load. Thus, an elevation of the outer margin of the foot leads to more pronation and distribution of the load away from the elevation towards the inner margin. A support of the medial arch does the opposite.
4. **Window oedema**: A simple circular cushion to offload an ulcer in the weight-bearing area facilitates the development of oedematous tissue filling the space inside the circle. This worsens the conditions needed for ulcer repair. The bone causing the prominence should therefore be supported, instead of using circular cushions (Fig. 19.5).

Many pitfalls are possible using cushioning material. Good education of all partners is needed, but is a good investment of time.

19.5.1 Techniques of Remote Padding

Some techniques are commonly used to offload prominences by remote padding. They are typically combined to achieve sufficient pressure relieve without overloading another region. The concepts are identical, whether they are used in insoles or integrated into dressings:

1. *Retrocapital Support*: In this case, a pad in the shape of a drop or a transverse bar is placed immediately proximal to the MTH. The less flexible the metatarsals are, the larger this support has to be, ranging from some centimetre to the

entire width of the sole. Produced in felt the height is of about 10 mm shrinking to 3–5 mm after some hours of use (Fig. 19.6). This element elevates the MTH and is used to offload it.

2. *Toe Balcony*: Toes which are able to bear load are elevated and thus enabled to sustain weight better (Fig. 19.7). This isn't possible in the case of clawed toes

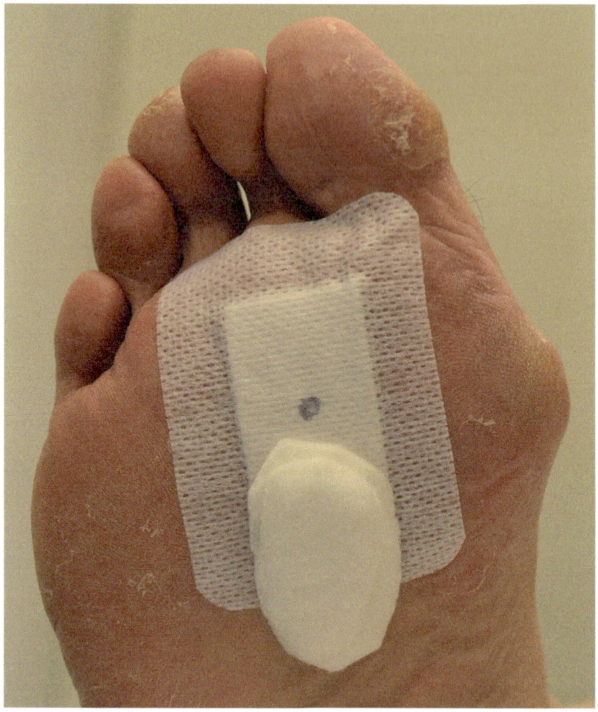

Fig. 19.6 Retrocapital support

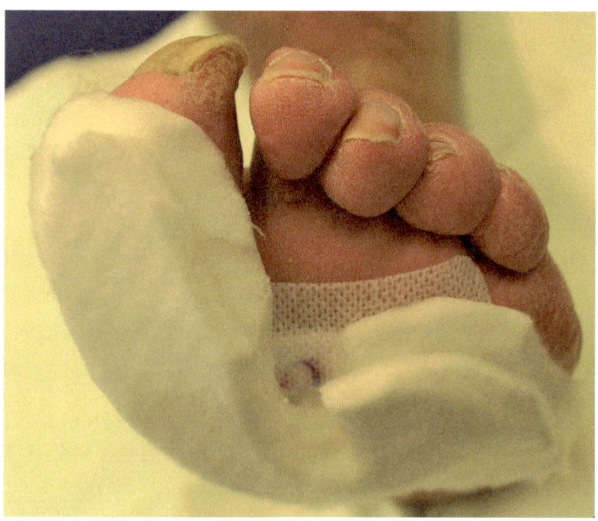

Fig. 19.7 'Toe balcony' beneath the hallux

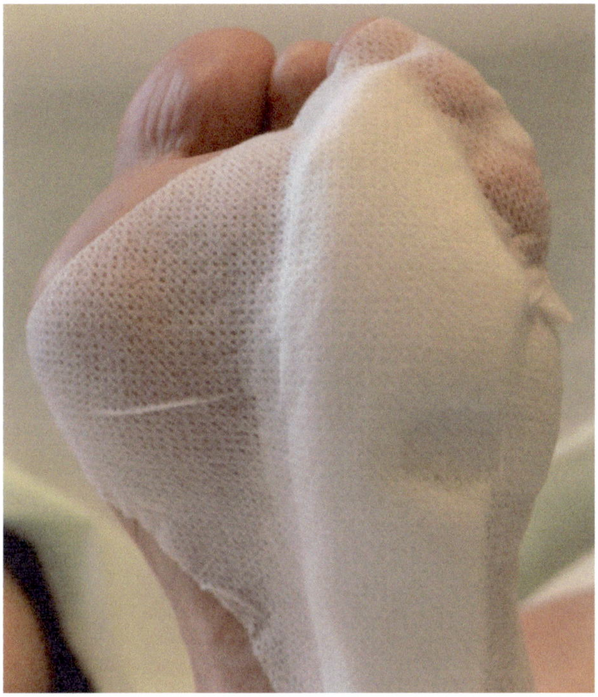

Fig. 19.8 Outer margin elevation combined with retrocapital support in case of an ulcer below the 5th MTH

because they are not able to bear weight. It is a measure often particularly effective when it supports the hallux.

3. *Outer Margin Elevation*: This pad elevates the 5th and to a lesser extent the 4th metatarsal bone by placing 5–10 mm of felt beneath these bones (Fig. 19.8). See also Chap. 14 for a step-by-step tutorial concerning the 4th or 5th MTH (Fig. 14.16a–f).
4. *Diagonal elevation of the outer margin*: This technique reduces load on the 5th MTK by lowering the first ray. The forefoot pronates, the foot plate unlocks and the foot becomes less rigid. To test the reaction of the foot to such an approach, the Coleman Bloc Test is useful. It should be especially considered when observing signs of overload on MTK 1 and 5 contemporarily (step-by-step tutorial in Chap. 14, Fig. 14.15a–l) (Fig. 19.9).
5. *Medial Arch Support*: The medial arch is covered with layers of felt of 20 mm or more in such a manner that the medial column is elevated (step-by-step tutorial in Chap. 14, Fig. 14.7a–n) (Fig. 19.10). This is useful in several entities concerning the first and 2nd ray (1, 3, 5 and 13).
6. *Medial and lateral Spacers*: Spacers can be placed to guarantee a certain distance between ulcers at the medial or the lateral outline of the foot and the shoe's inner lining. Made of relatively soft felt they should be 5–10 mm thick

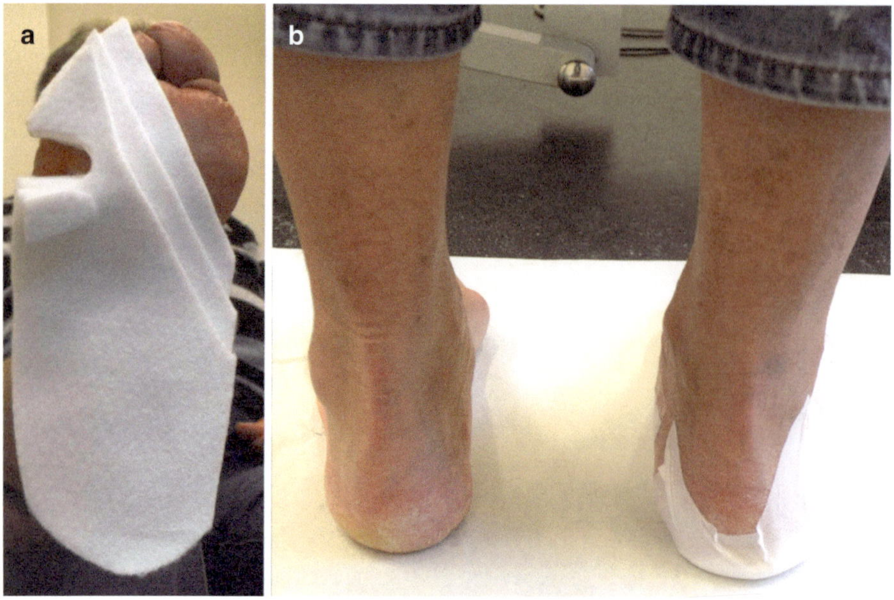

Fig. 19.9 (**a**) Diagonal elevation of the outer margin. This might be used to offload the first MTH and the 5th MTH. (**b**) It everts the heel and pronates the forefoot

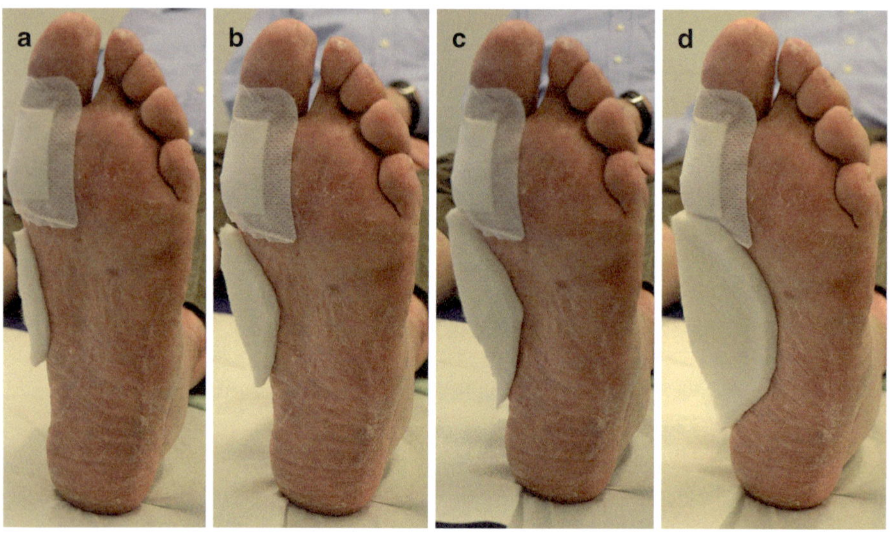

Fig. 19.10 (**a–d**) Support of the medial longitudinal arch

that may shrink to 3–5 mm when used. These cushions can provide one- (Fig. 19.11) or preferably two-point-support (Fig. 19.12). Spacers are used to protect prominences at the joints of the first or 5th MTH or at the base of the 5th

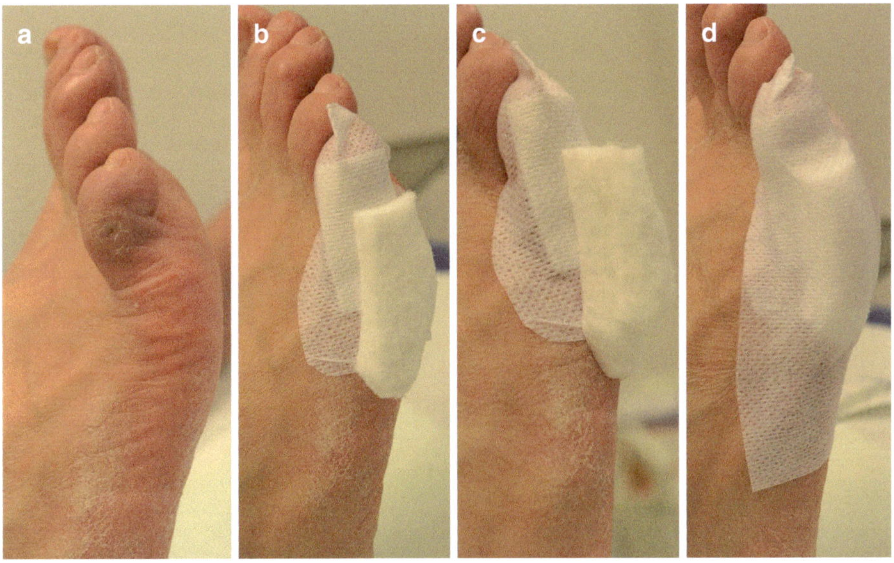

Fig. 19.11 (**a**–**d**) Protection of the 5th toe for lateral pressure by one support

Fig. 19.12 Spacer at the base of the 5th metatarsal using 2-point support

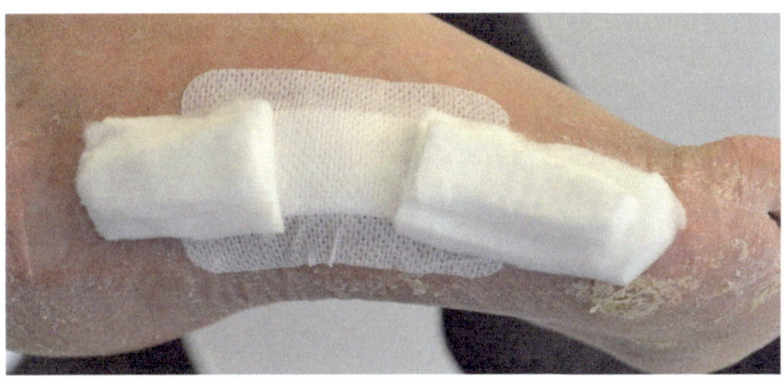

metatarsal and their prominences in non-weight-bearing areas described in chapters on entities 4, 10, 11, 12, 19 and 20. Spacers might also be used in unusual lesions (Fig. 19.13).

7. *Flexion fold spacer:* This is placed in the plantar part of clawed toes to straighten them and to elevate the toe in order to protect the tip of the toe. For this purpose, a strip 15–20 mm wide and 50–100 mm long of felt 5 mm thick is cut, rolled up and placed into the flexion fold of the clawed toe. The tip of the clawed toe should not touch the ground (Fig. 19.14). This spacer might be used in lesions of the tips of the toes (see chapter on entity 1 or 2).
8. *Instep spacer* is a spacer to protect the dorsal surface of the IP joints of the toes. To achieve secure distance it is necessary to avoid any contact with the shoe's upper. This is the case using four layers or more 5 mm each, which results in 7–10 mm in use (Fig. 19.15). People with neuropathy and critical PAD must not wear tight shoes. The spacers could compress the soft tissue and produce necro-

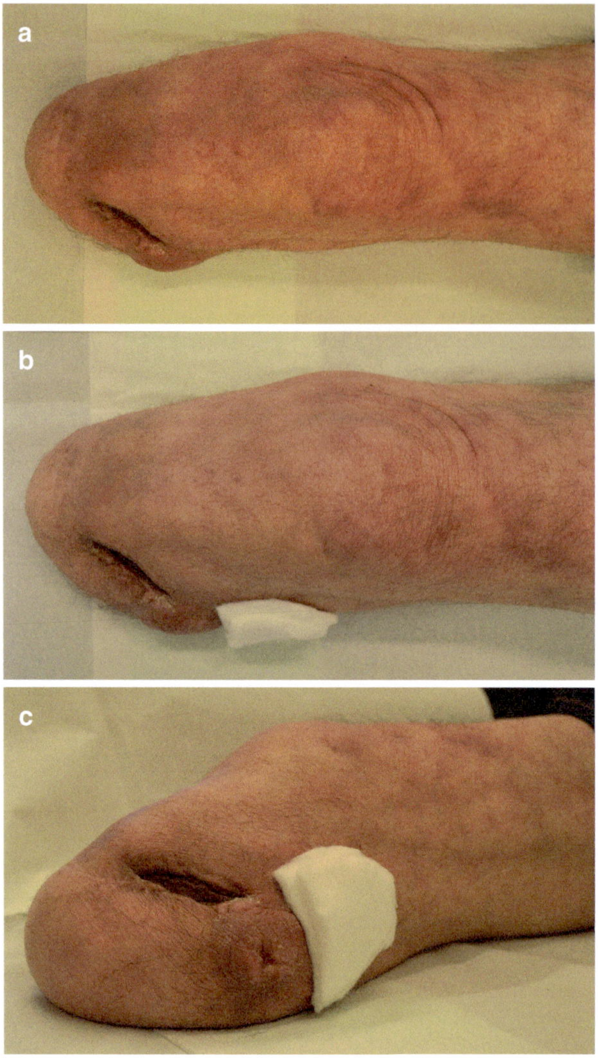

Fig. 19.13 (**a**–**c**) Spacer to offload an ulcer of the stump in a prosthesis, uninterruptedly used

sis if the patients with neuropathy don't use adequately wide shoes. For example, it would be extremely damaging to force the cushioned feet into the same shoes that had been the cause of the ulcer itself. The entities 7 and 8 profit from this type of protection.

9. *Coulisse cushion* for the space between Achilles tendon and malleoli: Felt 5–10 mm high fills this area (regio calcaneo-malleolaris) in such a way that a) compression also reaches these regions and b) extreme pressure exerted on the top of the malleoli is avoided (Fig. 19.16). This cushion is useful to treat and prevent lesions of this region and the top of the malleoli (entity 15 and 16).

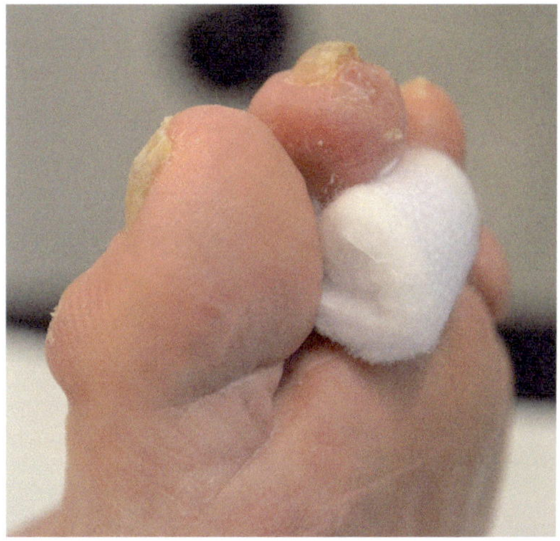

Fig. 19.14 Flexion fold spacer

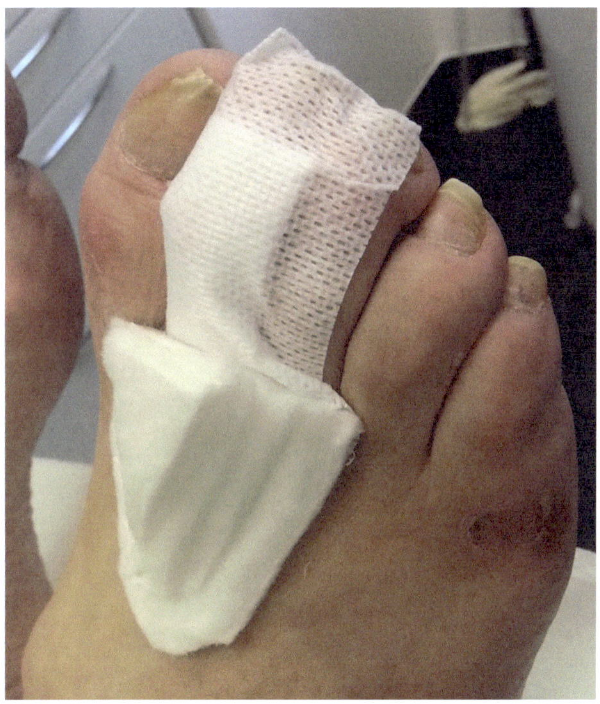

Fig. 19.15 Instep spacer

10. *Protection of the Tibialis-anterior tendon* (Fig. 19.17) avoids trauma of the tissue above the tendon. Its use is necessary in the case of very prominent tendons and warning signs such as redness.
11. *Calcaneal cushion*: The calcaneal tuberosity (entity 17) might be protected using a circular cushion made of felt with central window (Fig. 19.18). This is

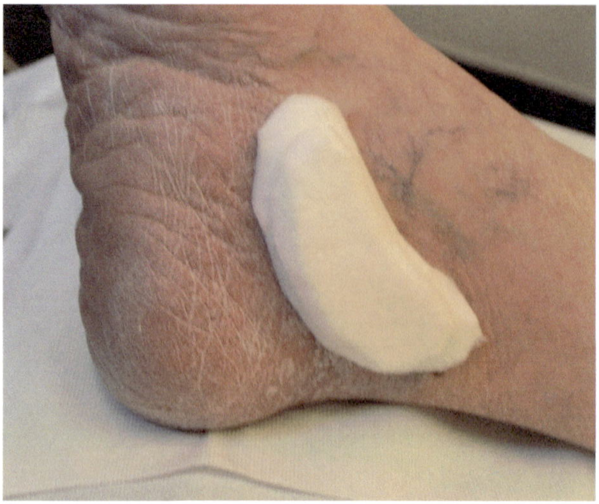

Fig. 19.16 Cushioning of the area between Achilles tendon and malleoli

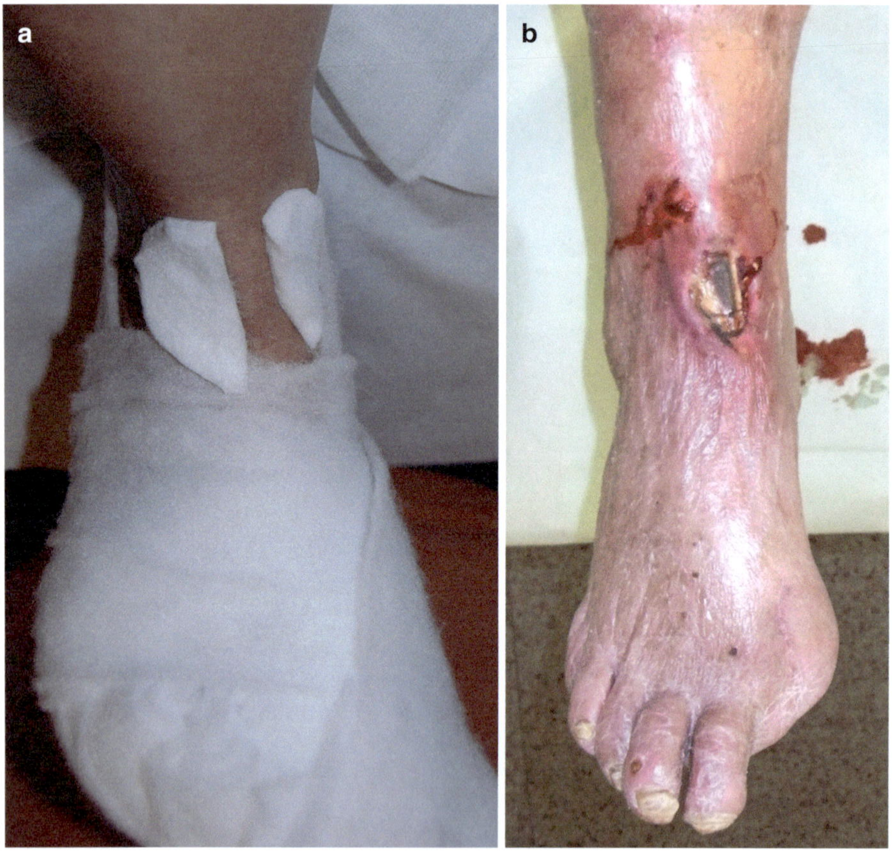

Fig. 19.17 (**a**) Pads to protect the tibialis anterior tendon. (**b**) Lesion due to compression bandages used to treat oedema

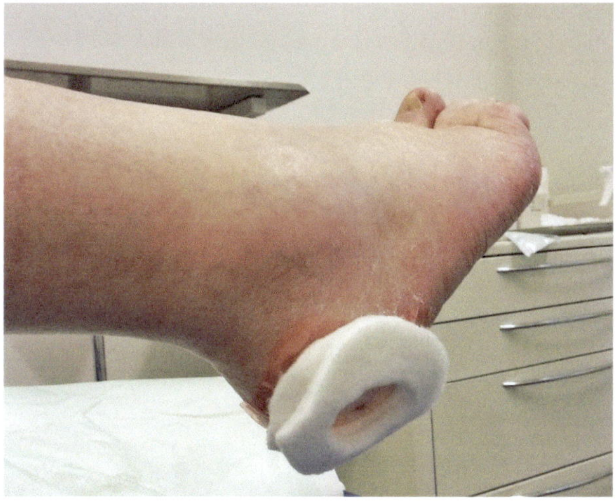

Fig. 19.18 Protection of the calcaneal tuberosity

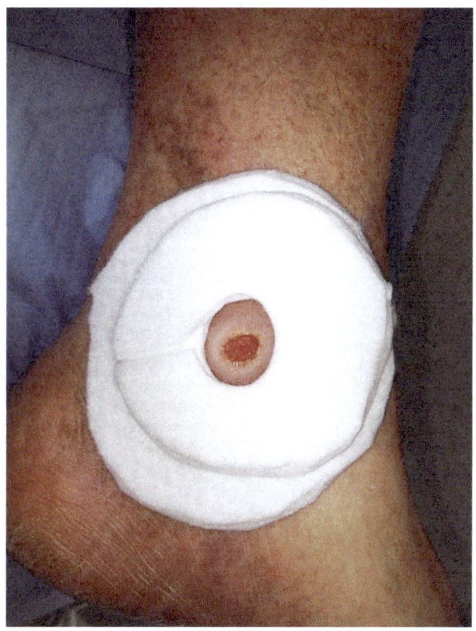

Fig. 19.19 Ankle protection

considerably less effective than more complex devices, but may provide minimum protection for patients who are mobile and feel clumsy wearing these devices.

12. *Ankle Protection*: Ulcers on top of the malleoli (entity 15) might be protected against the impact of collisions by rings of felt 10–15 mm high (Fig. 19.19).
13. *Hallux condyle pad* : The medial aspect of the bones forming the first IP joint might develop a prominent part (entity 3), that can be accommodated by a small but very effective pad (Fig. 19.20).

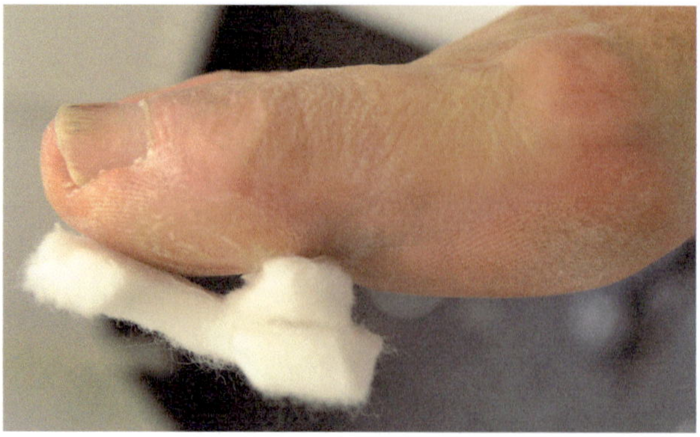

Fig. 19.20 Condyle pad to protect the first IP-joint

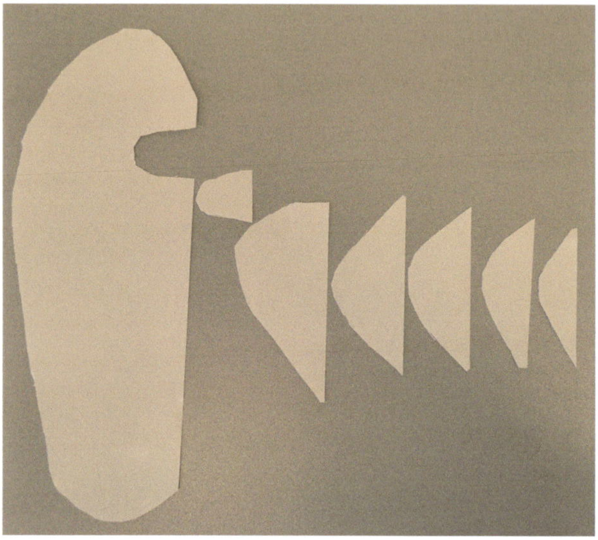

Fig. 19.21 Cutting patterns to help with the correct production of the pads. These samples are given to the patient accompanied by a detailed description

19.5.2 Preparation of Spacer Pads

After covering the ulcer with an adhesive dressing to avoid displacement later on, the cushion is applied and fixed. The plastic foil, that protected the adhesive surface of the felt, can be handed over to the patient as a template. At home, the shape of this template can be reproduced on the felt using a marker (Fig. 19.21). *Edges* in the weight-bearing areas are bevelled if it is intended to create a smooth transition from sustained areas to adjacent parts. If *more than one layer* is used, the smaller parts are used for the layers distant to the skin if this doesn't compromise the shape of the cushion. Edges at the margins of the sole do not need to be bevelled.

It's not always simple to create a cutout at exactly the right position. There are at least two possibilities to achieve correct placement. Marking with a lipstick is useful in this and other situations (Fig. 19.22). For this purpose, the ulcer is covered as usual and a mark of lipstick is placed on the dressing. To avoid contamination of the lipstick, a piece of lipstick can be cut off with the scalpel and applied. The foot is then placed in an offloading device and the area to offload is marked on the insole. For the purpose of remote cushioning by felt, it might be a quicker approach to place the nail of the left index finger on the area to offload (in case of lefthanders the right index finger). The felt is then held firmly between the index and the thumb in exactly the area to be cut away. The felt can be rotated until it has a position in which it can be cut easily (Figs. 19.23 and 19.24).

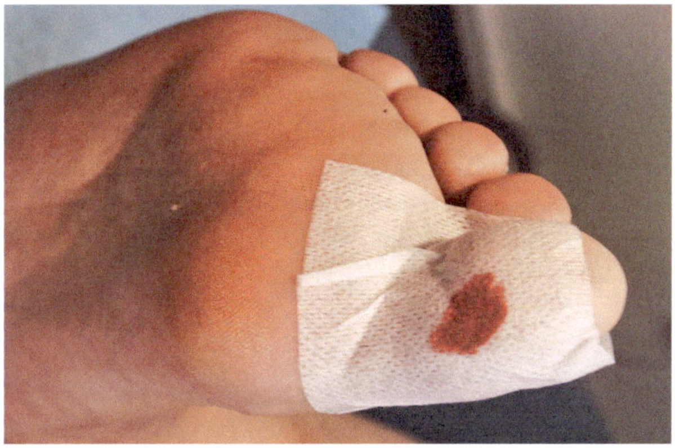

Fig. 19.22 Labelling with a lipstick

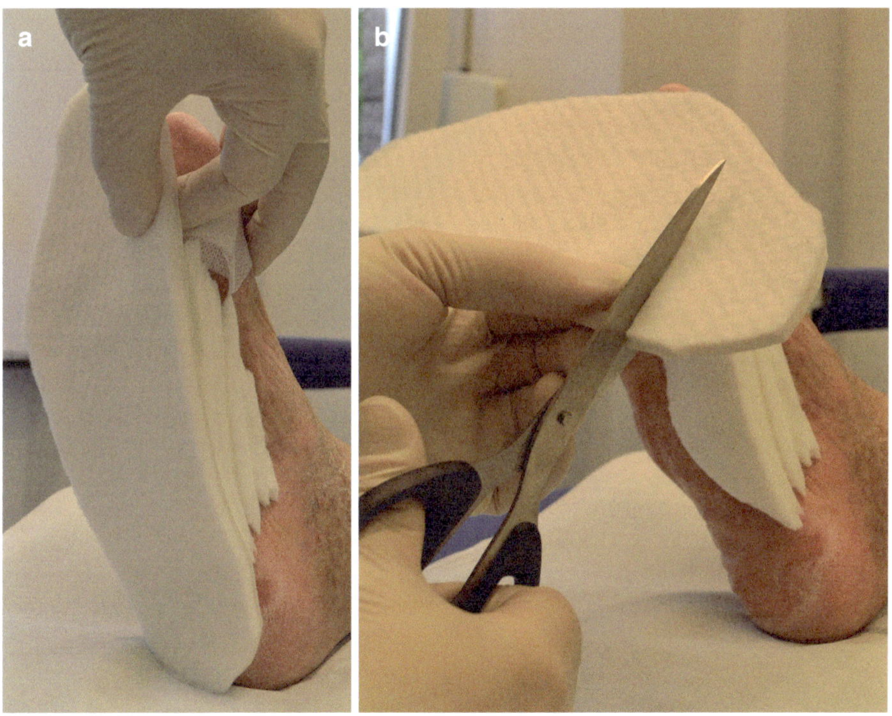

Fig. 19.23 Labelling the area to be removed and creating a cutout

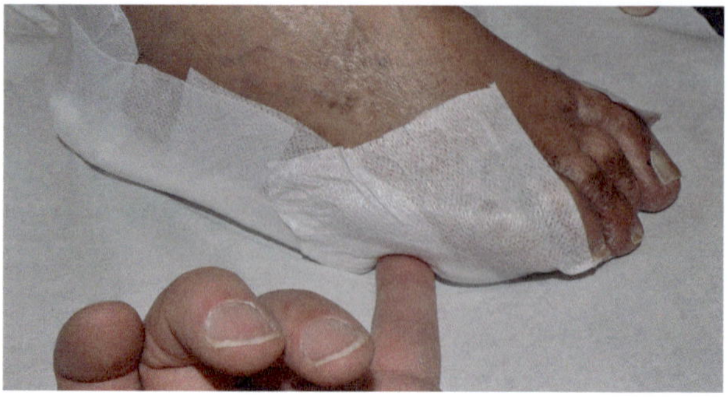

Fig. 19.24 Test of the efficacy of a diagonal elevation of the outer margin to offload the 5th MTH

The effect of the spacer varies depending on the properties of the spacer, its position, the flexibility of the foot and other factors such as the patient's weight. Therefore, it is necessary to test the effectiveness of the offloading construction in use. In addition to expensive pedobarographic plates, a simple test with the examiner's little finger is usually sufficient.

19.6 Selection of Prefabricated Devices

The choice is based on expediency, availability, usability and price. The purpose might be to offload an ulcer as much as possible or it may be the immobilisation of the joints of the foot, for example in case of a Charcot Foot.

Proof of efficacy of a device to offload plantar ulcers relies on measures made with pressure sensitive insoles. A range of devices are available [12, 13]. Ready-made shoes have been compared to orthopaedic footwear, half shoes, therapeutic shoes, *Removable Cam Walkers* (RCW), non-removable Walkers (e.g. instant Total Contact Cast (iTCC)) and non-removable TCC [14].

Published studies, looking at the degree of offloading provided by devices, have shown that the reduction in peak foot pressure is related to a reduction of the time to complete wound closure. The better the offloading works, the better the ulcer repair [15].

Usability dictates whether the patient can cope with his or her everyday life using the device. Factors of importance are the level of mobility required, the risk of falling, the speed at which the device can be applied and the overall ease of use. Uninterrupted use of the device depends on its usability, at least as long as it is removable.

Published research also shows a correlation between the proportion of time a device is used and the time needed to reach remission. The less a device is used, the longer it takes to close an ulcer [10].

Compared to a removable TCC, offloading (expressed in percentage of foot pressure reduction) provided by a Removable Cam Walkers is only slightly inferior [7]. And so if it is not possible for the patient to remove the walker, differences in ulcer repair compared to a non-removable TCC are very small [16, 17].

From a practical point of view, an important advantage of the TCC is that a TCC can be adapted to unconventional situations. These might be deformities, amputations, deformity of a limb, necessary corrections of position, or the integration of an external fixator for example. However, training should be done on less complex cases, and it should be ensured that full competency is attained prior to working with more complex pathology.

19.6.1 Groups of Devices

Some countries have a register of approved devices providing a long list of definitions, indications and descriptions but there is no international standard. In the following sections some of the most commonly used devices are described.

19.6.1.1 Surgical Shoe or Post-operative Shoe

Surgical or *post-operative shoes* are shoes that are so spacious that they can accommodate the foot along with any associated bandages and spacers. They protect against mechanical damage and dirt. In general, they lack an appropriate insole and don't offload. These shoes are thought best for people with reduced mobility when an exact match to the sole of the foot isn't needed and dressings together with the bandages are sufficient to achieve this goal. It is important to inform the patient that once they become more mobile these devices should not be considered as shoes without adding a different more appropriate insole (Fig. 19.25).

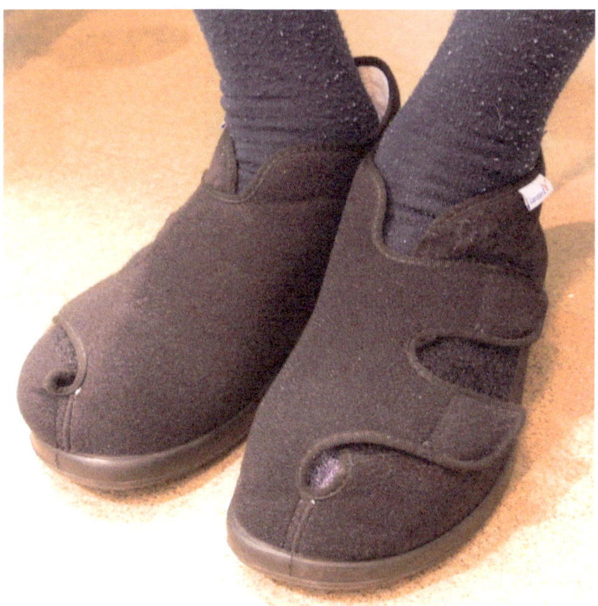

Fig. 19.25 Example of a surgical shoe

19.6.1.2 Therapeutic Shoe

Besides being appropriately roomy, therapeutic shoes also try to redistribute weight.

Therapeutic shoes for diabetic feet usually feature stiffened soles and rockers. They have insoles that should be supplied together with the shoe and cut individually or are manufactured by the orthotist (Fig. 19.26).

Partial sole shoes (*half shoes, wedge shoes)*, such as *forefoot offloading shoes* and *rearfoot offloading shoes* have been the standard devices for offloading neuropathic plantar ulcers during the latter part of the twentieth century. In recent years, they have been used less frequently for people with loss of protective sensation. When the patient is walking, forefoot offloading shoes should be used such that the affected foot is always placed in front of the healthy foot. The resulting small steps allow mobilisation for short distances only. Scuff marks often seen at the anterior edge of these shoes show that instead of offloading, there has been maximum loading because people have tried to walk normally and have placed the healthy foot in front of the diseased one. Moreover, the use of certain models has even been reported to precipitate the development of an acute Charcot foot. Rearfoot offloading shoes may lead to enlargement of an ulcer in an adjacent region in contact with the edge of the device. The authors use this kind of shoe only in exceptional cases.

19.6.1.3 Walkers

Walkers are devices which resemble total contact casts but without the need for a healthcare professional to master casting technique. They have therefore also been referred to as ***i**nstant **T**otal **C**ontact **C**asts (iTCC)* if rendered irremovable using cable ties or a casting tape and ***R**emovable **C**am **W**alkers (RCW)* if not. To adapt to the shape of the lower leg different methods are used to minimise in cast movement and achieve immobilisation (Fig. 19.27).

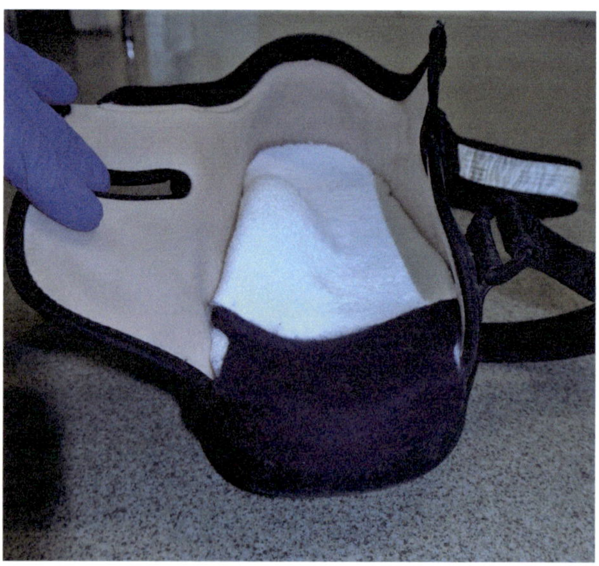

Fig. 19.26 Example of an individualised therapeutic shoe

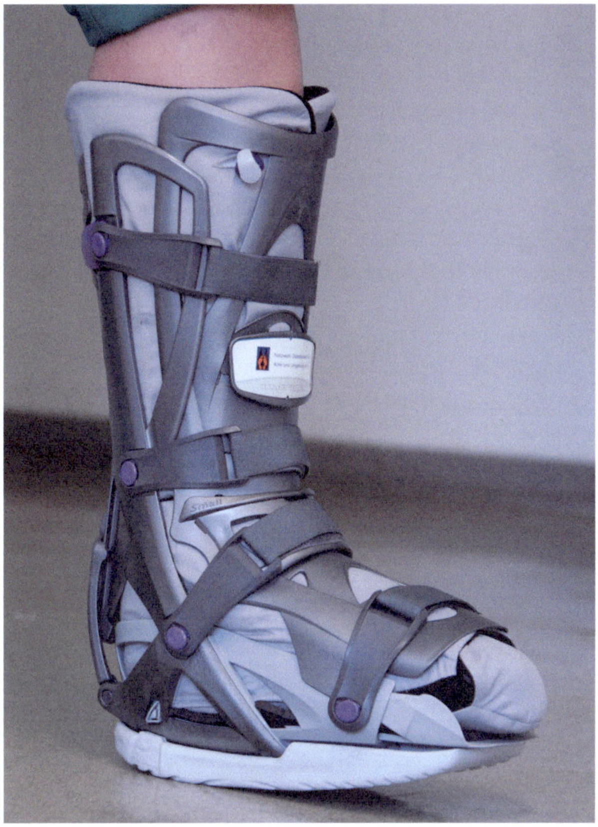

Fig. 19.27 Example of a Walker

19.7 Elements of Protective Footwear

The relationship of trust between the foot clinic and the shoemaker or orthotist is of the utmost importance given the complex clinical picture often seen with patients with DFUs. In different countries professional education and consultation style vary. These consultation styles universally try, however, to avoid collusion without blocking the desired aim to provide the best result for an individual patient.

Protective footwear for people with DFS combines supportive elements where needed with soft material wherever possible. The shoe is held firmly to the foot in two particular areas. Proximal to the MTH's, the foot becomes slimmer offering a sort of waist to hold shoes firmly to the foot. Strap fittings found on sandals as well as shoe-laces use this narrow part. The heel, however, appears similar to a sphere that can also be used to hold the foot. Using both areas, the shoe is held between instep, sole and heel. Pressure on the toes has to be avoided and therefore the toes must not be used to hold the shoe in place. Moreover, the toe cap has to be straight in the hallux area and must not push it laterally. Rigid materials aren't appropriate in the proximity of the toes and leather has to be particularly soft in this region [18].

Healthy footwear respecting the needs of the foot (Fig. 19.28) must fulfil certain criteria:

- The toe box must be sufficiently high and wide. It is rarely too high or wide. The part of the shoe that is used to prevent the foot from slipping forward must not restrict the toes but should fix the foot at the instep.
- The length of the shoe is sufficient if the space between the longest toe and the toe cap is the same size as the thumb of the patient. The minimum tolerance for propulsion of the foot in the shoe is about half the size of the patients thumb or 10–12 mm (1).
- It is important that sufficient width is available in the area of the MTH's and the toes. The width should not, however, be too great and should not allow lateral movements of the foot in the shoe (2).

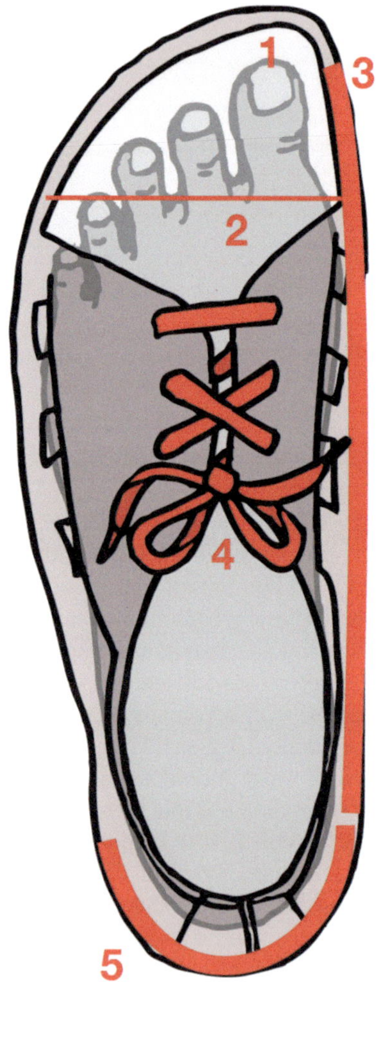

Fig. 19.28 Healthy footwear that respects the foot) must fulfil certain criteria

- The shape of the shoe has to accommodate the great toe's necessity to be directed straight forward and must not push the great toe laterally into a pointed shape. The medial part of the toe box should therefore be straight (3). The shape of the shoe hugs the shape of the foot. An insole adapted to the anatomy of the sole of the foot distributes the load evenly to a larger surface than a flat one.
- The shoe must be held in place between instep, heel and sole. Control of the position is achieved with the use of lacing or Velcro strips on the instep (4).
- The heel should be in tight contact with the shoe.
- The heel cap should be sturdy and softly padded (5).
- The heel spring should be of maximum 3.5 cm.
- The sole should allow for an unhampered gait cycle. Both the heel and the sole should be made of shock absorbing material.
- The upper should be made completely of breathable material that allows for a good internal climate. The materials must not contain PCP, Chrome 6, azo dyes or formaldehyde.

In some countries, a simple shoe made specifically for people with diabetes fulfilling these criteria is available in a prefabricated form with standard measures in width and length [19, 20].

A **customised shoe** is made using a last that has been customised according the shape and functional impairment of the foot of the patient. Such a last is not just a simple reproduction of the foot but should be able to create a shoe that is able to fit the changing shape of the foot during each phase of the gait cycle. This can be summed up by the sentence 'The shoe has to be tolerant, more than it has to be precise' (orthopaedic shoemaker Peter Brümmer, Cologne).

All types of shoes can be equipped with a curved sole ('*rocker bottom sole*' or '*roller*'). These soles are thicker than normal soles beneath the rear- and midfoot and become gradually thinner distal to the part of the sole that has to be offloaded. The curved shape brings about two features: firstly, it avoids some of the dorsiflexion of the MTP joints at heel-off. As a result, less dorsiflexion is required which is equivalent to a patial immobilisation. This helps to offload the MTHs. Secondly, part of the load exerted in front of the curve is converted into a torque which offloads this structure.

A ***sole stiffener*** leads to a rigid sole that can follow the movement of the foot during gait only if a curved 'rocker bottom sole' is added. The axis of this curve is oriented in the direction of walking (angle of abduction) and not along the axis of the shoe (Fig. 19.29). The central part is usually curved less which results in an almost flat surface beneath the midfoot. This is important for a secure stance. The more distal the start of the curved part of the sole is placed, the more secure the stance is. In addition, the more the proximal parts are curved, the easier it is to transit in the heel-off phase of the gait cycle and to move on. The orthotist should adjust the position and depth of the curved part of the sole in accordance with the walking and standing habits of the patient.

The *spring* describes how much the heel is higher than the ball of the foot in a shoe. Given the high frequency of a shortening of the calf muscles, a spring of a few

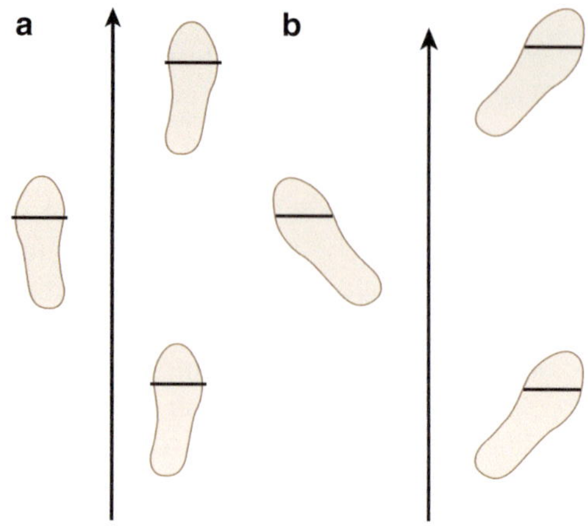

Fig. 19.29 Position of the axis of a rocker bottom sole

centimetres is often useful. If the spring becomes too high, which is sometimes the wish of some patients, the rear foot may not be retained in position and the foot slides forwards within the shoe. The elevation of the tip of the shoe in respect to the part below the MTH's is the toe spring.

An *arthrodesis cap* is a stiff part of the shoe reaching from the heelcap to the lower leg covering the ankle joint. It can only be used if the shoe shank reaches above the level of the ankle. It should help to avoid mobility in the ankle. This is often needed in inactive Charcot feet.

Standards and names of insoles vary. In its simplest form it may just be a flat, foam rubber material, sturdier in the heel region than in the forefoot region, whilst a more elaborate insole may consist of several layers of different hardness with a moulded surface. Insoles may be 'off the shelf' or, preferably for more complex cases, created for an individual with an increasing variety of techniques including 3 D printing.

Any type of insole could be placed in any type of shoe, but some combinations are not suitable. An insole could be elaborately manufactured and combine materials to support and relieve the foot in specific areas but will only work if the sole of the shoe is stiff and the position and shape of the foot does not change too much. The stiffened sole needs to have a rocker. The result may be a rigid, heavy and bulky shoe that may not be acceptable to the patient. This is not only because of design issues but also because walking may have become more difficult. For these reasons, very good offloading shoes may not be regularly worn by all patients. Compromises may thus be required; a shoe with less offloading is produced, but which is more acceptable to the patient, where the insole is less complex and the sole is more flexible perhaps and slightly curved. The resulting shoe will have more normal mechanical properties, weight and appearance. If more regularly worn, despite having slightly less offloading potential, then ultimately it could be more effective.

19.8 Summary

- **A life with DFS should be undisturbed by the disease as much as possible, and this should include continued mobility.**
- **This is best achieved by load redistribution which is the cornerstone for the prevention and treatment of the vast majority of cases of DFS.**
- **Load redistribution can be accompanied by joint immobilisation, if needed.**
- **Overprotection has to be avoided.**
- **It is important not only to study and teach these techniques, but also to create better methods to combine offloading standards with individual needs and ease of use for patients and providers.**

References

1. Armstrong DG, Lavery LA, Wu S, Boulton AJ. Evaluation of removable and irremovable cast walkers in the healing of diabetic foot wounds: a randomized controlled trial. Diabetes Care. 2005;28(3):551–4.
2. Lavery LA, Higgins KR, La Fontaine J, Zamorano RG, Constantinides GP, Kim PJ. Randomised clinical trial to compare total contact casts, healing sandals and a shear-reducing removable boot to heal diabetic foot ulcers. Int Wound J. 2015;12(6):710–5. https://doi.org/10.1111/iwj.12213.
3. Wu SC, Jensen JL, Weber AK, Robinson DE, Armstrong DG. Use of pressure offloading devices in diabetic foot ulcers: do we practice what we preach? Diabetes Care. 2008;31(11):2118–9. https://doi.org/10.2337/dc08-0771.
4. NICE. Diabetic foot problems: prevention and management; 2 Research recommendations. 2015. https://www.nice.org.uk/guidance/ng19/chapter/2-Research-recommendations. Accessed 27 Mar 2018.
5. Burnett O. Total contact cast. Clin Podiatr Med Surg. 1987;4(2):471–9.
6. Begg L, McLaughlin P, Vicaretti M, Fletcher J, Burns J. Total contact cast wall load in patients with a plantar forefoot ulcer and diabetes. J Foot Ankle Res. 2016;9:2. https://doi.org/10.1186/s13047-015-0119-0.
7. Piaggesi A, Macchiarini S, Rizzo L, Palumbo F, Tedeschi A, Nobili LA, Leporati E, Scire V, Teobaldi I, Del Prato S. An off-the-shelf instant contact casting device for the management of diabetic foot ulcers: a randomized prospective trial versus traditional fiberglass cast. Diabetes Care. 2007;30(3):586–90. https://doi.org/10.2337/dc06-1750.
8. Armstrong DG, Short B, Espensen EH, Abu-Rumman PL, Nixon BP, Boulton AJ. Technique for fabrication of an "instant total-contact cast" for treatment of neuropathic diabetic foot ulcers. J Am Podiatr Med Assoc. 2002;92(7):405–8.
9. Katz IA, Harlan A, Miranda-Palma B, Prieto-Sanchez L, Armstrong DG, Bowker JH, Mizel MS, Boulton AJ. A randomized trial of two irremovable off-loading devices in the management of plantar neuropathic diabetic foot ulcers. Diabetes Care. 2005;28(3):555–9.
10. Armstrong DG, Lavery LA, Kimbriel HR, Nixon BP, Boulton AJ. Activity patterns of patients with diabetic foot ulceration: patients with active ulceration may not adhere to a standard pressure off-loading regimen. Diabetes Care. 2003;26(9):2595–7.

11. Bus SA, van Deursen RW, Armstrong DG, Lewis JE, Caravaggi CF, Cavanagh PR, Foot International Working Group on the Diabetic. Footwear and offloading interventions to prevent and heal foot ulcers and reduce plantar pressure in patients with diabetes: a systematic review. Diabetes Metab Res Rev. 2016;32(Suppl 1):99–118. https://doi.org/10.1002/dmrr.2702.
12. Koller A, Kersken J. Hilfsmittel beim Diabetischen Fußsyndrom. Total Contact Cast und Orthesen. Orthopädie-Technik. 2013;7:1–6.
13. Morbach S, Müller E, Reike H, Risse A, Rümenapf G, Spraul M. Diabetisches Fußsyndrom. Diabetologie und Stoffwechsel. 2009;4(S 02):S157–65. https://doi.org/10.1055/s-0029-1224580.
14. Bus SA, Valk GD, van Deursen RW, Armstrong DG, Caravaggi C, Hlavacek P, Bakker K, Cavanagh PR. The effectiveness of footwear and offloading interventions to prevent and heal foot ulcers and reduce plantar pressure in diabetes: a systematic review. Diabetes Metab Res Rev. 2008;24(Suppl 1):S162–80. https://doi.org/10.1002/dmrr.850.
15. Armstrong DG, Lavery LA, Bushman TR. Peak foot pressures influence the healing time of diabetic foot ulcers treated with total contact casts. J Rehabil Res Dev. 1998;35(1):1–5.
16. Gutekunst DJ, Hastings MK, Bohnert KL, Strube MJ, Sinacore DR. Removable cast walker boots yield greater forefoot off-loading than total contact casts. Clin Biomech (Bristol, Avon). 2011;26(6):649–54. https://doi.org/10.1016/j.clinbiomech.2011.03.010.
17. Waaijman R, Keukenkamp R, de Haart M, Polomski WP, Nollet F, Bus SA. Adherence to wearing prescription custom-made footwear in patients with diabetes at high risk for plantar foot ulceration. Diabetes Care. 2013;36(6):1613–8. https://doi.org/10.2337/dc12-1330.
18. Tovey FI. The manufacture of diabetic footwear. Diabet Med. 1984;1(1):69–71.
19. Busch K, Chantelau E. Effectiveness of a new brand of stock 'diabetic' shoes to protect against diabetic foot ulcer relapse. A prospective cohort study. Diabet Med. 2003;20(8):665–9.
20. Uccioli L, Faglia E, Monticone G, Favales F, Durola L, Aldeghi A, Quarantiello A, Calia P, Menzinger G. Manufactured shoes in the prevention of diabetic foot ulcers. Diabetes Care. 1995;18(10):1376–8.

Internal Offloading 20

Internal offloading uses surgical measures to redistribute load or to change the position of inner pressure points. Some measures additionally remove damaged tissues or close wounds primarily.

The techniques in question have been developed to prevent pain caused by excessive stress. Some minor changes need to be made when using these techniques to treat people with reduced pain perception who develop ulcers. In general, this means to reduce the complexity of the surgical technique to core elements and to intensify aftercare if offloading is essential.

The methods proposed have been selected on the basis of the authors' personal experience. Their major benefits are assumed to be the prevention of amputations, recurrences and long recovery times alongside the associated consequences for patients and society. At present, these often simple but extremely effective procedures are rarely used.

Basic concepts and well-tried procedures are described in this chapter. In the chapters concerning the entities, these procedures are mentioned and explained in general terms in order to understand their indication and potential benefits regarding this particular entity. In this chapter, the whole procedure is described including relevant practical aspects. This should help when first using these techniques or when comparing alternative proceedings.

Surgical procedures that are not intended to reduce pressure on areas of the foot, such as amputation techniques, are not included in this chapter.

20.1 Overview

Deformities promote the development of foot ulcers. Acquired deformities are common because pronounced sensitive neuropathy is often associated with motor neuropathy, which is a major cause of acquired foot deformities. In rare cases, there may be congenital deformities as well.

D. Hochlenert et al., *Diabetic Foot Syndrome*,
https://doi.org/10.1007/978-3-319-92055-9_20

Limited joint mobility may also increase pressure. Unimpaired walking requires a flexible foot and joint stiffness automatically triggers unwanted forces.

Deformities as well as limited joint mobility increase pressure on osseous protuberances acting as hypomochlion (anatomical fulcrum, pivot point). The skin covering them is tightened and has to withstand transversal and vertical stress. If this stress exceeds resistance, tissue damage will occur.

If adequate nociceptive sensation exists, repeated overload causes pain. Compensation then is achieved by limping and other attempts to offload the overstressed parts. Foot and Ankle Surgeons have developed strategies to compensate for these painful impairments. Simultaneous neuropathies reduce the sensation of pain, stress is not avoided, and ulcers may occur. **Ulcers are the equivalent of pain in patients who do not feel pain**. The surgical strategies used to relieve pressure are essentially the same. However, instead of restoring the foot to its normal and thus painless state as far as possible, they aim to restore the damage-free function of the foot. In order to fulfil this task, less complex interventions are usually required. Nevertheless, since the main indicator for functional surgery is missing from the traditional point of view, this possibility is still largely overlooked.

Corrective interventions and protective footwear complement each other. The advantages of internal offloading are patient comfort and the uninterrupted presence of the offloading principle. After surgery, footwear might be changed from massive and obstructive protective shoes to less effective offloading which may be better integrated into a more normal life.

The benefit of internal offloading is self-evident, if it is used to prevent pain. Its use for prevention and therapy of diabetic foot ulcers instead is thought to require *external evidence* because the competing external offloading has been intensively investigated.

Studies investigating the benefits of surgical procedures used in the field of DFS often do not go beyond the level of case series. In particular, there is often no control group. For many procedures, the published case series are not focused on pressure relief in neuropathic patients, but have been performed to offload painful conditions in non-neuropathic patients. The review performed by the IWGDF 2015 revealed no conclusive evidence for or against surgical strategies in controlled trials [1]. Case series were not included as part of this review. There are several reasons for this lack of evidence. Firstly, the techniques are in continuous and rapid evolution because their use to prevent or close ulcers has only recently become widely known. Their rapid evolution makes it difficult to design long-term, randomised controlled studies meaningfully. Secondly, there is a cultural difference between surgical and medical disciplines. Standardisation of procedures and the conduct of proper controlled trials are essential for diabetologists in order to evaluate methods to prevent complications of diabetes. In the past, diabetologists had to face the problem that widespread drug therapy had to be abandoned after having proven ineffective or even harmful in large, multicentre controlled trials (RCTs). Surgeons become more directly aware of the impact of their efforts. They also vary their techniques based on personal experience. This makes it difficult to standardise procedures, to conduct multicentre studies and to learn from the result of a study. For example, it

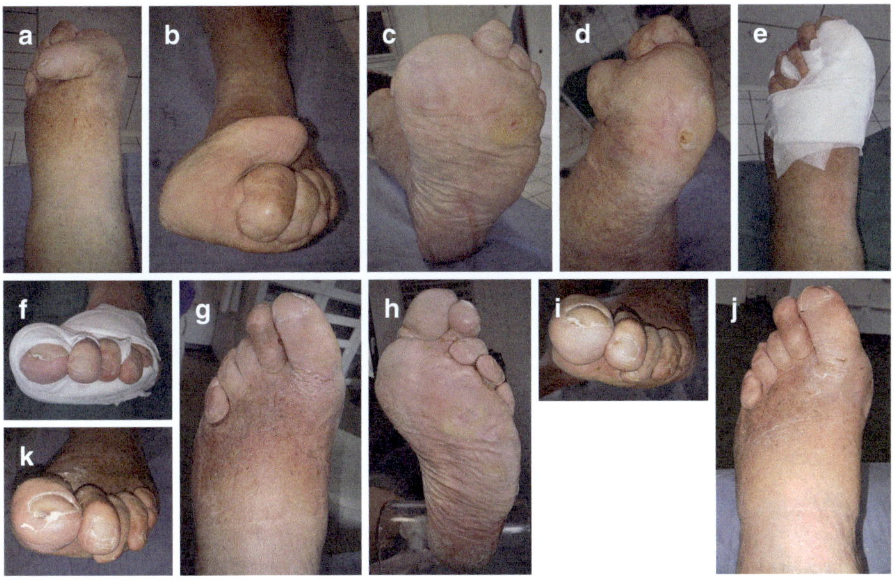

Fig. 20.1 Potential of minimally invasive surgery using only a cannula for blood sampling: (**a–d**) preoperative picture; (**e–f**) postoperative picture after tenotomy of the FHL-tendon, the extensor tendons (EHL and EHB) and a dorsal release of the 2nd MTP joint as well as tenotomy of the FDL- and FDB tendons of the 2nd toe in percutaneous technique (**g–i**) 7th day and (**j–k**) 4 weeks post-op

would be questionable whether the effect of a tenotomy of the long flexor tendon being performed on the 2nd toe could be transferred to tenotomies of the 5th toe. Or would results of openly performed operations be transferable to transcutaneously performed operations and vice versa?

Since the advantages of surgery exceed the risk in case series by far, and the personal experience of the authors is so convincing, they have made these procedures a part of the daily routine. **It may be recommended to consider their use at least when amputations are the alternative method and after recurrences that indicate a high risk of future amputations.** An argument in favour of using surgery at an early stage would be to prevent evolution to a state where amputation becomes unavoidable.

The wider use of surgery can be one key issue in the struggle to reduce the burden of the disease for people with DFS and for society (Fig. 20.1).

Missing this opportunity leads to a situation in which the number of amputations at the foot is high and has been increasing in many countries for decades. The alternatives are considered too dangerous, even though their worst complication would be precisely this amputation. As a consequence, there are two barriers to overcome: Firstly, surgeons have to be convinced to operate on people who don't complain of pain and to operate them even if wounds and diabetes are in place. Secondly, diabetologists tend to believe that the methods have not been tested well enough and are unfamiliar with their benefits.

Some methods require less blood supply than others. People with greater mobility need different measures than those who take only a few steps a day. Under certain circumstances time may be the most important factor. This is the case in patients with endocardial foreign material or valvular heart disease because this condition might be complicated by life-threatening endocarditis in patients with recurrent bacteraemia as a result of wounds in weight-bearing areas. In other situations, the need for rapid reintegration into working life may be the major concern.

The indication for surgery and the choice of the best method which is less invasive, but still functionally sufficient, needs to integrate information on biomechanical aspects, perfusion, desired mobility, implanted material, socioeconomic issues and general conditions.

These interventions must be integrated in an interdisciplinary, interprofessional and intersectoral strategy of shared care. Within a network of shared care, the surgeon has a key function by extending the treatment options to avoid amputations, to avoid hospital stays, to avoid recurrence and to accelerate wound closure which might be important in order to retain employment [2, 3].

Research and Professional education in this field are crucial in order to treat the enormous number of people in need. Aiming to apply internal offloading to the vast majority of these patients, the techniques used must be highly acceptable to them.

Minimally invasive techniques are also acceptable for people with important limitations. They therefore have decisive advantages in terms of acceptance, usability and benefits.

Surgeons who are dedicated to these patients should master minimally invasive methods and apply them to the vast majority. In several countries, the associations of foot and ankle surgeons have started to embrace this opportunity.

20.2 Special Aspects of Surgery Intended to Offload a Diabetic Foot

Many interventions can be done in an outpatient setting. In the case of adequate blood supply and controlled glucose metabolism, case series show complication rates no higher than those expected for people without diabetes [3, 4]. In general, local anaesthesia such as conductive anaesthesia (ankle block) is sufficient. An exception to this rule might be interventions in cases of severe infections requiring general anaesthesia or spinal anaesthesia. **Minimally invasive techniques** are often a good alternative to open surgery, especially in outpatient clinics. It is of great advantage if surgeons with a focus on the treatment of people with DFS are experienced in these techniques. Expensive equipment is required only for some of the interventions on bones or other procedures done in highly specialised centres. Needle tenotomies are amongst the most popular minimally invasive techniques and do not require any special equipment.

The indication is often seen as an alternative to conservative procedures, if these do not achieve adequate offloading. The decision to proceed to surgery should not be postponed because offloading devices are not being worn. This delay would result in continuing to go through endless loops of admonitions and failure. In finding the indication, '*optimised footwear*' means that there are no biomechanical flaws in the footwear that could be addressed, and every useful element is integrated.

In general, the **indication** is seen if an 'indicator lesion' occurs in an area where the intended intervention may reduce load.

An 'Indicator lesion' is

1. **a preulcerative lesion that recurs in optimised footwear or**
2. **an ulcer at a site which is not sufficiently offloaded in optimised offloading device or prognostically will not be sufficiently offloaded in optimised footwear after wound closure or**
3. **amputation is discussed as a possible therapy for this ulcer.**

'Optimised footwear/device' means that it is flawless from a biomechanical point of view and every useful element has been integrated. Optimising the patients attitude towards the footwear/device is NOT intended.

The interventions are regularly carried out **without blood arrest** because this is difficult to achieve due to medial arterial sclerosis and is not strictly necessary.

In general, the offloading device used before the intervention continues to be used, maybe after minor changes have been made.

The **suturing technique** to close an incision layer by layer may differ from procedures commonly applied in aseptic surgery. In interventions on the diabetic foot, the use of resorbable material for subcutaneous sutures is often be avoided. Resorbable material, which is covered by more superficial layers sutured one by one, would represent a foreign body for many weeks postoperatively. This would favour infections of the bacterially contaminated tissue and could not be removed without opening the whole site. The subcutaneous structures including joint capsules and muscle fasciae are adapted with non-absorbable suture material instead. These sutures start and end above the level of the skin. In this way, all foreign

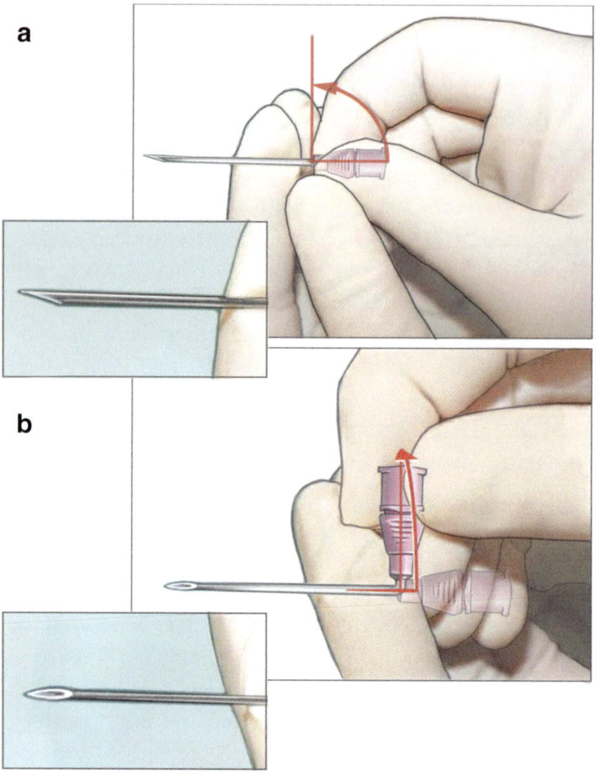

Fig. 20.2 The cannula is bent at the distal end (near the Luer-Lock) in such a way that the surgeon knows in which plane the cutting side of the grinded tip is located. Figure by kind permission of: Engels, G., H. Stinus, D. Hochlenert, and A. Klein. 2016. [Concept of plantarisation for toe correction in diabetic foot syndrome]. Oper Orthop Traumatol 28(5):323–334. doi:10.1007/s00064-016-0453-9

material will be removed on a regular basis. This removal can easily be anticipated if necessary.

It may be necessary to consider whether **anticoagulants or platelet aggregation inhibitors (PAI)** should be discontinued or not. This depends mainly on the possibility to mechanically compress the surgical site after the procedure and the trauma caused by the procedure. However, other factors may influence the decision: the possible consequences of a disruption of the preventive measures, the emotional impact this risk has on the patient, the surgeon's personal experience and practical issues. For most of the tenotomies performed by the authors, PAI is continued. Concerning coagulation, the aim is to control INR in such a way that anticoagulation is borderline insufficient by disrupting for some days. Other more traumatic interventions may require discontinuing the medication.

About a third of the patients have some degree of impairment of blood supply to the foot. Sufficient blood supply is crucial for a good outcome from surgical therapy. If necessary, revascularisation must be performed before corrective surgery. These considerations should be integrated in finding the best option for the patient: A) It must be born in mind that the some of the targeted structures such as superficial tendons are parsimoniously perfused and easy accessed. B) If the alternative is to leave it as it is: Many minimally invasive procedures require less additional blood supply than the ongoing traumas to the ulcer. C) If the alternative is amputation: A vascular disease may not justify the preference of an amputation at the foot over an inner offloading, since the necessary additional blood supply required is generally more intensive after amputation due to the more traumatic procedure.

Surgery is not generally contraindicated in people with impaired circulation, but requires careful and individual consideration.

In minimally invasive, transcutaneous techniques to sever tendons or to release contracted capsules, often a **simple blood sampling cannula** is used. This cannula is bent to mark the direction, in which the tip of the cannula is grinded (Fig. 20.2).

20.3 Perioperative Risks

Patients must understand the possible complications and other conditions that might complicate their daily life in order to give informed consent. In general, the possible risks of surgical interventions are infection, bleeding, nerve- and vascular damage, thrombosis and embolism. Specific complications in the field of internal offloading are as follows:

- So-called **transfer lesions** occur at primarily unaffected parts as a result of the load redistribution to them. The endangered areas must be monitored, and any possible overloads must be quickly eliminated before an ulcer occurs.
- **Aftercare** is intended to early recognise transfer lesions or local recidivism with the consequence of further interventions.
- **Loss of toes** may occur in case of impaired perfusion secondary to infections.
- Still **insufficient offload** despite successful operation with the need for further surgical correction may result.
- **Inability to take showers or baths** until wound closure is secure has to be respected.
- Patients with endocardial problems may develop **infective endocarditis** (IE) if wound infections and subsequently bacteremias occur. Prophylactic perioperative treatment with antibiotics (AP) is thought to prevent this risk. Guidelines have been changed substantially over the last decades and vary widely between the recommending institutions. Leading authorities in this ongoing discussion are the British NICE (National Institute for Health and Care Excellence), the

American AHA (American Heart Association) and the European ESC (European Society of Cardiology). While NICE doesn't recommend any routinely AP, AHA recommends prophylaxis for individuals at highest risk of an adverse outcome from IE (e.g., artificial heart valves) undergoing a high-risk procedure (such as on infected skin or musculoskeletal tissue) and ESC recommends it for those at highest risk of IE (e.g., native valve disease) undergoing a high-risk procedure perforating the oral mucosa [5]. Evidence is difficult to discuss as the disease is rare but dramatic. In people affected by DFS, bacteraemia might be common independent from an intervention because simply walking on the infected limb might cause the bacteria to spread. On the other hand, most of the patients with infected ulcers, if they are visiting a clinic, are undergoing antibiotic treatment. Individual consideration is therefore required.

20.4 Surgery on Soft Tissue

Soft tissue surgery involves anatomical structures apart from bones. At the foot, interventions are performed mainly on tendons, ligaments or joint capsules. The benefits can be seen particularly in the low incidence of complications. An additional advantage is their feasibility even in case of moderately impaired blood supply. This is possible because tendons and ligaments are in any case sparsely perfused and repair processes after interventions on them do not require significantly increased blood supply (see also Sect. 20.2 in this chapter).

20.4.1 Tenotomy of the Long Flexor Tendons of the Toes

The *Tenotomy of Flexor hallucis longus—Tendon* (FHL) and the *Tenotomy of the Flexor digitorum longus—Tendon (*FDL*)* are used to offload the tips of flexibly clawed toes [4]. These are loaded by plantarisation due to hyperflexion of the distal phalanx or the torsion of the 5th toe (see also Chap. 2, Sect. 2.7.4, Chaps. 6, 7, and 13). After this procedure, the distal phalanx can no longer be plantarflexed. Instead of its tips, the plantar pulp is again exposed to pressure. Or in case of a torsion, the toe is de-rotated. Lesions located at the plantarised parts of the toes often close rapidly after such an intervention, even if they have been present for a long time.

Indication: This procedure offloads plantarised parts of the toes: the tip of the toe or the lateral aspect of the minor toe in clawed toes and the medial aspect of the hallux. The indication has to be actively sought because it might be a functional deformity leading to the plantarisation that is not apparent at rest. Therefore, if the deformity is not static (present at rest), people suffering from 'indicator lesions' at the tip of the toes or the lateral aspect of the 5th toe or the medial aspect of the IP joint of the hallux have to be examined with tests such as the 'claw test' (see details in Chap. 3, Sect. 3.4.1.3) to reveal the underlying functional plantarisation. This is essential even if a possible culprit is found in form of inadequate footwear. Otherwise, the possibility of a definitive correction of plantarisation might be overlooked. Impaired blood supply is not an absolute contraindication, but requires careful evaluation. An ankylosis (fusion of bones) makes the intervention pointless, but other causes of a rigid toe can be addressed by additional, contemporarily executed, minimally invasive techniques such as a capsule release.

Procedure: The tendon might be reached without uncovering deep tissue using a blood sampling cannula. Alternatively, access is possible through a small, longitudinal, lateral or medial incision. It is up to the surgeon to choose the preferred way. Transverse incisions have been abandoned after the experience of dehiscence due to postoperative stretching of the skin on the plantar surface of the toe. The tenotomy should selectively be done on the long flexor tendon (FDL). The short tendon should not be cut as in this case the extensor tendons lack a balancing counterpart. The resulting extension of the PIP may induce an upright toe (*cocked-up toe*). This complication is avoided by overextending the clawed toe in the DIP joint while simultaneously applying dorsal pressure to the PIP joint to find the tensed FDL tendon immediately under the skin (Figs. 20.3, 20.4, and 20.5).

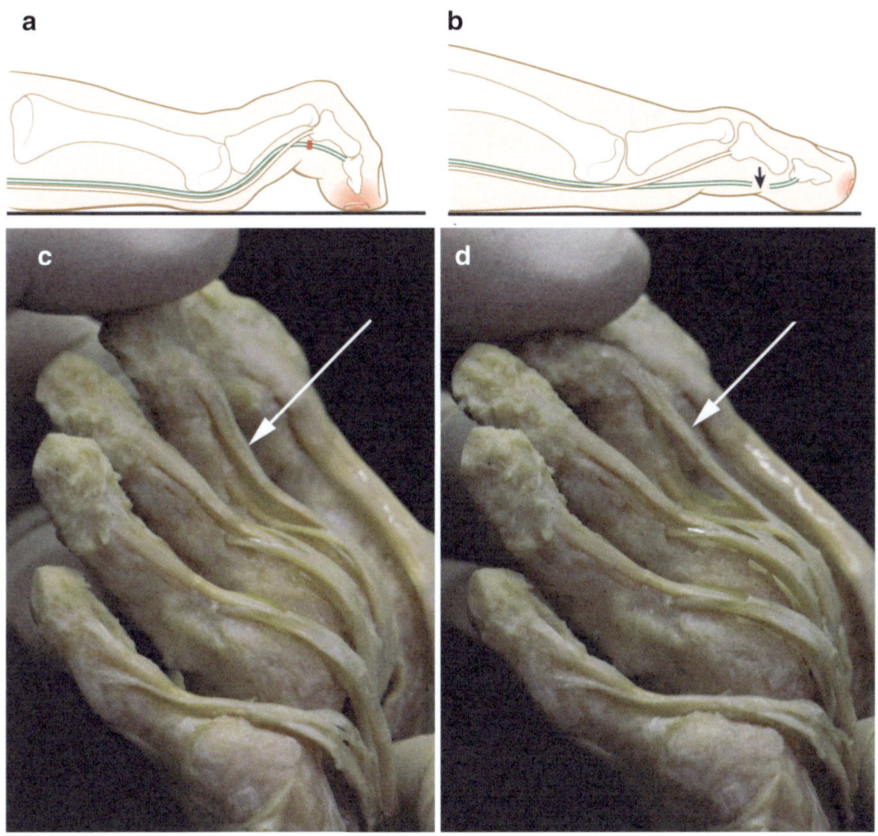

Fig. 20.3 (**a**, **b**) Schematic representation of a tenotomy of the FDL tendon. (**c**) Anatomical representation in neutral and (**d**) in overextended position of the 2nd toe. The shift of the FDL tendon (arrows) to a more plantar (superficial) position due to overstretching can be easily recognised (arrow in **d**)

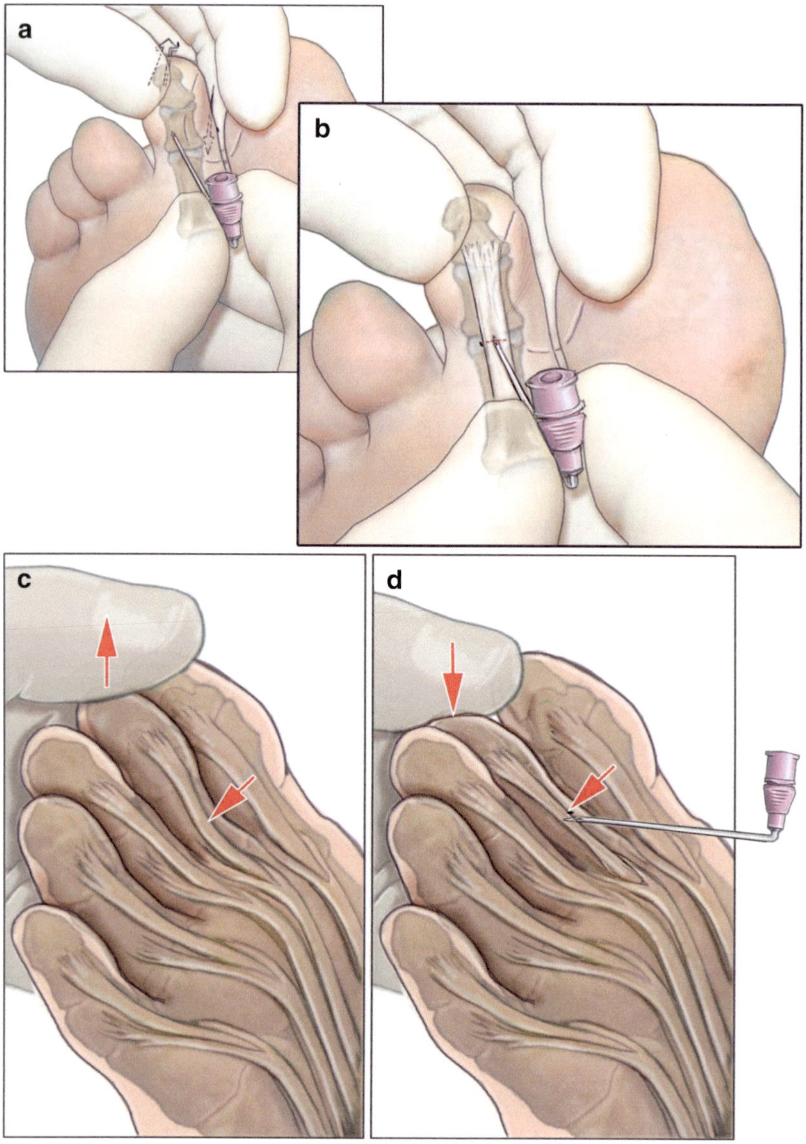

Fig. 20.4 (**a**) The middle finger of the hand holding the toe presses the toe in the area of the proximal interphalangeal (PIP) or interphalangeal (IP) joint in plantar direction. The thumb overstretches the distal phalanx in the DIP or IP joint pressing the plantar side of the distal phalanx in opposite direction. This ensures that the long flexor tendon moves beneath the plantar skin of the toe. (**b**) Now the cannula is introduced centrally and slightly proximal to the flexion fold of the distal joint. (**c**) By loosening the thumb for a short moment, the tip of the cannula can be placed between skin and tendon. The flexor digitorum longus (FDL) or flexor hallucis longus (FHL) tendon is then tenotomised carefully. (**d**) The thumbs pressure on the distal phalanx is slowly increased again and the tendon is stretched. Figures by kind permission of: Engels, G., H. Stinus, D. Hochlenert, and A. Klein. 2016. [Concept of plantarisation for toe correction in diabetic foot syndrome]. *Oper Orthop Traumatol* 28(5):323–334. doi:10.1007/s00064-016-0453-9

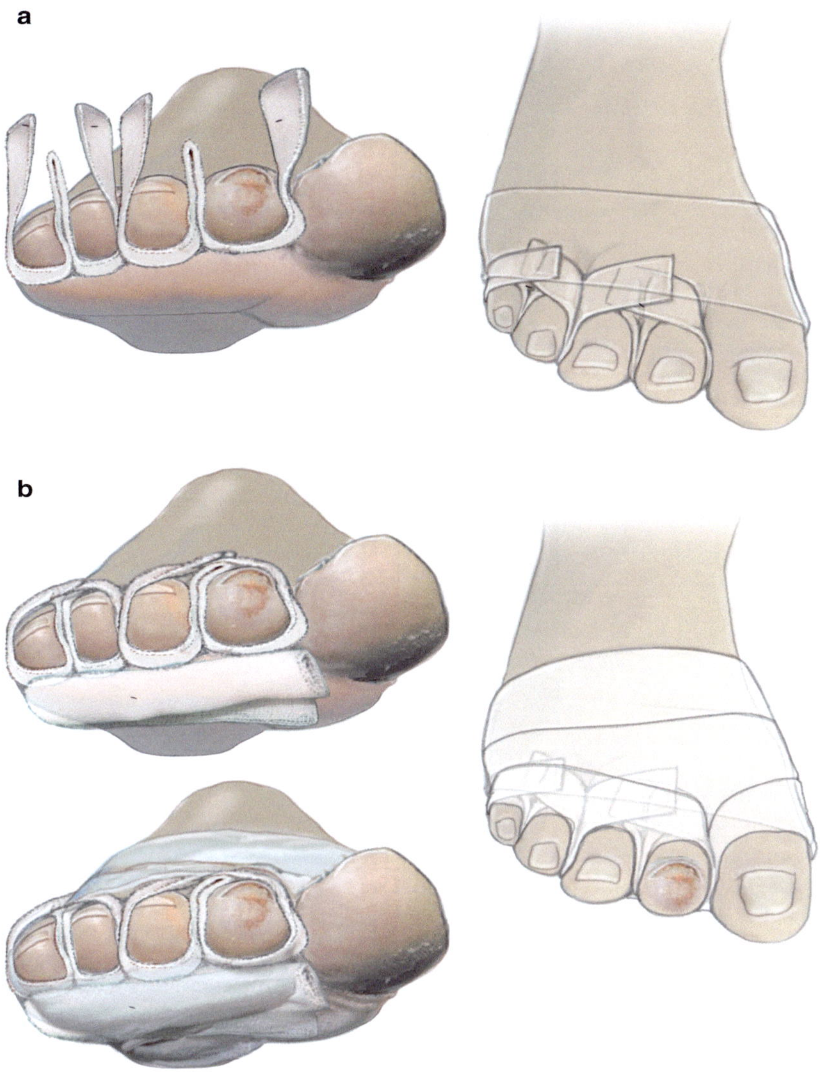

Fig. 20.5 (**a**) After a short compression of the puncture site, the initial bleeding of the skin vessels stops. The *redressing bandage* is applied with a compress (10 × 10 cm) which is unfolded (10 × 20 cm) and then folded longitudinally twice (3.3 × 20 cm). As a loop, it holds the operated toe and the neighbouring toes in a dorsal position and is fixed to the back of the foot with an elastic plaster. (**b**) In addition, another compress is rolled up, inserted into the flexion folds of the toes and fixed with an elastic bandage. Figures by kind permission of: Engels, G., H. Stinus, D. Hochlenert, and A. Klein. 2016. [Concept of plantarisation for toe correction in diabetic foot syndrome]. *Oper Orthop Traumatol* 28(5):323–334. doi:10.1007/s00064-016-0453-9

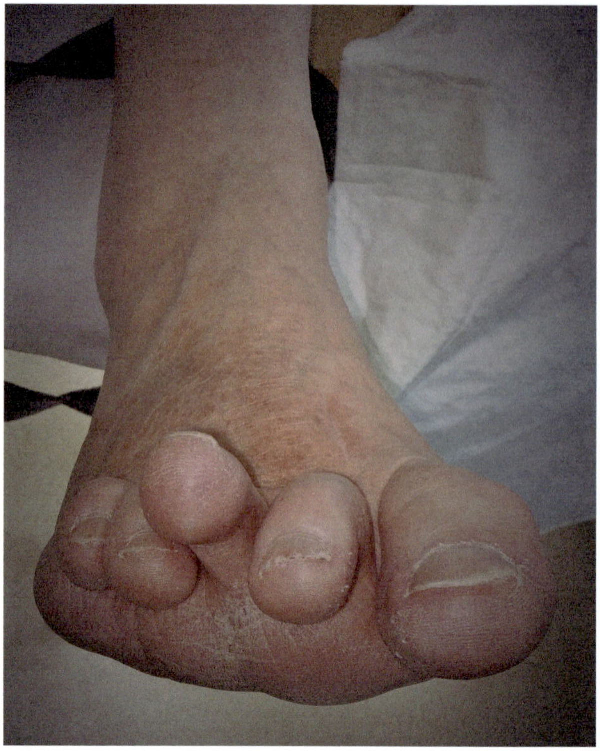

Fig. 20.6 Cocked-up-toe

Aftercare: Redression bandages are applied for a few days to dorsalise the distal phalanx as described above. Controls are carried out after 1–2 days, after 1, 3 and 8 weeks and then every 3 months to detect incipient transfer lesions or insufficient functional correction.

Specific risks:

- 'Cocked-up toe' (Fig. 20.6) occurs if the flexor digitorum brevis's tendon is accidentally or intentionally severed. At the hallux, this deformity is possible due to other causes, but not as a complication after tenotomy of the FHL tendon. In case this complication occurs, the extensor digitorum longus tendon (EDL) has to be severed too, which in general causes no additional problems.
- Deformities and limitation in active movements of the toe
- In rare cases unsteady gait in case of pronounced polyneuropathy

Evidence: A study with a control group does not exist, but there are many case series. Systematic reviews [6, 7] show good results in terms of wound closure and new ulcers. The mean duration to postoperative wound closure was 29.5 days, with an overall healing rate of 97%. The rate of ulcer recurrence was 6%. None of the prophylactically operated toes developed ulcers. The complication rate was generally low, transfer lesions ad adjacent MTHs have been reported by several authors. One case series explicitly treated patients with impaired blood supply due to PAD and good results could be achieved [8] (Fig. 20.7).

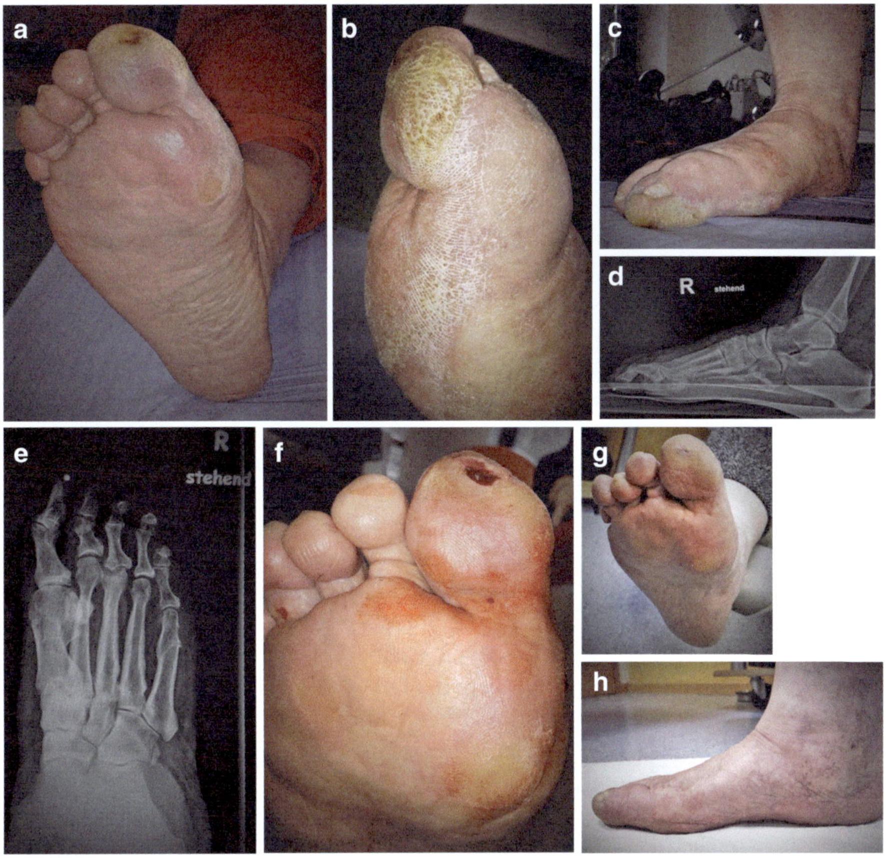

Fig. 20.7 (**a**–**c**) preoperative finding, the lesion has been present for 9 months (**d**, **e**) radiological finding in offloading; ulcer marked by external pellet (**f**) postoperative finding after tenotomy of the FHL and FDL tendon of the 4th toe (**g**, **h**) postoperative finding after 4 weeks

20.4.2 Lengthening of the Extensor Tendons of the Toes

An excessive dorsiflexion of the toes at the MTP joint displaces the MTH in plantar direction. An example of this type of deformity is represented by the toes of a pes cavus. The pathophysiological concept is discussed in Chap. 2, Sect. 2.7.3.1 (see Figs. 2.54, 2.56, 2.57, 2.60) and for further aspects of the typical lesions Chaps. 11 and 14.

At the hallux this may induce plantar lesions in projection to the medial sesamoid bone. This hypomochlion is exposed to extreme peak pressures. The elongation of the extensor tendons allows for a stretching of the MTP joint and thus the straight alignment of the toe.

This has several beneficial consequences:

- Firstly, the wound is stretched less and the edges move closer to each other.
- Secondly, the ulcer shifts out of the immediate pressure zone into a more proximal position, which often allows the defect to close rapidly.

- Thirdly, this shift conveys less damaged tissue beneath the internal pressure point and partially restores the protective function of the fat pad and the plantar plate. These cushions increase the contact surface and reduce peak pressure.
- And fourthly, a reduction of the peak pressures is also determined by less pressure on the MTH from above. The MTH may shift dorsally by a few millimetres, which is often decisive.

Similarly, a lengthening of the extensor tendons of the 2nd to 5th toe can reduce an overstretching in the respective MTP joint and avoid peak pressures beneath the MTH. Without pressure due to a dorsally displaced toe, the MTH is then again able to avoid pressure by moving in dorsal direction. In addition, soft tissue is relocated and wound edges are approximated in the same way as described for the hallux.

Sometimes, an additional dorsal capsule release is required to mobilise the toe and to allow the proximal phalanx to return to its original position.

If this intervention was carried out on claw toes as a single procedure, pressure on the tips of the toes would increase significantly. Therefore, this intervention is usually combined with a tenotomy of the long flexor tendon.

Indication: Excessive dorsiflexion of the toes at the MTP joint with consecutive 'indicator lesions' at the dorsum of the PIP joint or beneath the MTH might indicate this intervention. An ankylosis of the MTP joint cannot be corrected this way, but other causes of rigidity can be resolved contemporarily (e.g. by dorsal capsule release). This possibility can be ascertained by radiography in advance. Thus, a fixed MTP joint rarely limits the indication.

Procedure (Fig. 20.8): The intervention is performed under local anaesthesia and is initiated by two longitudinal incision at the distal and intermediate part of the dorsum of the foot parallel to the EHL tendon. After careful preparation of the tendon, it is incised transversally in half at both sites. The two incisions of the tendon are made in opposite direction to sever each fibre of the tendon only once. The tendon is then lengthened by a forced plantar flexion of the toe and a simultaneous active extension. The distance between the two cuts determines the extent to which the tendon might be lengthened before it is completely severed. It is not necessary to sew the tendon. The term '*Z-plasty*' is often used to describe this type of tendon lengthening which is also used for other tendons such as the Achilles tendon.

In people with markedly reduced mobility, an extension of the tendon can also be performed using a percutaneous technique. After an infiltration anaesthesia, the EHL tendon is also partially severed at different points with a blood sampling cannula so that it can be extended. However, the risk of a complete dissection of the tendon is high in this procedure.

Aftercare: Plantarising redression bandages are applied for 6 weeks. Check-ups take place after 1–2 days, after 1, 2, 3 and 8 weeks and then every 3 months in order to detect transfer lesions or insufficient functional correction. The suture material is removed after 10–14 days.

Specific risks of the operation that must be explained to obtain informed consent are:

- Deformities and limitation in active movement of the toe and, in rare instances, unsteady gait if polyneuropathy is markedly pronounced.

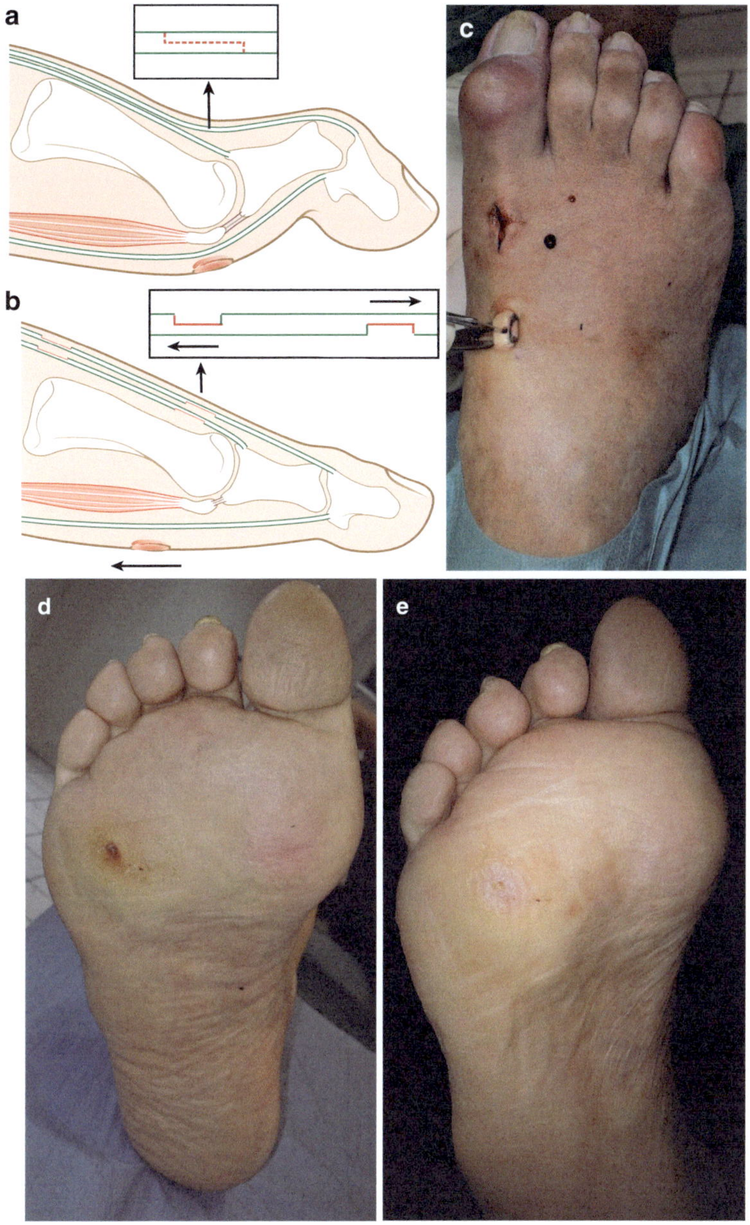

Fig. 20.8 (**a**, **b**) Schematic representation of the relocation of the plantar soft tissue. Shift of the plantar lesion from beneath the sesamoid bone to a more proximal position by a lengthening of the extensor tendon with a Z-plasty (**c**) intraoperative picture. (**d**–**g**) Case history of a combined procedure with tenotomy of the FDL and FDB tendons and simultaneous tenotomy of the extensors of the lesser toes and release of the dorsal capsule of the 2nd to 5th MTP joint. This patient showed recurrent plantar lesions at the 4th MTH in orthopaedic bespoken shoes over the years. After the intervention, the patient was without recurrence for 5 months. (**d**, **e**) day of the operation (**f**, **g**) 2nd postoperative day

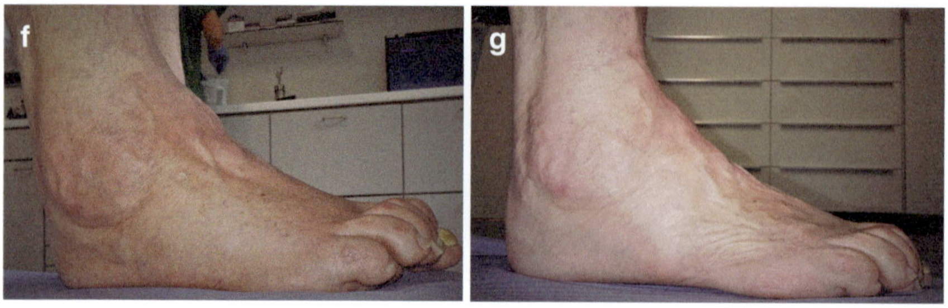

Fig. 20.8 (continued)

Evidence: This procedure is used as part of more complex methods in case reports [9], but to our knowledge it has not been reported as used for diabetic feet.

20.4.3 Combined Interventions on Soft Tissue

As described above, the lengthening of the extensor tendons is often combined with a tenotomy of the long and sometimes the short flexor tendons. For example, hammer toes might be straightened in this way if the PIP joint and the MTP joint retain a certain degree of flexibility. If these joints are rigid and the stiffness is not caused by a connection between bones, the capsules might also be released. This involves a **plantar capsulotomy of the PIP joint** or a **dorsal release of the MTP joint**.

In the treatment of a hallux valgus deformity, a so-called '**lateral release**' of the first MTP joint is regularly used together with other procedures [10]. Three elements are usually combined in the 'lateral release': the conjoined tendon (adductor hallucis tendon and the tendon of the lateral head of the FHB) and the deep transverse metatarsal ligament (which inserts into the lateral (fibular) sesamoid) are severed and the lateral joint capsule is released. This frees the hallux from its attachments to the more lateral parts of the forefoot and therefore allows its straighter alignment. This can also be done transcutaneously using a needle-technique.

In a hallux valgus deformity compromising the 2nd toe positioned as '**superductus**' or '**infraductus**' (see also Chap. 2, Fig. 2.35), a combination of tenotomies may be helpful. In this case, the FHL and the EHL are severed and a percutaneous lateral release of the first MTH is performed contemporarily. This reduces the bowstring-effect to such an extent that wound closure might be achieved. One of the standardised procedures to correct a hallux valgus deformity might be performed later on, if this is considered useful in view of age and mobility (Fig. 20.9).

Combinations might also include interventions on bones (Fig. 20.10).

A resection of the PIP joint is necessary if it is opened dorsally by an ulcer. Further indications for a resection of the PIP joint are the ankylosis in flexed position or ulcers at an extremely long 2nd toe. If the latter was treated with tenotomies alone, the toe would become even longer and thus exposed to injuries.

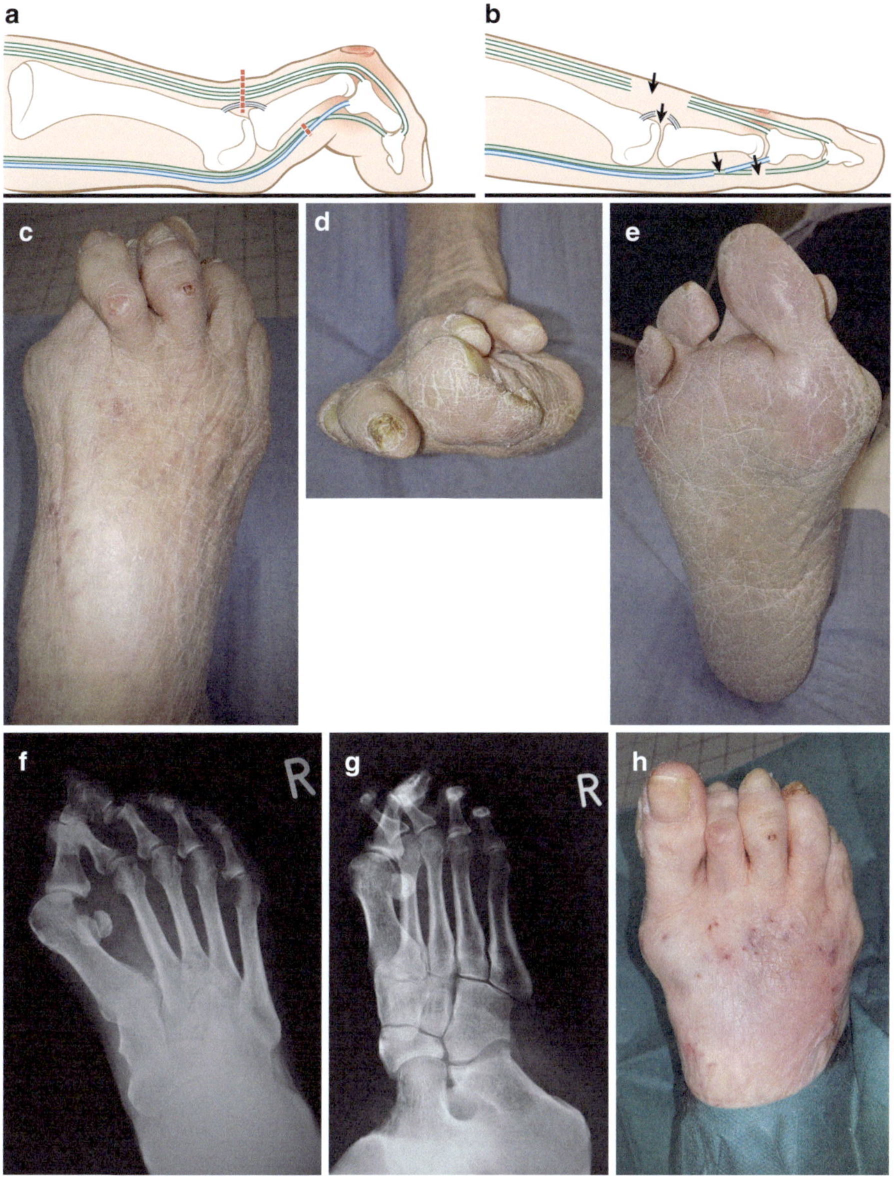

Fig. 20.9 (**a**, **b**) Schematic representation of the effect combining a tenotomy of the FDL and the FDB with a lengthening of the extensor tendons to offload a lesion at the PIP joint dorsally (**c**–**e**) clinical picture of a hallux infraductus (**f**, **g**) radiological finding (**h**–**j**) intraoperative situation after tenotomy of the extensor and flexor tendons of all toes, a lateral release of the hallux and a dorsal release of the 2nd to 4th MTP joints, (**k**, **l**) the postoperative radiological picture, (**m**) after 3 weeks

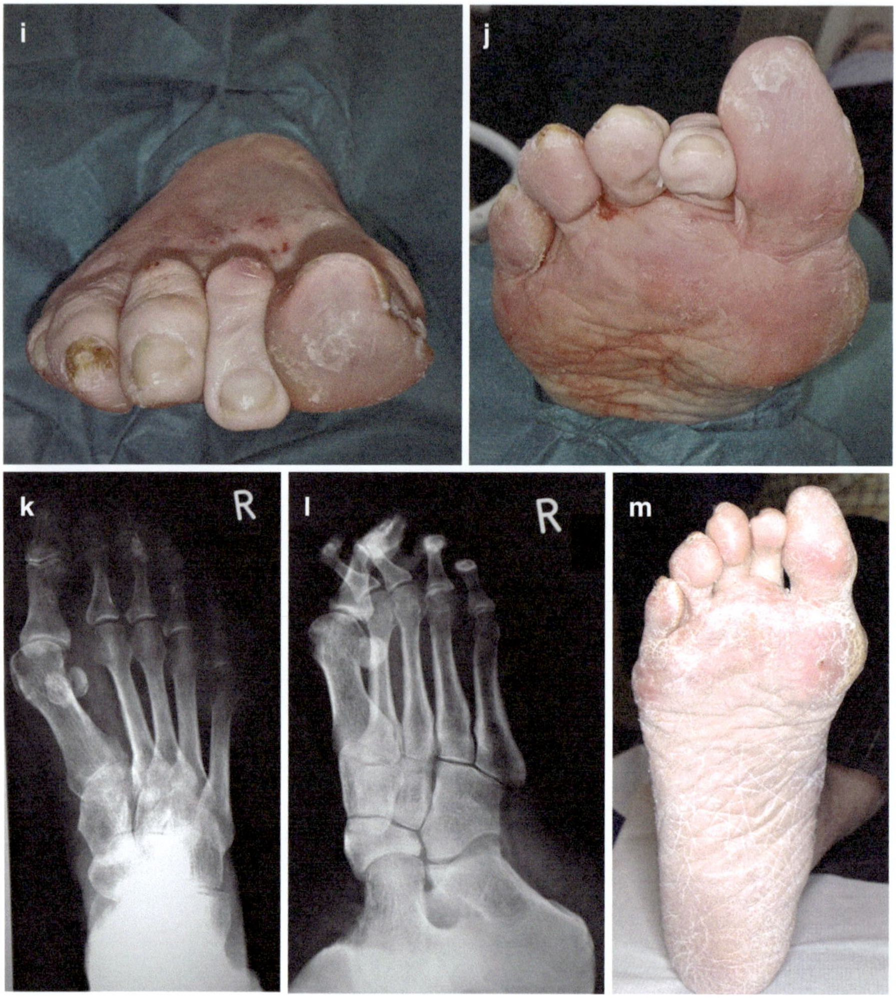

Fig. 20.9 (continued)

20.4.4 Jones Procedure

Another possibility to offload a lesion in projection to the first MTH is to proximalise the tendon of the EHL, known as 'Jones Procedure'. This is particularly useful in the case of a pes cavus with a hallux usually in zig-zag position. Such a malalignment increases the pressure on the plantar soft tissues in the area of the sesamoid bone complex.

Indication: A chronic overload of the first MTH, especially in case of a pes cavus, that has induced an indicator lesion, might be an indication for this procedure. The prerequisite is a sufficient mobility of the first ray at the first TMT joint (metatarso-cuneiforme I), MTP joint and IP joint (Fig. 20.11).

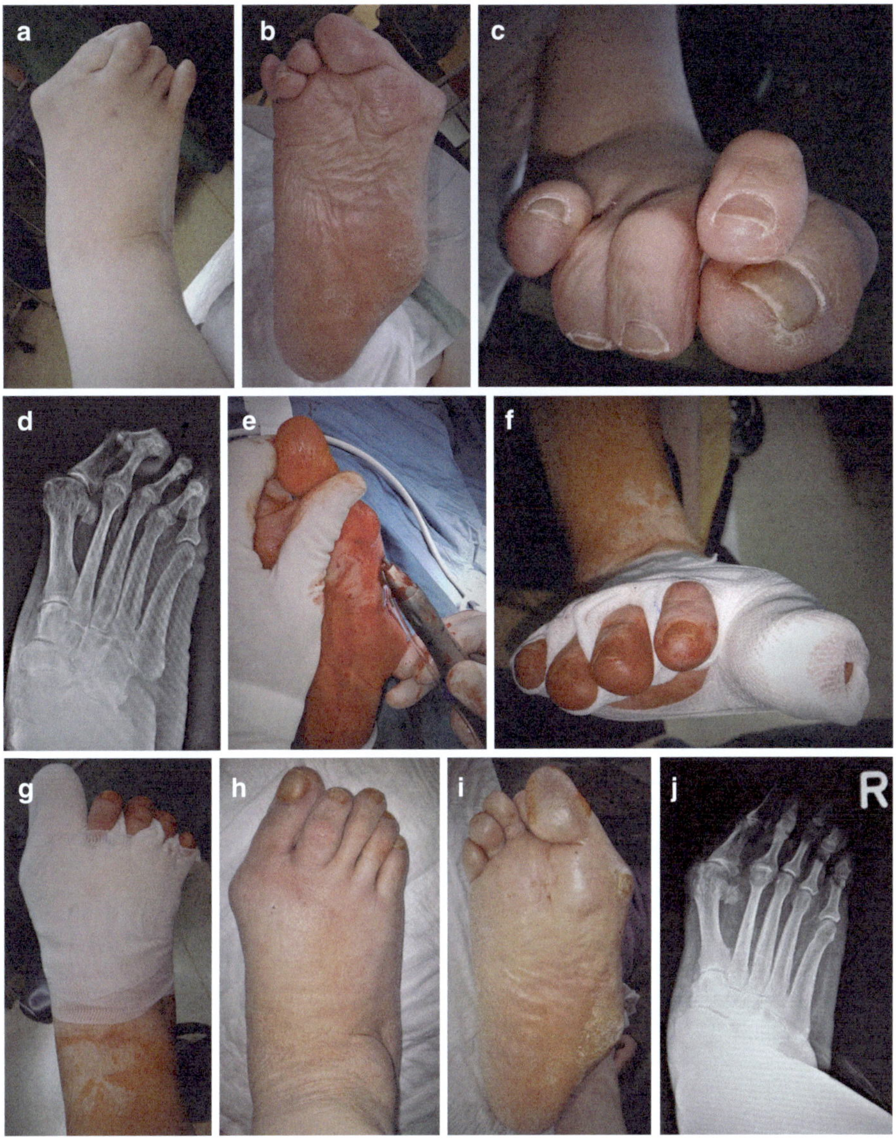

Fig. 20.10 Combined intervention on tendons and bone, anaesthesia by ankle-block, percutaneous tenotomy of the EHL-, FHL tendons as well as FDL-, FDB- and EDL tendons of the 2nd to 5th toe, percutaneous lateral release and minimally invasive ablation of a 'pseudoexostosis' of the first MTH (**a**–**d**) preoperative, (**e**) intraoperative (**f**, **g**) postoperative picture (**h**–**j**) 4 weeks later

Procedure: The access is at the dorsum of the foot. The long extensor tendon is prepared and severed distally near its insertion. A transversal hole is drilled in the distal metatarsal bone and the tendon is passed through the hole. The tendon is then dorsally sutured to itself. This procedure may be combined with an arthrodesis of

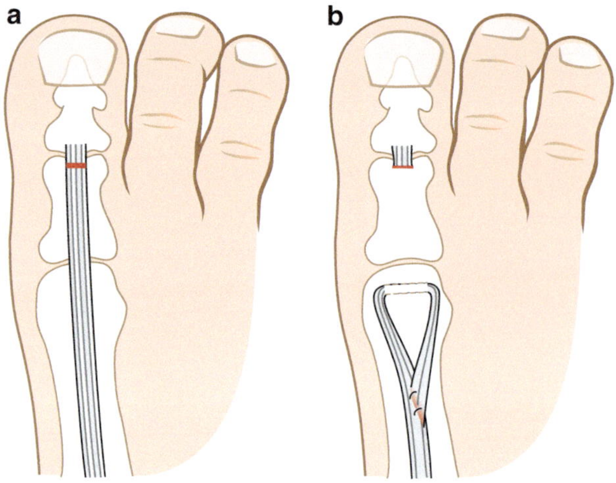

Fig. 20.11 (**a**, **b**) Schematic representation of the proximalisation of the long extensor tendon (EHL) according to Jones

the IP joint to ensure stronger plantar flexion of the entire toe or with other interventions (see subheading 'Evidence' below).

Aftercare: The desired effect of this procedure is an active elevation of the first metatarsal and a flexion of the hallux resulting in a considerable relief of the first MTH. This should be supported and controlled in aftercare. A redressing bandage should be applied for 6 weeks. Controls are necessary after 1 day and after 1, 2, 3, 6 and 8 weeks and then every 3 months thereafter to detect transfer lesions or insufficient functional correction in time. The suture material is removed after 10–14 days.

Specific risks:

- Deformities
- Limitation in active movement of the toe, in rare cases unsteady gait in the case of pronounced polyneuropathy
- Dislocation of the foreign material
- Rupture of the suture of the tendon

Evidence: A cohort study of 26 people with diabetes and chronic ulceration under the first MTH were treated by a modified Jones procedure including an extensor hallucis longus transfer and a flexor hallucis longus transfer. If that was functionally insufficient, the tendon of the long fibular muscle was transferred to the lateral margin of the foot. If the ankle dorsiflexion was <5° with the knee extended, a gastrocnemius recession was performed. Evaluation showed wound closure on average after 4.4 weeks (2–8). In the follow-up period averaging 39.6 months (12–61) after surgery there was no recurrence of ulceration under the first MTH [11] (Fig. 20.12).

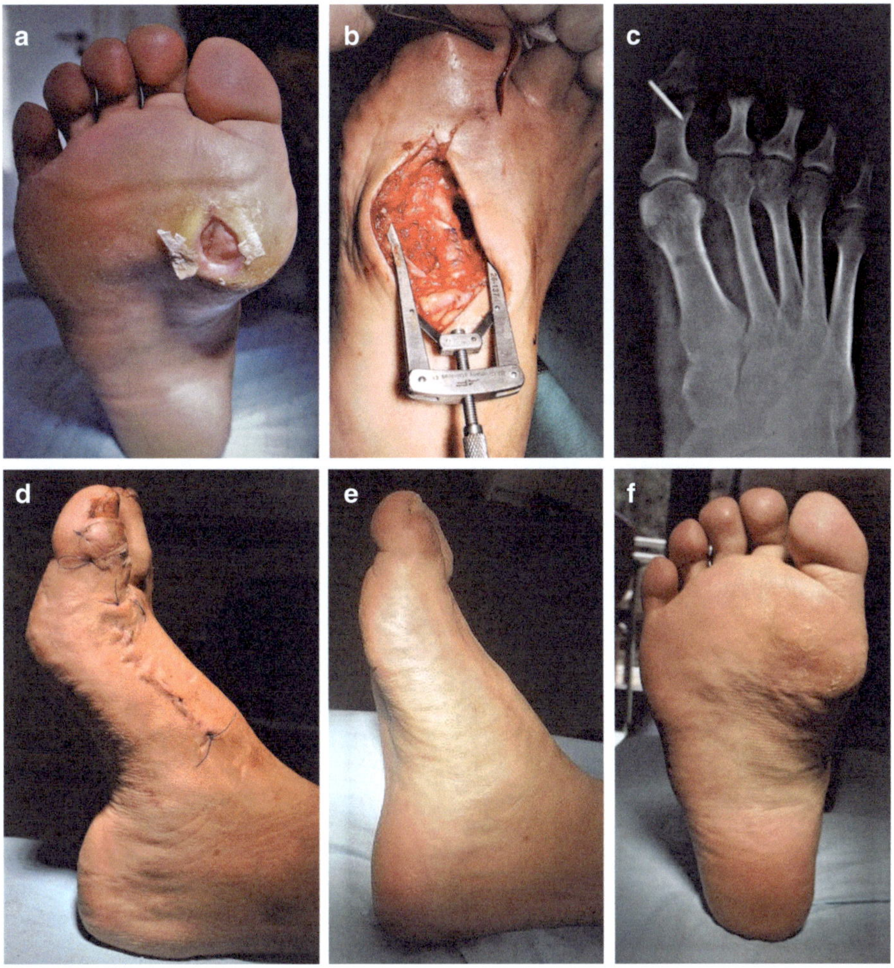

Fig. 20.12 Case history of a 26-year-old woman affected by type 1 diabetes and having a history of a surgical treatment of a spinal lipoma which resulted in a neurogenic pes cavus. For many years lesions at the first MTH occurred. She works as a hairdresser and adequately offloading shoes are not acceptable; (**a**) initial picture (**b**) intraoperative aspect, Jones procedure and ATL are done simultaneously (**c**) postop. X-ray image (arthrodesis of the IP joint) (**d**) Findings at the 2nd post-operative day (**e**, **f**) 9 months after surgery, wearing sneakers with soft, custom-made insoles

20.4.5 Achilles Tendon Lengthening (ATL)

A high percentage of people with diabetes show a clinically significant shortening of the triceps surae in the calf, also known as '*Shortening of the Achilles Tendon*'. This might increase forefoot plantar pressure and prolong the duration of high plantar pressure at the forefoot. As a consequence, surgical elongation of the Achilles tendon may reduce plantar pressure at the forefoot [12].

Traction at the Achilles tendon while the foot is plantarflexed induces an inversion of the calcaneus and the subtalar structures are locked. If this occurs too early during the gait cycle, the subtalar structures are locked prematurely. In other words, the foot becomes rigid earlier while walking and is then stiffened in an inverted position.

Indication: The indication is found at clinical examination. An equinus foot deformity, that cannot be compensated sufficiently by conservative methods and has given way to indicator lesions might be an indication for an Achilles tendon lengthening.

Procedure: The procedure is simple, can be performed under local anaesthesia and involves two or three percutaneous incisions at different heights and in opposite directions. The distal cut is performed laterally, the others each opposite to the distally adjacent one. With three incisions the recommended distance is 4–5 cm. With two cuts the distance slightly greater. The suralis nerve and the Vena saphena parva must be considered. The extent of length gained depends on the extent the foot is dorsiflexed after the cuts are applied. The desired length is reached when the foot is extended (=dorsiflexed) at 5–10°. If the Achilles tendon dysfunction is due solely to a contracture of the gastrocnemius muscle, the intervention can be limited to this more superficial muscle. This is known as 'gastrocnemius release' or 'Strayer procedure' or 'gastroc recession' or 'gastroc slide'. The decision is made based on the Silfverskjöld-Test (see Chap. 3, case history: Fig. 3.14) (Figs. 20.13 and 20.14).

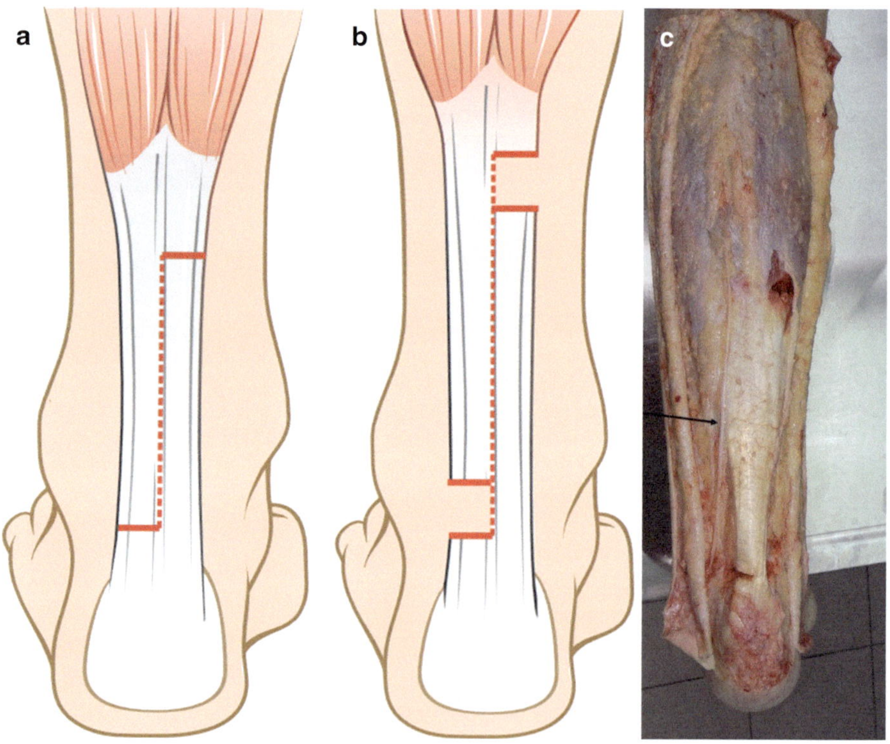

Fig. 20.13 (**a–c**) Schematic representation and anatomical preparation for the technique using two cuts, the course of the sural nerve is marked with an arrow

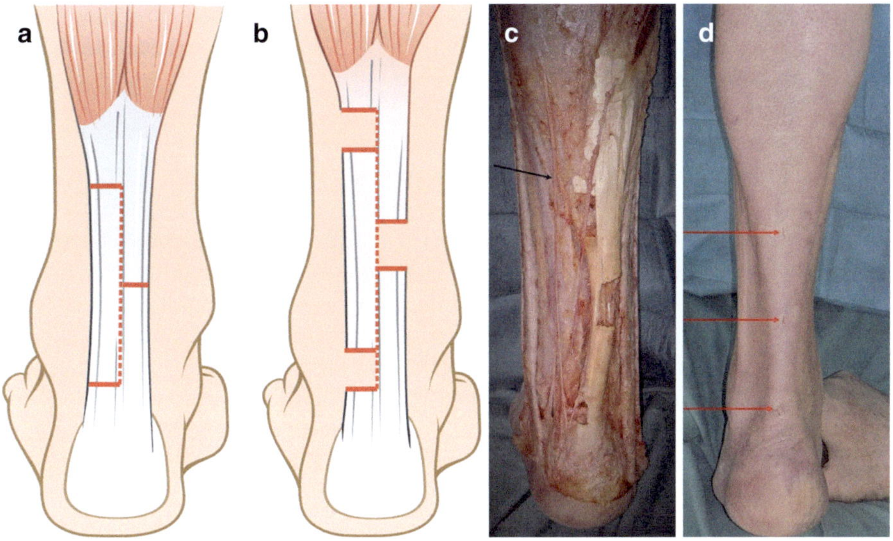

Fig. 20.14 (**a–c**) Schematic representation and anatomical preparation for the technique using three cuts, the course of the sural nerve is marked with an arrow. (**d**) Incisions marked with an arrow

Aftercare: A functionally satisfactory result of this procedure requires a reliable protection against further unintentional extension of the tendon. This is achieved by using a total contact cast (TCC) that has to be worn unconditionally and uninterruptedly for 6 weeks. After gastrocnemius release, protection is necessary for 4 weeks. Compression therapy with two short-stretch bandages can be considered for 14 days after surgery. A complete severance of the tendon should be avoided as this would result in a high risk of overloading the heel. The suture material can be removed after 10–14 days. At this point, it is possible to obtain measurements needed to purchase the most appropriate shoe.

Specific risks:

- Rupture of the tendon with high risk of plantar ulcer of the heel.
- Damage to the vena saphena parva or the nervus suralis.
- The cast must be kept in place 24 h a day for 6 weeks without interruption. A non-removable TCC is most appropriate to ensure this with absolute certainty.

Evidence: A randomised controlled trial in patients with neuropathic ulceration of the plantar aspect of the forefoot, diabetes mellitus and limited ankle dorsiflexion (≤5°) compared TCC alone with TCC after ATL. The researchers found a faster wound closure (100% against 88%) and fewer recurrences after 7 months (15% against 59%) [12]. Other authors put emphasis on the need to prevent excessive lengthening and by that transfer lesions at the heel [13, 14]. They also report a generally low number of recurrences and side effects [15, 16].

A case series of 11 people treated with gastrocnemius-soleus recession as the sole treatment of diabetic midfoot ulcers showed 10 wound closures. The last person achieved wound closure after an additional midfoot fusion. At follow up (at average 36 month) one major amputation due to a new ulcer and two deaths for medical reasons independent of DFS occurred [17].

20.4.6 Tibialis Anterior Tendon Transfer or Split

Lesions in the plantar or lateral-plantar area of the 5th MTH are particularly associated with a supination of the forefoot, an inversion of the mid- and hindfoot and an overload of the lateral margin of the foot. This might be due to a muscle imbalance characterised by a weakness of the fibularis muscles with simultaneous predominance of the tibialis anterior muscle. A transfer of the tibialis anterior tendon completely ('transfer') or half ('split') to the lateral side of the foot is used together with other tendon transfers to correct deformities. This has been reported as beneficial for children [18]. To our knowledge, the use of this method to correct an imbalance in people with DFS has not yet been described.

Indication: Chronic overload of the outer margin due to an insufficient action of the fibularis muscles, that had induced indicator lesions.

Procedure (Fig. 20.15): Under conduction anaesthesia, a medial longitudinal incision is made above the distal part of the tibialis anterior tendon near its insertion and the tendon is exposed. Now a longitudinal incision is made ventrally above the ankle joint where the tendon is palpable. The tendon is prepared and exposed also at this site. In the 'split' procedure, a longitudinal incision is made in the tendon at the proximal access. A strong filament is introduced through this incision and is passed alongside the tendon to reach the distal access. The filament is now pulled through the tendon to the distal access to split it. The medial part of the tendon is wrapped with suture material close to the insertion and then severed as near as possible to the insertion. The medial part of the tendon is now extracted through the proximal access. Subsequently, the fibularis tertius tendon is exposed via a third, lateral access. The part of the tibialis anterior tendon that is now available at the proximal access is channelled below the retinaculum musculorum extensorum and passed through the lateral access. The foot is placed in a neutral position on the sagittal plane and in eversion. The part of the tibialis anterior tendon is located beneath the fibularis tertius tendon and sutured to this tendon using non-absorbable material or anchored directly to the bone. Skin closure is performed as usual. Above the tendon transfer at the lateral access, a continuous subcutaneous suture is additionally applied transcutaneously (see details of the suture technique in Sect. 20.2 in this chapter).

Aftercare: Postoperative checks after 1, 3, 7 days and 2, 4 and 6 weeks. The suture material is removed after 10–14 days. Follow-up treatment uses a TCC or other non-removable knee-high device for 6 postoperative weeks. At this point, it is possible to obtain measurements needed to purchase the most appropriate shoe. A perioperative antibiotic therapy for 7 days might be considered.

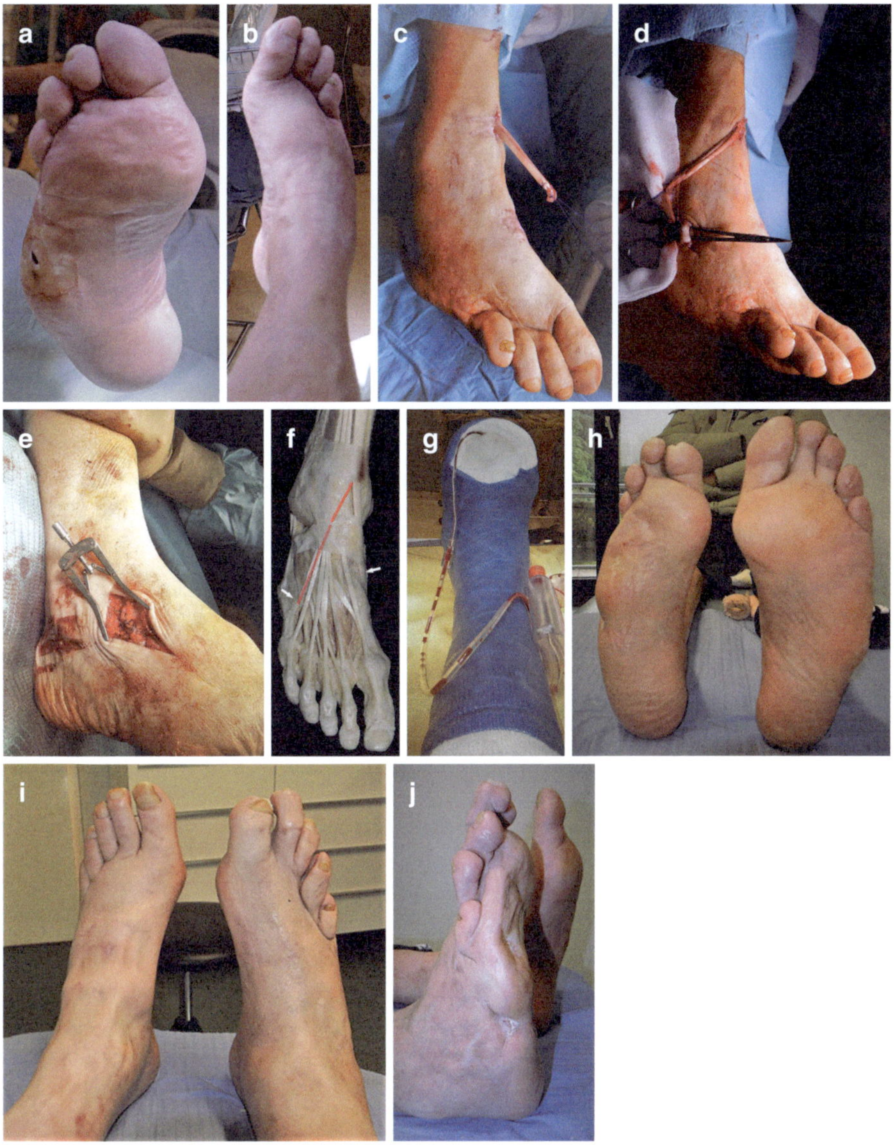

Fig. 20.15 Tibialis anterior transfer (**a**, **b**) preoperative situation (**c**) the tibialis anterior tendon is medially severed (**d**) lateral transfer of the tibialis anterior tendon, the fibularis tertius tendon is displayed with a forceps (**e**) the tibialis anterior tendon is sutured beneath the tendon of the fibularis tertius. (**f**) Representation of the transfer in the anatomical preparation. The red line represents the course of the tibialis anterior tendon after transfer (**g**) postoperative offloading in TCC for 6 weeks (**h**–**j**) clinical situation 32 months after surgery

Specific risks: The tendon may rupture in the region of the insertion. An infection of the non-absorbable suture material may occur. Therefore, an ulcer-free foot is preferred at the time of the operation. This is usually achieved by preoperative use of a TCC. Its use can be continued postoperatively.

20.4.7 Lengthening of the Tibialis Anterior Tendon According to Ponseti

The procedure was originally introduced by Ignacio Ponseti (1914–2009) in the middle of the last century as tenotomy of the Achilles tendon for the therapy of children's clubfoot. Thereafter, also to describe other interventions on tendons to correct foot deformities, his name has been used. To our knowledge, the adaption of the technique to correct overload in diabetic feet by an intervention on the tibialis anterior tendon has not been published yet.

Indication: The indication is given by an 'indicator lesion' on the plantar or latero-plantar side of a supinated foot (especially at the MTH), if the supination is due to imbalance. This imbalance is due to a combination of excessive tension of the tibialis anterior tendon and reduced tension on the fibularis tendons. The strength of this procedure is that it causes little trauma, which is important for non-revascularisable PAD. The disadvantage is the possibility of a tear in the tendon leading to an impaired gait. The best procedure for the patient in view of age, comorbidity and mobility is chosen.

Procedure (Fig. 20.16): In the course of the tibialis anterior tendon between the medial insertion and slightly proximal to the retinaculum musculorum extensorum, the tendon is weakened at different levels using a blood sampling cannula in such a way that an extension of the tendon is achieved. The positive result is immediately visible, as the foot it is no longer pulled into an inverted position when actively dorsiflexed, but is now lifted laterally via the EDL tendon.

Aftercare: Immobilisation is assured in a TCC for about 2–3 weeks. In the case of reduced mobility, a tape bandage may also be sufficient. The shoes should be adjusted with a slight elevation of the outer margin. Postoperative check-ups are necessary on the first and 3rd day, then after 2 and 6 weeks.

Specific risks: A rupture of the tendon is possible, but this is usually not associated with a relevant problem in people with reduced mobility. Local haemorrhage may occur, so a mild compression dressing is recommended for 1 day.

20.5 Bone Surgery

The methods of bone surgery for the treatment of people with Diabetic Feet differ largely due to the presence or absence of bone infection. Combined treatments including interventions on bone have proven to be beneficial compared to conservative treatment alone [19]. In case of osteitis, surgery is performed to remove tissue considered to be necrotic. In the absence of bone infection, surgery is used to redistribute weight or to relieve the inner pressure point.

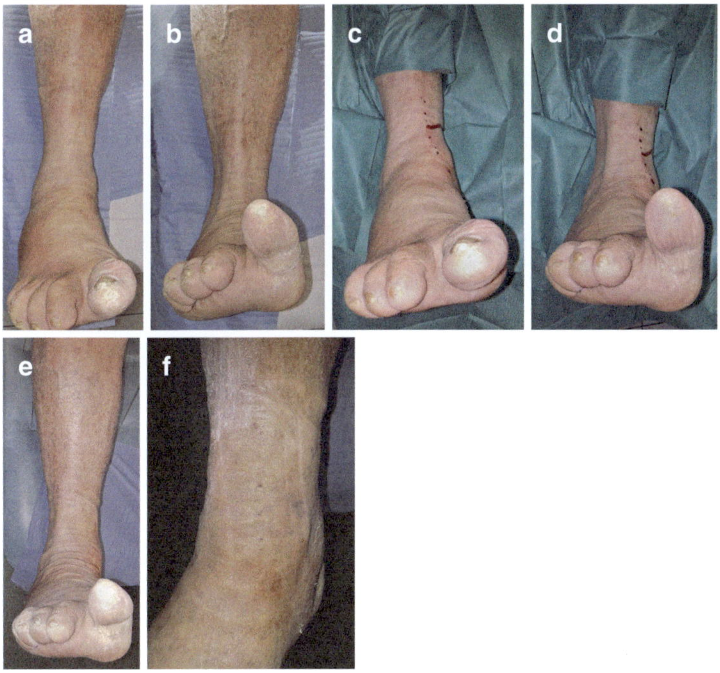

Fig. 20.16 Lengthening of the tibialis anterior tendon according to Ponseti (**a**) preoperative relaxed (**b**) preoperative active dorsiflexion (**c**) postoperative relaxed (**d**) postoperative active dorsiflexion (**e**) first postoperative day, active dorsiflexion (**f**) first postoperative day, local findings at the site of percutaneous prolongation

Specific risks of surgery on bones exceeding the general risks described above and necessary to communicate in order to obtain informed consent are:

- Perioperative wound infections that compromise wound repair are more common after interventions on bone than after those on soft tissue. The more proximally they are located, the more dramatic the consequences might be. Ascending infections through compartments are possible and might lead to other operations and sometimes amputations. Infections of the operation site are even more common if a bone infection already exists before the intervention.
- Perioperative antibiotic prophylaxis or treatment might be considered in view of the risk of infection at the site of surgery and the risk of infective endocarditis (see also Sect. 20.2 in this chapter).

The measures discussed here are intended to avoid amputation, and the maximum risk in most cases would be precisely this, amputation. These concerns should therefore not cast doubt on the indication itself but help to choose the appropriate perioperative management.

Aftercare usually considers the following aspects: Depending on the presence (or not) and conditions of a plantar wound and the required intensity of the offloading, therapeutic shoes, orthosis or TCCs might be used. The suture material is removed after 12–14 days. In the case of infection it is removed immediately. Clinical control takes place after 1 day and again after 2–3 days, after 1, 2 and 8 weeks and then every 3 months to detect infections, transfer lesions or insufficient functional outcome. Depending on the condition of the wound more frequent controls may be necessary. As aftercare is often very similar, in the following paragraphs only additional aspects are described.

20.5.1 Surgery of Osteitis

In order to avoid unnecessary amputations, it is important to distinguish between infected and necrotic bone. Inflammation is the reaction of vital tissue and therefore it is not necessary to remove bone that is inflamed due to an infection. A vision of bone surgery in the diabetic foot with the objective of controlling the infection might be misleading if it resulted in the removal of bone that would be restorable by offloading and antibiotic therapy.

A distinction between infected bone and necrotic bone might be useful because tissue repair is possible in both states, but will be much easier to achieve in non-necrotic tissue. Necrotic bone could be determined histologically. A clinical assessment can be made taking as criteria resistance to mechanical strain or tendency to bleed if scratched. A cancellous bone easily removable with a curette without bleeding could be considered necrotic in this respect. The regional limit of an infection in the bone is even more difficult to determine. Imaging examinations like MRIs may show some inflammatory reaction even in more distant parts of the bone. The margins of surgical cuts often show microbiological growth even if the lesion is healing without antibiotics at the time when the result of the microbiological examination arrives. As an indication of the best level of resection, the criterion **'infected bone'** might lead to exaggerated removal and be too ambiguous to be of any use.

As an alternative to resection, in some countries, long-term antibiotic treatment is preferred. In other countries, surgery is used to remove bone thought to be necrotic and in a third group of countries surgery is used to remove bone thought to be infected [20–23]. In order to decide in which cases, to what extent and at what point of time surgery might be helpful, the criterion of **'necrotic bone'** could be helpful to determine the optimal pathway.

Surgery of osteitis is particularly useful if it combines the removal of necrotic bone with internal offloading. Examples are:

- the removal of the apical tuberosity combined with a tenotomy of the FDL/FHL or
- the removal of an infected IP joint or MTP joint combined with tenotomies of flexor tendons and lengthening of extensor tendons.

Case series demonstrate the often possible selective removal of bone to avoid amputation [24, 25].

20.5.1.1 Removal of the Apical Tuberosity

A resection of an osteolysis of the apical tuberosity through an oval excision of the existing lesion together with a tenotomy of the FHL or FDL tendon seems to be a natural response to this type of lesion.

Indication: Deep ulceration of the tip of the toe with exposed bone.

Procedure: Depending on the position and shape of the lesion, an oval excision is performed with its larger diameter in the transversal or sagittal plane. In the author's experience, postponing wound closure to the time after conditioning the wound surface leads to good results. This requires a few days of offloading and treatment with antibiotics. Tenotomy of the flexor tendon is equivalent to an immediate offloading which leads to a rapid decline in the signs of infection in the area which is no longer traumatised. Therefore, this intervention should be done without delay. If vascular supply is insufficient, this should be corrected in advance (Fig. 6.9a–l).

Aftercare: This is the same as described for the tenotomy of the FDL/FHL. Antibiotic therapy is usually needed for about 5 days. After closure of a wound by suturing its margins, the wound has to be checked every 1–5 days. If signs of infection arise, the suture material has to be removed.

Specific Risks: Besides the risk of infection as described above, this intervention has no specific risks beyond the risks of the tenotomy of the FDL/FHL, which is usually performed at the same time.

Evidence: In combined interventions together with tenotomies of the long flexor tendon in a case series of 15 patients with osteomyelitis [3], wound closure occurred in all patients, in 72.2% without further interventions.

20.5.1.2 Resection of the PIP joint

In surgery of claw toes, various procedures have been developed that include a resection or arthrodesis of the PIP joint. These interventions tend to be complex and involve implant of foreign material. Thus, they are not suitable for the treatment of an infected joint. In a traditional view, these lesions are treated with amputations. Avoiding foreign material and combining arthroplasty with tenotomies to straighten the toe, an arthrodesis might be a valuable alternative to amputation. We were not able to find published data on this type of intervention.

This resection is also used to treat interdigital ulcers or ulcers at the 5th toe if they have opened an IP joint at its medial or lateral side. These situations do not relate to specific problems apart from the general aspects discussed above.

Indication: The indication usually is seen in cases of lesions caused by an overstretched MTP joint. Therefore, this intervention is usually combined with other measures which together aim to correct the overload caused by the deformity of the toe. The deformed toes may also feature several pressure points that are at risk of ulceration and require treatment. In claw toes, for example, dorsal lesions involving the PIP joint might occur together with lesions of the apical tuberosity or beneath the MTHs. In these cases, a combined removal of the PIP joint and the apical tuberosity might be a good alternative to the often performed amputation of the toe. At the same time several areas can be relieved of excessive pressure combining interventions on bones and tendons. This might avoid a '*Vacuum-Phenomenon*' and the associated complications which are often seen after amputation.

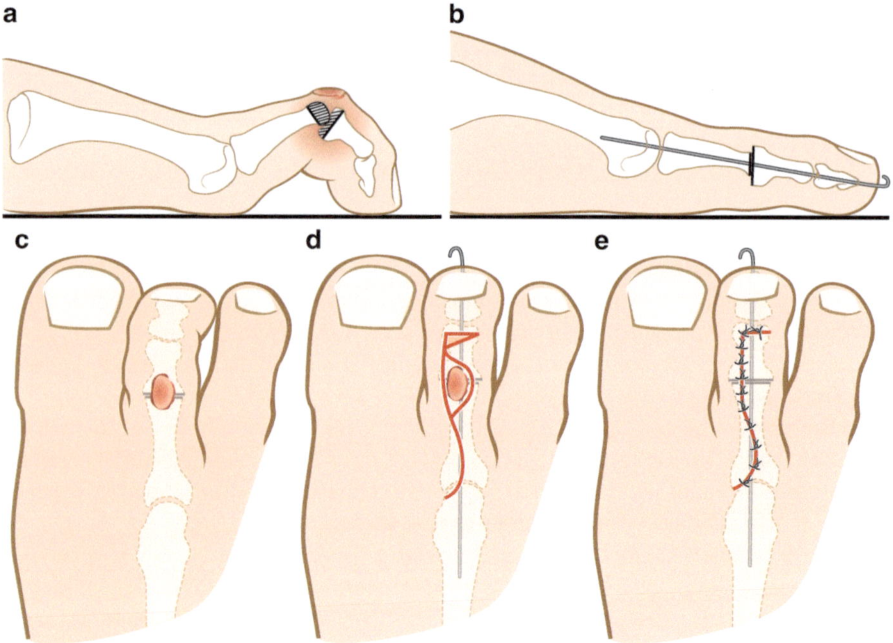

Fig. 20.17 Schematic representation of a PIP joint-resection with excision of a dorsal lesion, modified Z-plasty of the skin and osteosynthesis with Kirschner-wire. Kirschner-wire is not necessary in most cases

A combined resection of the MTP joint and the PIP joint might be used if the joints are fused and therefore soft tissue interventions are unsuitable (Figs. 20.17 and 20.18).

Procedure: Access includes an incision of the skin at the dorsum of the toe in the most appropriate direction in dependence of the shape of the ulcer. This incision sometimes is extended proximally reaching the MTP joint and distally to the oval excision of the lesion. If the extensor tendon is compromised, necrotic tissue is removed longitudinally. If the damage is more extensive, the tendon is severed transversally. The joint is exposed by the use of a Hohmann retractor to avoid damage of nerves and vessels. The head of the proximal phalanx and the basis of the intermediate phalanx are removed using the Lambotte chisel at the level of cancellous bone. The flexor tendon is attached by a percutaneous, U-shaped suture from distal to proximal using non-absorbable material. The skin is then closed by means of a modified Z-plasty. Sometimes, a release of the MTP joint together with the mobilisation of the plantar plate might be useful. A temporary arthrodesis by use of Kirschner-wire (1.6–1.8 mm) should only be used in exceptional cases.

Aftercare: Redressing bandages dorsalise the medial and distal phalanx in respect to the proximal phalanx. They are applied until stable wound closure has occurred. Therapeutic footwear with sufficient space is used for offloading.

Specific Risks:

- Risk of infection, especially if osteosynthesis is achieved by temporary use of a Kirschner-wire.

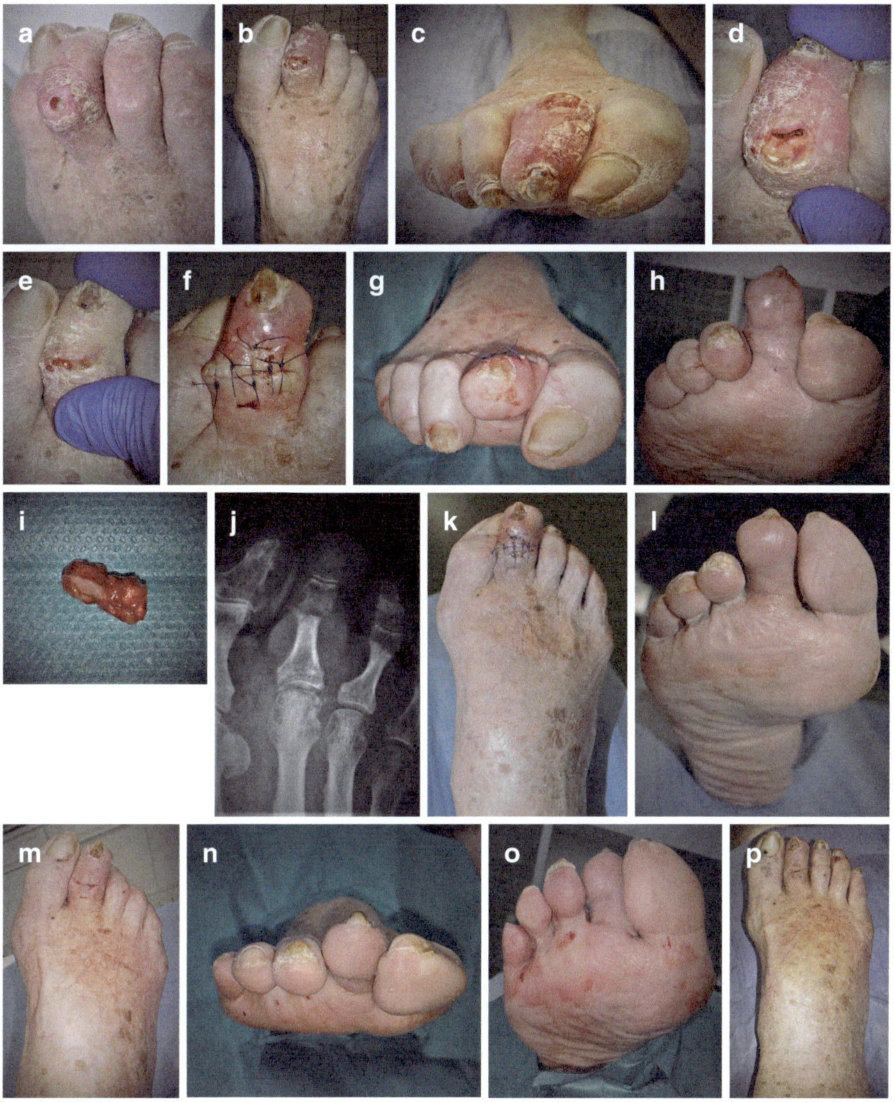

Fig. 20.18 Example of a resection of the PIP joint in a patient with a dorsal ulcer at the PIP joint, open capsule and osteonecrosis. (**a**) Initial lesion (**b**, **c**) after 3 month of conservative treatment an infection occurred with consecutive indication of amputation of the toe by three clinics, which the patient refused. (**d**) Passive plantarflexion (**e**) passive extension (dorsiflexion); Therapy: tenotomies were done on all extensors and flexors of the toe, a dorsal release of the MTP joint and a resection of the osteonecrosis; the sutures converge the edges (**f**–**h**) postoperative picture (**i**) parsimoniously removed head of the proximal phalanx (**j**) postoperative radiography (**k**, **l**) picture at the 5th postoperative day and (**m**–**o**) 2 weeks later the patient returned for tenotomy of the FDL- and FDB tendon of the 3rd to 5th toe and the FHL tendon; (**p**) 3 weeks after the resection of the 2nd PIP joint and 1 week after tenotomy of the flexor tendons 3–5 and the FHL tendon

20.5.1.3 Resection of the Metatarsophalangeal Joint (MTP joint)

Indication: In the case of plantar wounds involving MTP joints, a resection of the joint might be useful. A distal resection of 2/3 of the metatarsals has long been popular in many countries. After these interventions, difficulties in tissue repair and wound closure have been frequent due to the large wounds. Therefore, many surgeons now prefer more distal resections. These are often performed at the level of the cancellous bone of the articulation, which in most cases is not infection-free. However, this does not seem to jeopardise the surgical outcome. After a resection at the level of the metaphysis, the remaining metatarsal bone might deteriorate resulting in the radiological exam as characteristic 'candy stick'-appearance. The risk of such a degeneration is avoided if the resection is performed at the level of the cancellous bone.

If the joint is not opened by the ulcer, the authors' preference would be for other interventions with less impact on biomechanical issues like combined tenotomies of the extensor and flexor tendons and a dorsal release of the MTP joint or a dorsal closing wedge osteotomy.

Procedure: Access is from the dorsal side of the foot (dorsomedial or dorsolateral). The operation itself is performed in the usual way. The resection edges of the bone are located in the cancellous bone and are bevelled at the plantar edge.

Aftercare: As described above in the context of bone surgery, checks are carried out by X-ray after 2–3 days and 6–8 weeks in order to exclude an ongoing or progressive osteitis. The contiguous MTHs are particularly at risk.

Specific risks:

- Risk of deterioration of the remaining metatarsal bone.
- Transfer lesions under the adjacent MTHs

20.5.1.4 Resections in the Area of the IP Joint of the Hallux

These resections concern the medial condyle of the proximal phalanx of the hallux or of an accessory sesamoid bone within the FHL tendon. In the case of limited mobility of the first MTP joint (hallux limitus or rigidus) the hallux is not able to fulfil passive dorsiflexion as much as needed, and the IP joint takes on this movement (see Chap. 2, Sect. 2.7.4.3 and Chap. 9). The IP joint is normally unable to extend (=dorsiflexion), but in this situation is forced to overextend. The plantar aspect of the IP joint and especially the condyle of the proximal phalanx is therefore subject to unusual exposure and pressure. Sometimes, an accessory sesamoid bone in the FHL tendon at the level of the IP joint might be relatively large and act as an adjunctive hypomochlion. The localisation of the lesion might be positioned centrally or medially depending on the extent in which a torsion of the hallux occurs contemporarily. In general, it only becomes clear during the operation which structure is the pressure point and should be removed. The removal of the medial condyle or of an accessory sesamoid bone within the FHL tendon selectively corrects the inner pressure point. The intervention is supposed to facilitate wound closure and to avoid recurrence. We weren't able to find published data on this procedure when used to treat DFS.

Indication: If an overload of the medio-plantar or plantar side of the IP joint of the hallux leads to an 'indicator lesion', it may be worth considering this procedure.

The IP joint is usually not opened. An exposed surface of the joint is therefore rarely a problem for this intervention.

Procedure (Fig. 20.19): The access is achieved through a medial incision on the IP joint. The bundle of vessels and nerves should be protected while opening the capsule. The medial condyle is uncovered. The condyle might be surprisingly large. It is removed using the Lambotte chisel. After this, the FHL tendon can be explored

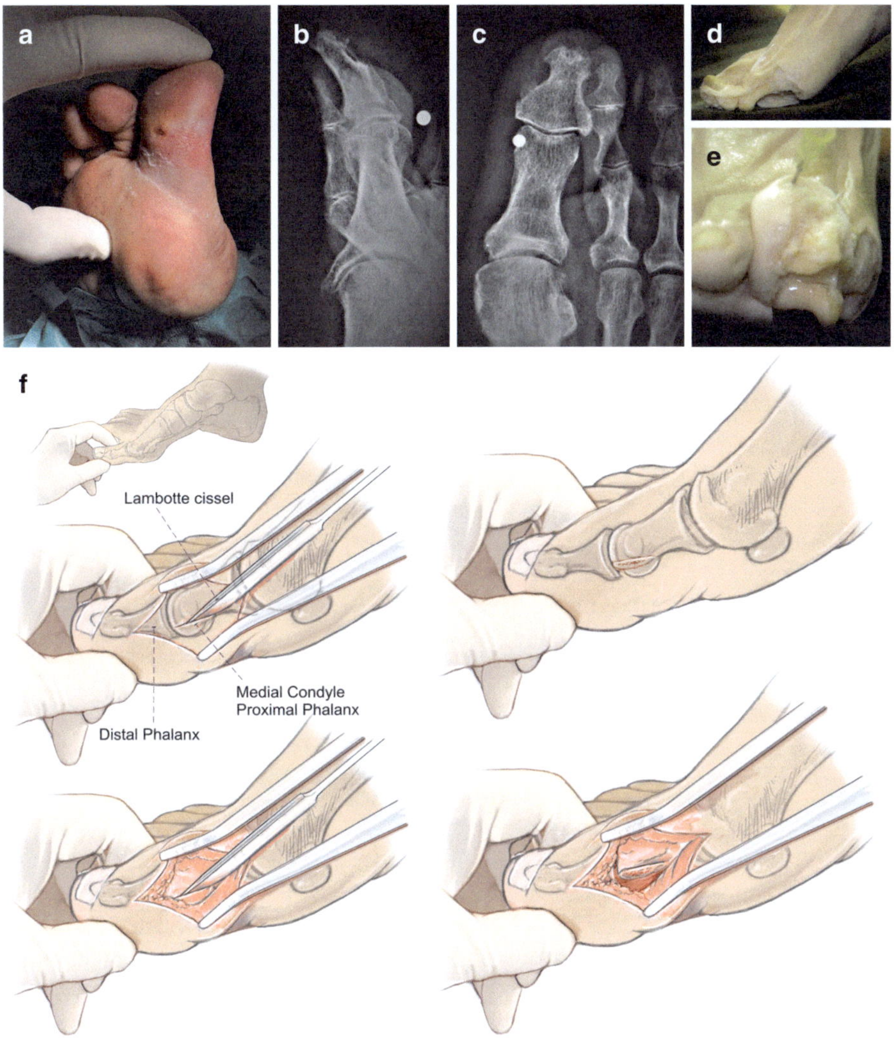

Fig. 20.19 (**a**) Preoperative condition with Hallux rigidus and lesion beneath the medial condyle at the head of the proximal phalanx (**b**, **c**) preoperative radiological findings (**d**, **e**) anatomical picture of a similar finding (**f**) surgical procedure, schematic, Figures by kind permission of [3]: (**g**) removed medial condyle of the proximal phalanx (1), removed accessory sesame bone of the FHL tendon (2), removed plantar fibrous changes (3) (**h**) postoperative finding

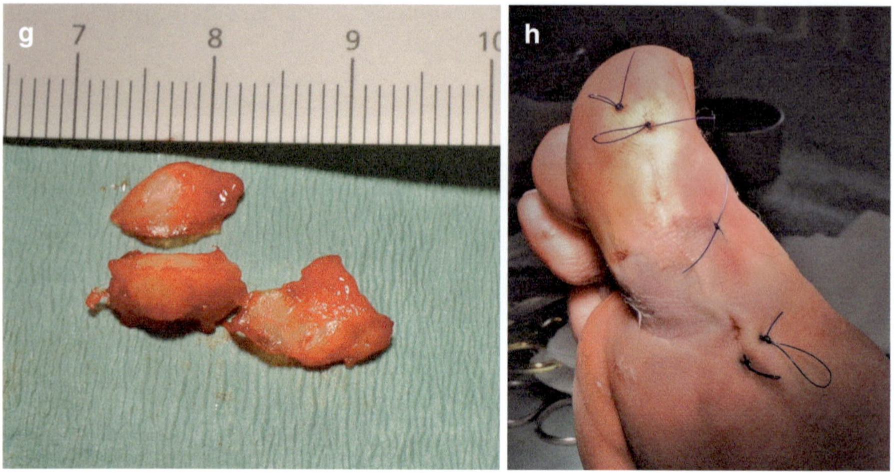

Fig. 20.19 (continued)

and if an accessory sesamoid bone is present, it may be removed (example Fig. 7. 10a–c). In this case, the accessory sesamoid bone can be removed through the same incision (example Fig. 9.3a–c). The ulcer is closed with a transcutaneous continuous suture using non-absorbable material and a suture for the skin (see details of the suture technique in Sect. 20.2 in this chapter). Sometimes, a redon-drainage is placed.

Minimally invasive surgery might represent a good alternative for this procedure.

Aftercare: As described above in relation to bone surgery, checks are carried out by X-ray after 2–3 days.

Specific risks: This intervention has no specific risks beyond the risks of bone surgery depicted above.

20.5.2 Rearrangements of Bones to Offload Lesions

20.5.2.1 Dorsal Closing- Wedge-Osteotomy of the 2nd to 5th MTH

This intervention has been known for many years and has several names ('dorsal open wedge resection', 'dorsiflexion osteotomy'). The description 'open' or 'closed' might be confusing as the wedge has an angle that is open in dorsal direction but is removed to permit closure of the gap. Although this procedure has been widely used for decades, we weren't able to find case series in people with diabetes. A similar, minimally invasive procedure (Distal Metatarsal Diaphyseal Osteotomy = DMDO) had excellent results in a case series [26].

Indication: An 'indicator lesion' beneath a prominent condyle of a MTH would indicate the usefulness of this procedure. On the other hand, at the 5th MTH with a (slightly) supinated foot, the authors' preference would be for the sole resection of the condyle and/or one of the interventions on the tendon to reduce supination. If the ulcer had already opened the articulation, the authors would prefer a resection of the MTH to the wedge osteotomy.

Procedure: The bone is accessed from dorsum. A wedge with its wider part in dorsal direction is sawn or chiselled in the cancellous bone at the transition between metaphysis and the head. The plantar cortex is left unaffected. Applying pressure, the head is pushed slightly upwards, the wedge closes and the metatarsal bone becomes slightly shorter. Both functional effects result in offloading of the MTH. The fragments remain together and don't need foreign material to assure osteosynthesis. In order to adjust the toe in a straightened position, a lengthening of the extensor tendons and sometimes a resection of the base of the toe's proximal phalanx might be necessary. In particular, markedly overstretched toes can block the surgical access to the MTH. The plantar plate should be preserved and the bone free of infection (Fig. 20.20).

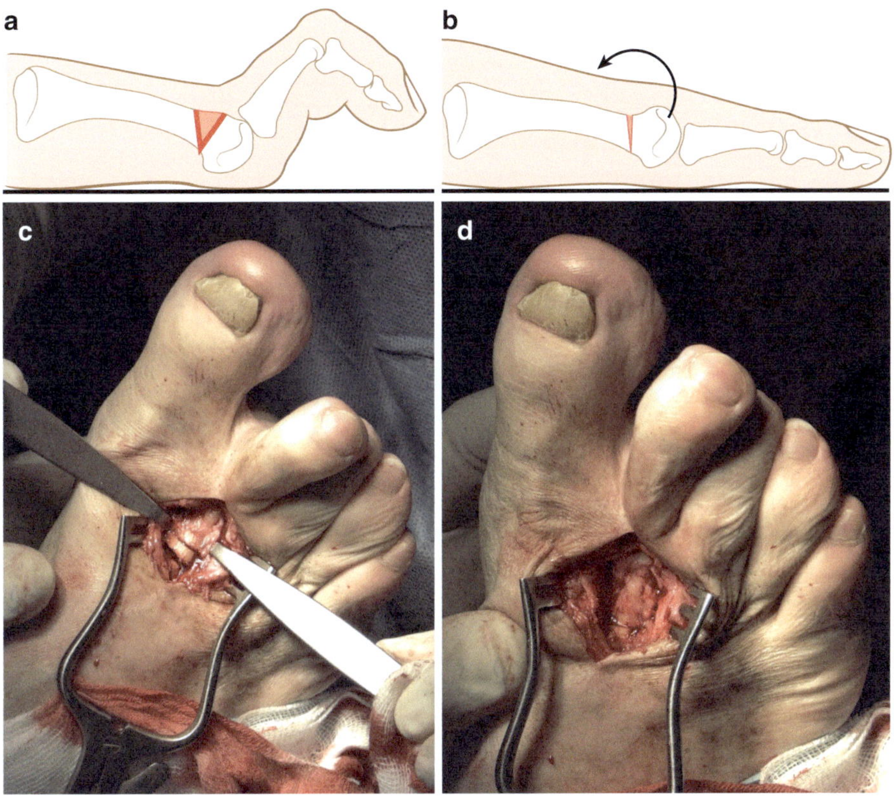

Fig. 20.20 (**a** and **b**) schematic representation of the dorsalising removal of a wedge in the distal metatarsal bone and reposition of the MTP joint to offload a plantar ulcer, (**c** and **d**) are intraoperative pictures, in (**c**) the wedge is cut but not yet removed, in (**d**) it is removed and the gap is closed by applying pressure at the head from the plantar side (**e**) radiologic picture after intervention

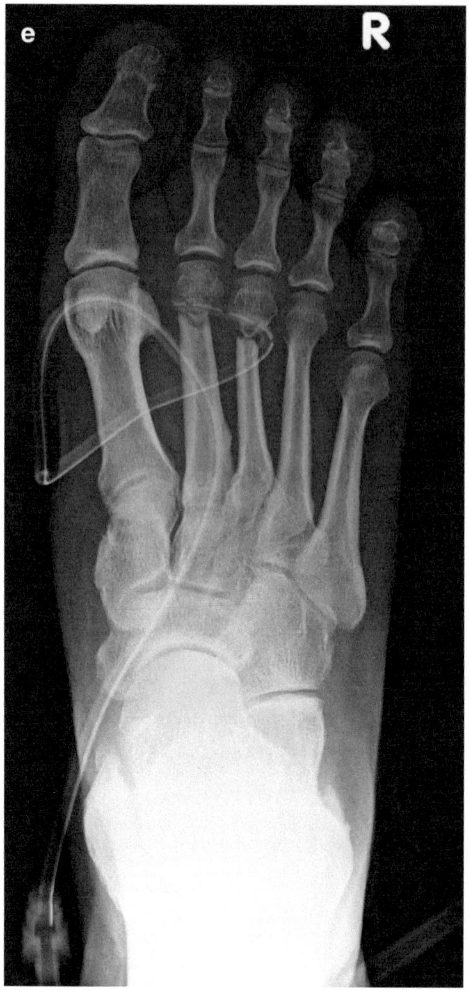

Fig. 20.20 (continued)

Aftercare: As described above concerning bone surgery. Checks are performed by X-ray after 2–3 days.

Specific risks: This intervention has no specific risk beyond the risks of bone surgery described above.

20.5.2.2 Resection of the Condyle of the 5th MTH

This intervention removes the hypomochlion selectively and is less invasive than a resection of the entire 5th MTH.

The lateral condyle of the 5th MTH is often slightly more pronounced than the medial one. It might be further exposed in a supinated foot due to the rotation around the sagittal axis. This is the case, for example, in a pes cavus together with marked dorsiflexion in the MTP joint which further exposes the condyle of the MTH. The removal of this prominence results in an effective displacement of the inner pressure point (see Chap. 14 and Fig. 14.1c).

The removal of the entire MTH has shown beneficial aspects as it was associated with less re-ulceration than conservative treatment [27]. The assumed benefits of the more selective removal of the lateral condyle are as follows: preserved weight-bearing, at least equivalent avoidance of re-ulceration and more rapid wound closure.

Indication: An 'indicator lesion' beneath a prominent lateral condyle of a (slightly) supinated foot might indicate the intervention. If the ulcer had already opened the articulation, the authors' preference would be for a resection of the MTH.

Procedure: Access to the joint is best laterally above the joint. The joint capsule is prepared and opened by a longitudinal incision taking the vessel-nerve cord into account. The MTH is prepared and the lateral condyle is removed using the Lambotte chisel. The joint capsule is sutured using a transcutaneous suture with non-absorbent material. In rare cases, a redon drainage is put in place (10CH). Thereafter, skin is also sutured (see details of the suture technique in Sect. 20.2 in this chapter).

If marked dorsiflexion of the toe in the MTP joint is present, an intervention on the tendons might help to achieve an orthograde position of the toe and allow the MTH to shift dorsally.

This intervention might benefit from a minimally invasive technique (Fig. 20.21).

Aftercare In addition to the above-mentioned principles, an X-ray inspection after 2–3 days is recommended.

Specific risks: This intervention has no specific risk beyond the risks of bone surgery depicted above.

20.5.2.3 Valenti Resection Arthroplasty

This procedure, also known as 'cheilectomy' or 'Valenti procedure' is widely used to correct hallux limitus as a cause of pain in patients without neuropathy see also Chap. 9). Its results have been documented in case series [28, 29]. For the treatment of this dysfunction in neuropathic patients we were unable to find even a case series. As this intervention offloads the IP joint in case of a hallux rigidus, it is supposed it helps to close ulcers at this location and prevent recurrence.

Indication: This procedure is used in the case of a Hallux rigidus and consecutive plantar indicator lesion of the skin above the IP joint (see also Chap. 9, Fig. 9.1).

Procedure: Access to the joint is made dorsomedially. The joint capsule is exposed and longitudinally incised. Osteophytes are removed. A V-shaped wedge (angle of approximately 45°) with parts belonging to the dorsal MTH and the proximal phalanx is removed. The sesamoid bones are mobilised, and the joint capsule is positioned between both bones or sutured. In the intraoperative situation, the dorsal extension of the toe should be at least 75° in relation to the neutral position. Usually a redon drainage is needed. The plantar parts of the joint and the windlass mechanism must be preserved carefully (see Fig. 9.6a–d).

Aftercare: In people without neuropathy the joint has to be mobilised by means of painful physiotherapy during aftercare. A person who has no perception of pain will mobilise early and powerfully and therefore avoid this disadvantage. Other aspects are as described above concerning bone surgery. Checks are performed by X-ray after 2–3 days.

Specific risks: This intervention has no specific risk beyond the risks of bone surgery depicted above.

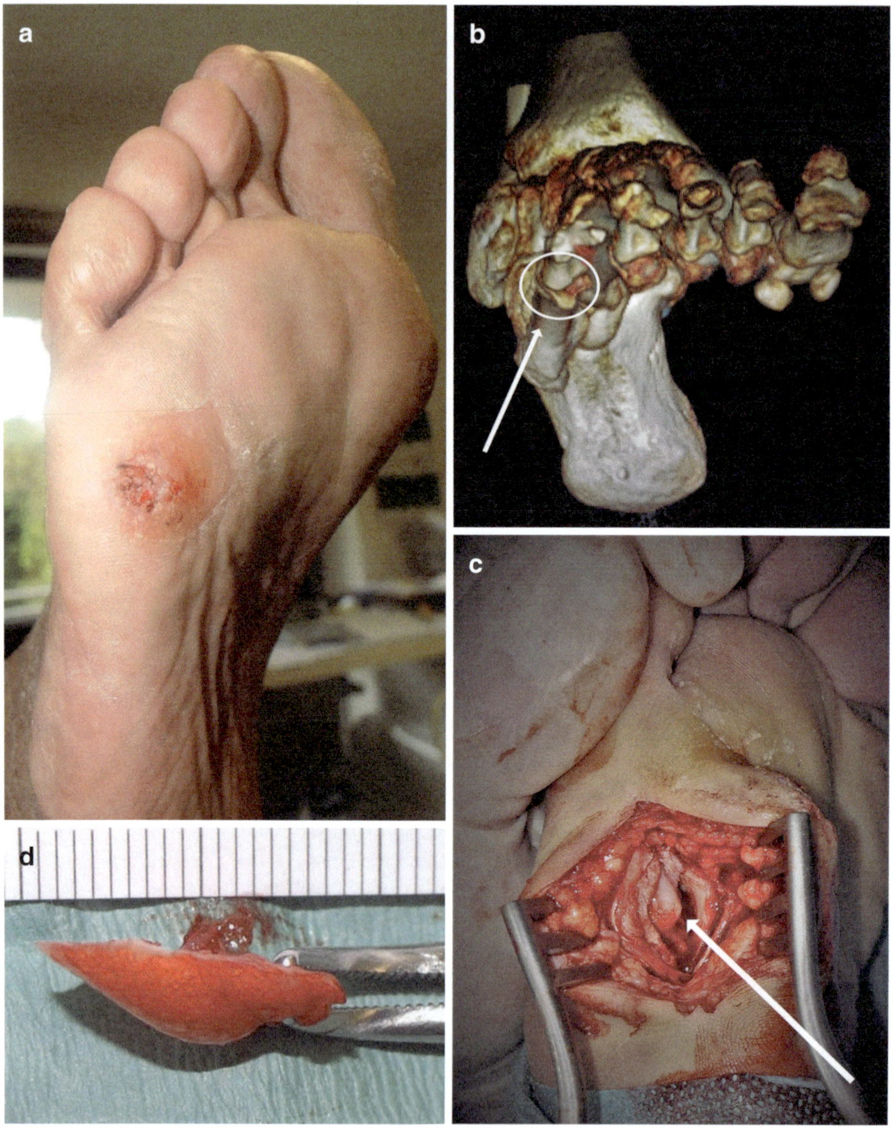

Fig. 20.21 Resection of the lateral condyle of the 5th MTH (**a**) clinical picture for overview (**b**) CT reconstruction (**c**) site of the intervention (**d**) removed condyle (**e**, **f**) result post-OP; the lateral condyle is marked by an arrow in (**b** and **c**)

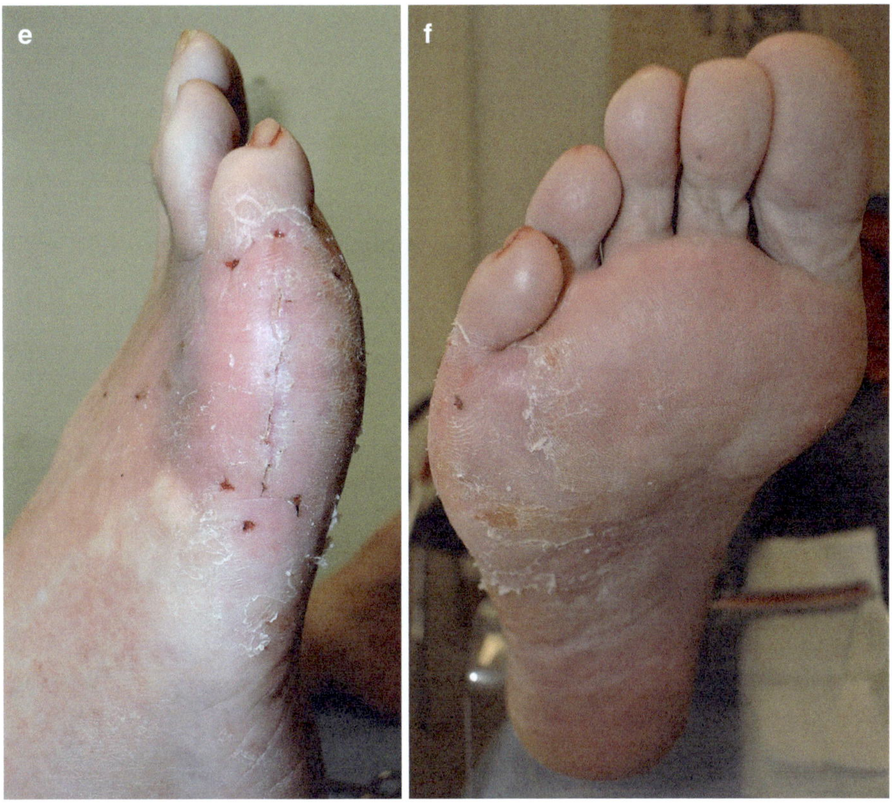

Fig. 20.21 (continued)

20.5.2.4 Resection of the Medial Sesamoid Bone

The sesamoid bones together with their ligaments are important for a powerful plantarflexion of the hallux during propulsion. The FHL tendon runs between the two sesamoid bones and therefore is protected and able to pull the toe downwards, even during propulsion. It prevents the tendon from being blocked. The removal of the medial sesamoid bone will reduce this ease of motion and therefore other methods should be preferred if available and sufficiently effective. This resection has been used to treat osteonecrosis of the sesamoid bone [30] and is supposed to be effective in offloading the tissue above this prominence.

Indication: An indication might be an 'indicator lesion' at the medial sesamoid bone in a pes cavus with lowered first MTH and zig-zag deformity of the hallux. In this case, lengthening of the Achilles tendon combined with an elongation of the EHL tendon and sometimes of the FHL might be sufficient. During aftercare, a shoe with diagonal elevation of the outer margin might be used. If there is a recurrence, the sesamoid bone can be removed (see also Figs. 14.1a, 14.1b, 14.6a, b, and 14.7a–g). This step-by-step approach should not result in a dangerous delay. The next step should be considered right from the start because the joint can usually not be saved once it has been opened by an ulcer.

Procedure: Access is from the medial side of the joint. The capsule of the MTP joint is prepared and longitudinally incised whilst paying attention to not compromise the vessel-nerve cord. The sesamoid bone is then liberated from the plantar parts of the capsule. After removal of the bone the capsule is closed with a transcutaneous suture using non-absorbent material (see Sect. 20.2 in this chapter). Plantar defects of the capsule, if existing, are sutured too. Sometimes, a redon-drainage (10CH) must be used and then the skin is also closed.

As an alternative the medial sesamoid bone might be partially removed using minimally invasive techniques.

Aftercare: As described above concerning bone surgery. Checks are performed by X-ray after 2–3 days.

Specific risks: This intervention has no specific risk beyond the risks of bone surgery depicted above.

20.6 Summary

- **Each surgical procedure on diabetic feet has specific prerequisites. The experienced surgeon chooses between procedures considering perfusion, the desired grade of mobility and other general conditions.**
- **There are many alternatives to amputation and fear of complications is not justified, because the maximum complication is exactly this, amputation.**
- **If more than one method is possible, the least invasive method, but one that still provides sufficient offloading is preferred.**
- **These interventions have high potential because they usually eliminate overloading permanently and have low rates of complication. Nevertheless, they are not regularly included in the therapy planning and rarely used due to the lack of experienced surgeons and the lack of knowledge by diabetologists.**

20.7 Recommended Literature

De Prado, Ripoll, Golanó: Minimally Invasive Foot Surgery

Presentation of innovative procedures of minimally invasive surgery of deformities of the foot. Excellent photos taken whilst perfoming the operations on cadavers describe the techniques very convincingly, 2009 Barcelona

Banks, Downey, Martin, Miller: McGlamry's Forefoot Surgery

Comprehensive standard reference concerning forefoot surgery, Lippincott Williams & Wilkins, 2004—620 pages

Thomas Zgonis (Editor): Surgical Reconstruction of the Diabetic Foot and Ankle

Comprehensive overview of procedures of surgical therapy including surgical care for the Charcot Foot, the infected Charcot Foot, reconstructive surgery and therapeutic footwear. Many easily understandable schematical and clinical pictures. 2009 Wolters Kluwer, ISBN 978-0-7817-8458-0

References

1. Peters EJ, Lipsky BA, Aragon-Sanchez J, Boyko EJ, Diggle M, Embil JM, Kono S, et al. Interventions in the management of infection in the foot in diabetes: a systematic review. Diabetes Metab Res Rev. 2016;32(Suppl 1):145–53. https://doi.org/10.1002/dmrr.2706.
2. Engels G. Ambulante chirurgische prozeduren bei diabetischem fußsyndrom diabetes. Stoffwechsel und Herz. 2010;19(2):111–5.
3. Engels G, Stinus H, Hochlenert D, Klein A. Concept of plantarization for toe correction in diabetic foot syndrome. Oper Orthop Traumatol. 2016;28(5):323–34. https://doi.org/10.1007/s00064-016-0453-9.
4. van Netten JJ, Bril A, van Baal JG. The effect of flexor tenotomy on healing and prevention of neuropathic diabetic foot ulcers on the distal end of the toe. J Foot Ankle Res. 2013;6(1):3. https://doi.org/10.1186/1757-1146-6-3.
5. Thornhill MH, Dayer M, Lockhart PB, Prendergast B. Antibiotic prophylaxis of infective endocarditis. Curr Infect Dis Rep. 2017;19(2):9. https://doi.org/10.1007/s11908-017-0564-y.
6. Bonanno DR, Gillies EJ. Flexor tenotomy improves healing and prevention of diabetes-related toe ulcers: a systematic review. J Foot Ankle Surg. 2017;56(3):600–4. https://doi.org/10.1053/j.jfas.2017.02.011.
7. Scott JE, Hendry GJ, Locke J. Effectiveness of percutaneous flexor tenotomies for the management and prevention of recurrence of diabetic toe ulcers: a systematic review. J Foot Ankle Res. 2016;9:25. https://doi.org/10.1186/s13047-016-0159-0.
8. Rasmussen A, Bjerre-Christensen U, Almdal TP, Holstein P. Percutaneous flexor tenotomy for preventing and treating toe ulcers in people with diabetes mellitus. J Tissue Viability. 2013;22(3):68–73. https://doi.org/10.1016/j.jtv.2013.04.001.
9. Blank HA. Extensor release. J Foot Surg. 1978;17(2):58–9.
10. Hromadka R, Bartak V, Bek J, Popelka S Jr, Bednarova J, Popelka S. Lateral release in hallux valgus deformity: from anatomic study to surgical tip. J Foot Ankle Surg. 2013;52(3):298–302. https://doi.org/10.1053/j.jfas.2013.01.003.
11. Dayer R, Assal M. Chronic diabetic ulcers under the first metatarsal head treated by staged tendon balancing: a prospective cohort study. J Bone Joint Surg Br. 2009;91(4):487–93. https://doi.org/10.1302/0301-620X.91B4.21598.
12. Mueller MJ, Sinacore DR, Hastings MK, Strube MJ, Johnson JE. Effect of Achilles tendon lengthening on neuropathic plantar ulcers. A randomized clinical trial. J Bone Joint Surg Am. 2003;85-A(8):1436–45.
13. Colen LB, Kim CJ, Grant WP, Yeh JT, Hind B. Achilles tendon lengthening: friend or foe in the diabetic foot? Plast Reconstr Surg 131 (1):37e-43e; 2013. https://doi.org/10.1097/PRS.0b013e3182729e0b.
14. Holstein P, Lohmann M, Bitsch M, Jorgensen B. Achilles tendon lengthening, the panacea for plantar forefoot ulceration? Diabetes Metab Res Rev. 2004;20(Suppl 1):S37–40. https://doi.org/10.1002/dmrr.452.
15. Laborde JM. Neuropathic plantar forefoot ulcers treated with tendon lengthenings. Foot Ankle Int. 2008;29(4):378–84. https://doi.org/10.3113/FAI.2008.0378.

16. Lin SS, Lee TH, Wapner KL. Plantar forefoot ulceration with equinus deformity of the ankle in diabetic patients: the effect of tendo-Achilles lengthening and total contact casting. Orthopedics. 1996;19(5):465–75.
17. Laborde JM. Midfoot ulcers treated with gastrocnemius-soleus recession. Foot Ankle Int. 2009;30(9):842–6. https://doi.org/10.3113/FAI.2009.0842.
18. Mulhern JL, Protzman NM, Brigido SA. Tibialis Anterior Tendon Transfer. Clin Podiatr Med Surg. 2016;33(1):41–53. https://doi.org/10.1016/j.cpm.2015.06.003.
19. Piaggesi A, Schipani E, Campi F, Romanelli M, Baccetti F, Arvia C, Navalesi R. Conservative surgical approach versus non-surgical management for diabetic neuropathic foot ulcers: a randomized trial. Diabet Med. 1998;15(5):412–7. https://doi.org/10.1002/(SICI)1096-9136(199805)15:5<412::AID-DIA584>3.0.CO;2-1.
20. Aragon-Sanchez FJ, Cabrera-Galvan JJ, Quintana-Marrero Y, Hernandez-Herrero MJ, Lazaro-Martinez JL, Garcia-Morales E, Beneit-Montesinos JV, Armstrong DG. Outcomes of surgical treatment of diabetic foot osteomyelitis: a series of 185 patients with histopathological confirmation of bone involvement. Diabetologia. 2008;51(11):1962–70. https://doi.org/10.1007/s00125-008-1131-8.
21. Game FL, Jeffcoate WJ. Primarily non-surgical management of osteomyelitis of the foot in diabetes. Diabetologia. 2008;51(6):962–7. https://doi.org/10.1007/s00125-008-0976-1.
22. Senneville E, Lombart A, Beltrand E, Valette M, Legout L, Cazaubiel M, Yazdanpanah Y, Fontaine P. Outcome of diabetic foot osteomyelitis treated nonsurgically: a retrospective cohort study. Diabetes Care. 2008;31(4):637–42. https://doi.org/10.2337/dc07-1744.
23. Uckay I, Gariani K, Pataky Z, Lipsky BA. Diabetic foot infections: state-of-the-art. Diabetes Obes Metab. 2013. https://doi.org/10.1111/dom.12190.
24. Faglia E, Clerici G, Caminiti M, Curci V, Somalvico F. Feasibility and effectiveness of internal pedal amputation of phalanx or metatarsal head in diabetic patients with forefoot osteomyelitis. J Foot Ankle Surg. 2012;51(5):593–8. https://doi.org/10.1053/j.jfas.2012.05.015.
25. Tamir E, Finestone AS, Avisar E, Agar G. Toe-sparing surgery for neuropathic toe ulcers with exposed bone or joint in an outpatient setting: a retrospective study. Int J Low Extrem Wounds. 2016;15(2):142–7. https://doi.org/10.1177/1534734616636311.
26. Biz C, Gastaldo S, Dalmau-Pastor M, Corradin M, Volpin A, Ruggieri P. Minimally invasive distal metatarsal diaphyseal osteotomy (DMDO) for chronic plantar diabetic foot ulcers. Foot Ankle Int. 2018;39(1):83–92. https://doi.org/10.1177/1071100717735640.
27. Armstrong DG, Rosales MA, Gashi A. Efficacy of fifth metatarsal head resection for treatment of chronic diabetic foot ulceration. J Am Podiatr Med Assoc. 2005;95(4):353–6.
28. Nicolosi N, Hehemann C, Connors J, Boike A. Long-term follow-up of the cheilectomy for degenerative joint disease of the first metatarsophalangeal joint. J Foot Ankle Surg. 2015;54(6):1010–20. https://doi.org/10.1053/j.jfas.2014.12.035.
29. Roukis TS. The need for surgical revision after isolated valenti arthroplasty for hallux rigidus: a systematic review. J Foot Ankle Surg. 2010;49(3):294–7. https://doi.org/10.1053/j.jfas.2010.02.001.
30. Mauler F, Wanivenhaus F, Boni T, Berli M. Nonsurgical treatment of osteomyelitis of the hallux sesamoids: a case series and literature review. J Foot Ankle Surg. 2017;56(3):666–9. https://doi.org/10.1053/j.jfas.2017.01.025.

Fundamentals of Local Treatment 21

This chapter describes local therapy of ulcers both in terms of medical management and surgical procedures. The natural process of tissue repair and wound closure is poorly understood. The possibilities for accelerating this process without surgery are limited. Thus, mechanisms of tissue repair are presented here in basic terms. Methods of plastic reconstructive surgery are presented in more detail because they offer the opportunity to really change the natural course of an ulcer and may avoid amputation.

We have deliberately not used the word '*healing*' because lack of recognition as a lifelong disease is one of the major problems in organising care for people with DFS. The word 'healing' suggests that the problem has disappeared and nothing special needs to be taken into account thereafter.

21.1 Overview

There are only a few randomised controlled trials concerning the patient-relevant endpoint 'wound closure'. The planning and implementation of this type of study is very difficult. The closure of ulcers is similar to a relay race. The baton is carried by a multitude of simultaneous and sequential processes, reaching from limiting the initial damage to the final stage where the skin covers the defect and is able to withstand pressure. To test the effectiveness of just one measure which is thought to support one single process, it would be necessary to standardise all accompanying factors and investigate a large number of test candidates, in order to average out the effect of the other measures and the natural variance. Recently, one such study has been published in favour of a dressing that inhibits lytic enzymes [1], but patients have been highly selected and the result has not yet been confirmed. Because there are no such studies for most questions of this type, therapists need to rely on their experience and intuition. They observe the process of tissue repair and wound closure and eliminate anything which might prevent them from taking place. Many different materials are available that show small differences in features which don't

D. Hochlenert et al., *Diabetic Foot Syndrome*,
https://doi.org/10.1007/978-3-319-92055-9_21

lead to different indications. In choosing the right materials it is more important to avoid a few major errors than to find the 'best material'.

The guidelines on which this advice is based are the 'IWGDF guidance on the use of interventions to enhance the healing of chronic ulcers of the foot in diabetes' [2], 'Practical Guidelines on the Management and Prevention of the Diabetic Foot' *2011* [3], the 'National Guidelines for Treatment of the Diabetic Foot' [4] and the guidelines 'Local Therapy of Chronic Ulcers in Patients with the Risk of Peripheral Arterial Disease, Diabetes mellitus, Chronic Venous Insufficiency' [5].

21.2 Subdivisions

A distinction is traditionally made between 'primary' (per primam intentionem or p.p.) and 'secondary' (per secundam intentionem = p.s.) wound closure. Primary wound closure takes place when the edges of the defect are close together and there is no substantial infection. In this case, the closure takes place almost entirely without leaving a scar. By contrast, secondary wound closure takes place when the defect is larger or when infection is present. In both situations, as a first step the defect is filled with scab, which is then substituted by granulation tissue, which is substituted later by a scar (Fig. 21.1). Minimal defects allow primary closure which results in a limited amount of granulation tissue and therefore minimal scar tissue as end product.

The processes of tissue repair can best be observed in the case of secondary wound closure, as this is more time-consuming, and the repair process is openly visible. This is divided into phases in order to simplify the progression on a chronological basis (Fig. 21.2). The problem here is that the different phases can appear

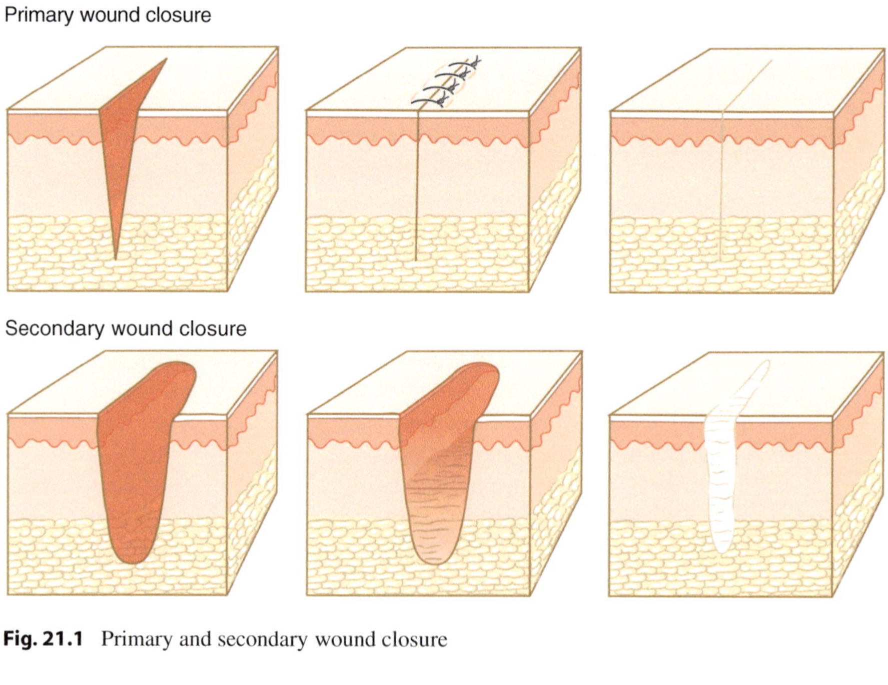

Fig. 21.1 Primary and secondary wound closure

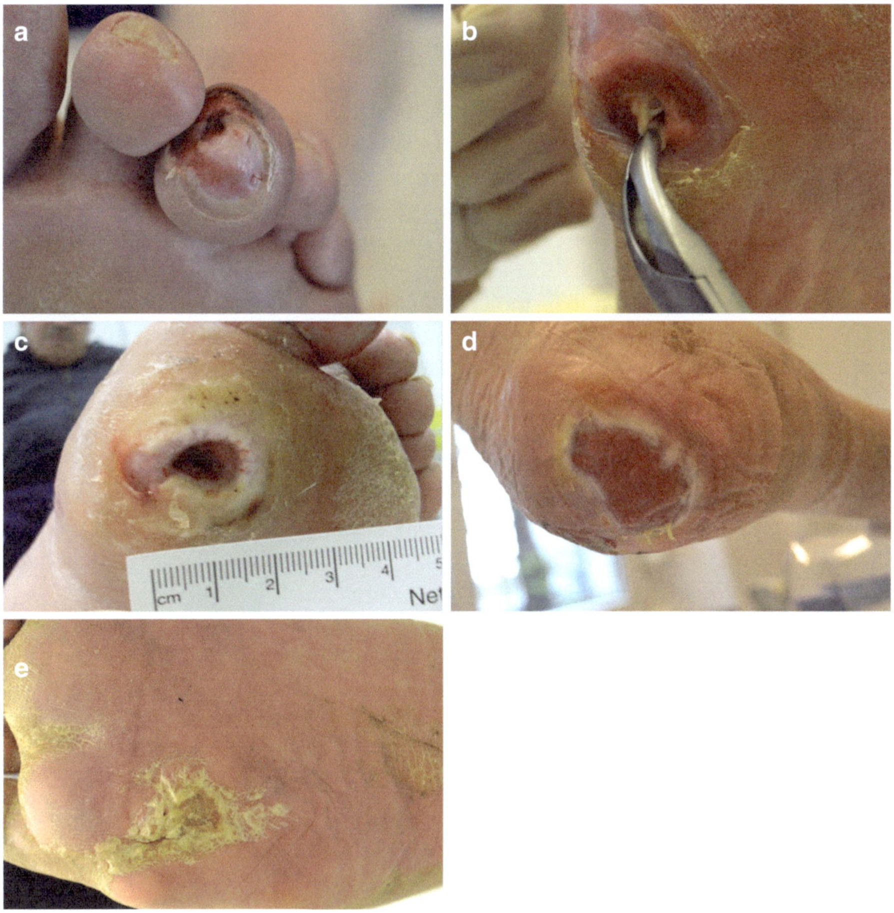

Fig. 21.2 Examples of ulcers in the various phases of repair; (**a**) infection phase in the mediodorsal part of the ulcer, no demarcation of the borders; (**b**) infection phase with demarcation, allowing the complete removal of all necrotic tissue with the use of Luer forceps; (**c**) ulcer maintained unrepaired by constant trauma, which can be recognized by the punctate bleeding within the edges. The wound closure stops during the granulation phase; (**d**) heel lesion in the epithelisation phase with granulation tissue at skin level; (**e**) plantar scar with hyperkeratosis

simultaneously at different sites of an ulcer. In addition, this classification is an extreme simplification of a series of overlapping processes. Nevertheless, to make the principal processes easier to understand and to support the search of therapeutic alternatives tissue repair is presented in phases in this book.

21.2.1 Phase 1: Inflammatory Phase, Cleansing Phase

The ulcer contains foreign bodies, deposits of blood with erythrocytes, leucocytes and thrombocytes as well as traumatised tissue. Some of this compromised tissue is dead, and some can be revitalised. Microorganisms can spread undisturbed in devitalised regions. The tissue which is still vital forms a boundary and brings white blood cells into this border region, especially granulocytes, monocytes and macrophages. The vital tissue can soon be clearly distinguished from the devitalised tissue. Autolytic enzymes released from dead, local cells and enzymes from migrating granulocytes/macrophages behave in a similar way to digestive enzymes in the stomach and the intestine. They cause devitalised organic structures to liquefy. In excess, these enzymes can affect the intact skin surrounding the ulcer and cause the ulcer to spread. These enzymes also play a role in the further phases of tissue repair and are summed up under the term MMPs (**M**atrix-**M**etallo**P**roteases) due to the presence of a metal atom in their molecular structure. In the first phase, in addition to autolytic debridement, their task is to open the basal membrane and to stimulate cell migration. Excess effects should be prevented by their inhibitors, or TIMP's (**T**issue **I**nhibitors of **M**etallo**P**roteinases), [6–8]. One study has shown a decrease in time to wound closure using a substance that inhibits MMP's [1]. This suggests that MMP's might play a major role in preventing a wound from closing.

In some presentations, the inflammatory phase is divided into two parts. The exudative phase comprises the first few hours after the damage with the development of a wound scab. The second, resorptive phase describes the subsequent days with autolytic processes and the start of granulation tissue growth.

Possible influences: A moist condition stimulates enzymatic autolysis. Autolytic debridement can be complemented by mechanical or biosurgical debridement, thus shortening the inflammatory phase.

With appropriate therapy, the inflammatory phase could last no longer than 3–5 days.

21.2.2 Phase 2: Granulation Phase

The ulcer is filled with blood vessels which appear on the surface like a layer of small elevations (grains of corn = granula) and is therefore referred to as granulation tissue. Its purpose is to rapidly form a surface at the same level as the surrounding area and to enable epithelisation. In a later step, this surrogate tissue is completely replaced by fibroblasts and their product, collagen, which results in a white scar. This means that in the area of weight-bearing it is not the best option to allow deep ulcers with large surface areas to close by granulation. In such a situation, reconstructive surgery e.g. with a local flap may be more suitable. Apart from this exception, granulation is a welcomed precondition for subsequent epithelisation. In this phase, the MMPs have the task of enhancing vessels to start growing.

Possible Influences: A moist condition is also necessary for the growth of granulation tissue [9]. An ulcer which remains very damp for a long time, e.g. around the edges of a fistula, may even lead to hypergranulation. In this case, the overwhelming granulation extends above the level of the skin blocking epithelisation. The protruding granulation tissue can simply be cut away. Apart from brief haemorrhage, which is easily stopped, no complications are to be expected. The granulation tissue can also be put under pressure by the use of short stretch bandages. The important point here is to find and eradicate the cause of this ongoing inflammation and enhanced secretion. The cause might be, for example, an infected bone sequestrum in deep, inaccessible parts of the ulcer.

21.2.3 Phase 3: Epithelisation Phase

Epithelisation requires less moisture. In this phase, the wound contraction causes the margins to be drawn to the centre. In superficial wounds, epithelial cells spread from sweat glands, hair follicles, and sebaceous glands that had survived in the wound. This is not possible for deep ulcers, where migration of epithelial cells starts only from the edges and takes more time. New skin appears as a pale pink seam. In some cases, white patches may also be visible in the ulcer. These are islands of epithelial tissue with keratinized squamous cells, which hasten the closure of the ulcer (Fig. 21.3).

The development of granulation tissue is, in general, followed seamlessly by epithelisation, so that the two processes are often combined and referred to as the 'Proliferation phase'.

Possible Influences: In the epithelisation phase it is better for the ulcer not to be too moist, without drying out entirely. In addition, the surface of the ulcer should be at the same level as its margins. Oedema of the edge of the ulcer with a deep step to the granulating base of the ulcer impedes epithelisation. For this reason, it may be necessary to use bandages and apply pressure to the ulcer if there are signs of oedema at the edge of the ulcer.

21.2.4 Phase 4: Remodelling: Stabilisation of the Skin and Scar Development

After initial closure of the ulcer, which is recognisable by the lack of secretion on the dressing and the lack of scabbing of the wound, the ulcer is not yet able to withstand pressure. It may take months until the skin has achieved its final level of

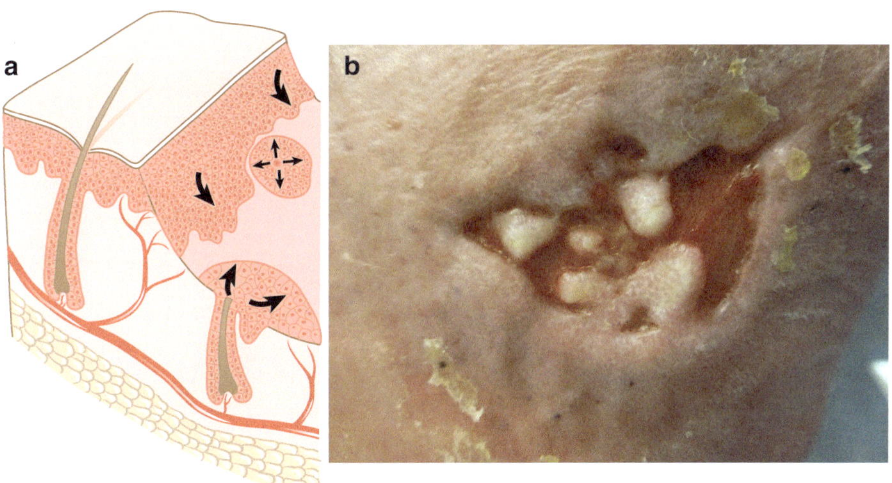

Fig. 21.3 Epithelisation (**a**) ways of propagation during epithelisation (**b**) islands of skin accelerate epithelisation

resilience and in general this is not the same as the original resilience of the skin at the site. Depending on the degree of pressure to which the foot will be subjected, the former ulcer area may be regarded as relatively stable after 2–4 weeks of remodelling. The feet may then be loaded again under close control and wearing protective footwear [10].

21.2.5 Regulation of Wound Repair

The regulation of wound repair is not fully explained. Lytic enzymes (MMPs), their inhibitors (TIMP's) and growth factors participate. Growth factors are thought to be involved in a variety of tasks:

- Regulation of cell migration
- Control of infection
- Coordination of tissue growth, regression and remodelling
- Stimulation of the production of collagen
- Promotion of capillary spreading

Therapy with single growth factors has not fulfilled expectations. The main reason for this is thought to be the fact, that tissue repair and wound closure are regulated by equally important processes of growth and degeneration which require a coordinated interaction of enzymes, inhibitors, and growth factors in chronological order. At present, there is no reliable way of determining which factors are lacking and which are in surplus at a given point in time. For this reason, a targeted regulatory intervention is still not possible [11].

21.3 Debridement

Debridement is the removal of all non-vital materials from the ulcer and of hyperkeratosis from the skin surrounding the ulcer. It has various functions:

- It allows an assessment of the ulcers characteristics.
- It creates the precondition for a biopsy or a deep swab.
- It can shorten the time to wound closure, since removal of debris relies not only on autolysis.
- It improves the chances of repair:
  - Reduction of the breeding ground for bacteria and the amount of pathogenic agents
  - Removal of mechanical threat due to necrotic tissue in the ulcer
  - Relief of pressure on the growth area at the edge of the ulcer
  - Improvement of accessibility for topical therapies on the surface of the ulcer

Debridement can be performed mechanically, biosurgically, autolytically or by other less common means. Surgical debridement is a variation on mechanical debridement, which is performed by the operating surgeon. Sometimes, ulcer cleansing, which does not extend to the intact tissue, is differentiated from debridement, which goes further.

Surgical debridement is the most invasive form. Its primary goal is to remove all dead material from the ulcer. For this reason, it also affects small parts of healthy tissue. Various instruments are used, in particular the scalpel. It requires sufficient anaesthesia, although the amount of anaesthesia may be reduced due to neuropathy. There may be bleeding that will stop on compression after a short time. In general, there is also a conversion of the ulcer from chronic to acute state. This lays the foundation for the physiological tissue repair and the closure of the ulcer (Fig. 21.4). It represents the most effective form of debridement and is considered to be the basis for a stage-adapted ulcer therapy [12–15]. For many reasons, for example the inability of the patient to undergo anaesthesia, this type of procedure may not be possible.

Less invasive methods of *simple mechanical debridement* range from the use of abrasive gauze to the use of sharp instruments ('sharp debridement'), e.g. scalpels, ring curette or sharp spoons. A simple mechanical debridement can often be performed without any anaesthesia. If pain perception is not completely lost, topical local anaesthetics might be used. The time required for the local anaesthetic to work must be taken into account (Fig. 21.5). Mechanical debridement may be necessary during dressing changes in order to remove any remaining necrotic tissue, if present.

Biological debridement (biosurgery) describes the treatment of the ulcers with sterile maggots, currently in particular the species Lucilia sericata. The cleansing of

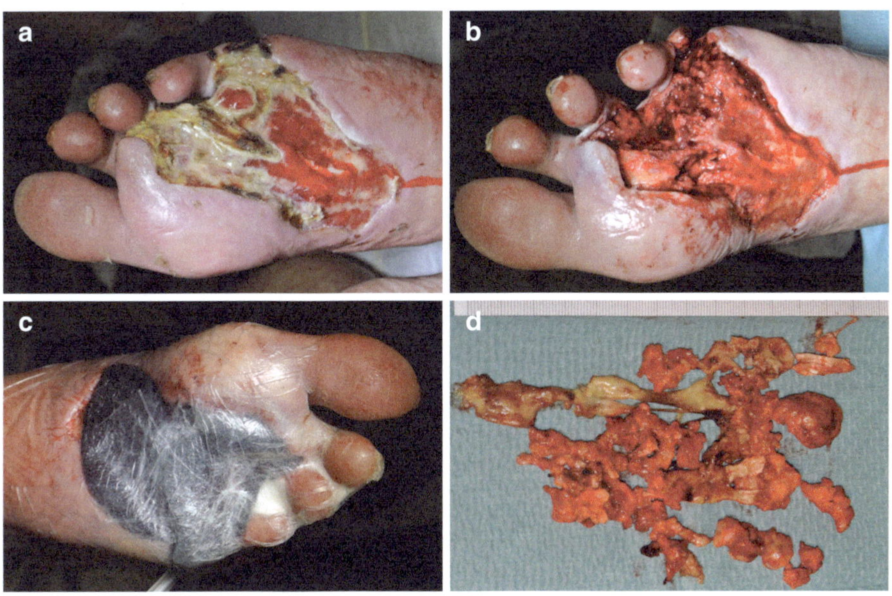

Fig. 21.4 (**a**–**d**) Plantar ulcer before and after surgical debridement and appliance of a negative pressure bandage

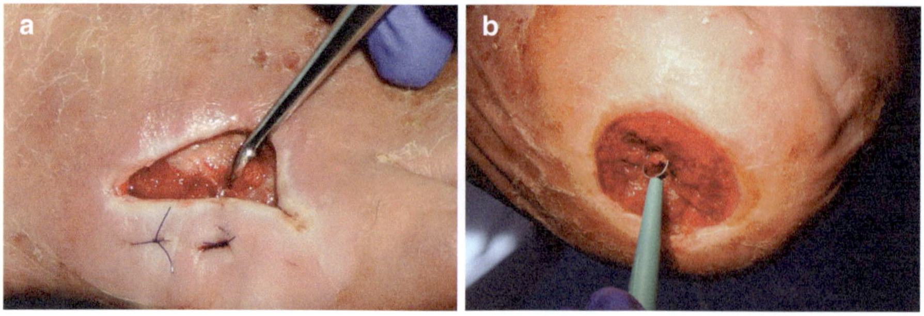

Fig. 21.5 (**a**, **b**) Debridement with sharp spoon and ring curette

Fig. 21.6 Treatment with maggots in a biobag after 3 days of application

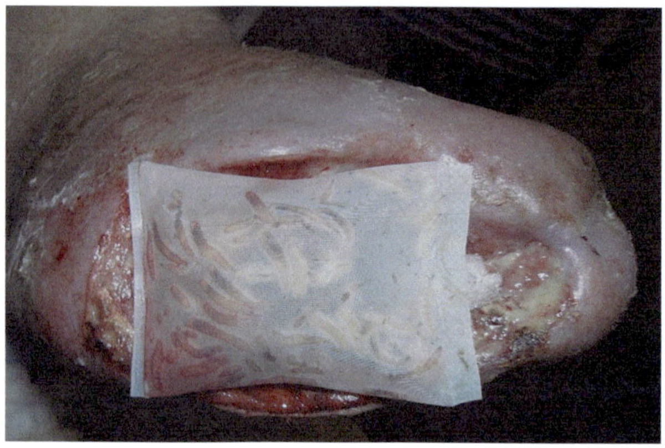

infected ulcers using maggots was described by W.S. Baer, who started treating ulcers systematically which were bacterially affected in cases with chronic osteomyelitis in 1928 and later published the results [16].

The digestive secretions of the maggots lead to a selective necrolysis in the ulcer resulting in a border zone necrosectomy, in general without causing bleeding. The effect of the digestive secretions has in large part not been investigated and the supposed benefits are not proven [17–19].

This form of treatment may be carried out as a so-called 'free-range treatment' or in special 'biobags' (Fig. 21.6), a bag-like convenience product. The recommended dosage is approximately 5–10 maggots per cm^2 ulcer area.

In the case of *Lavage techniques,* fluids are used, either in a bath or applied specifically at the ulcer itself. This is carried out as a low-pressure rinse or at very high pressure as a water jet cutting technique, which can also achieve a necrosectomy. These procedures have not yet been widely implemented and have not been adequately investigated, particularly in view of undesired effects, such as infiltration of deeper layers of tissue structures by microorganisms [13, 20].

Enzymatic debridement employs enzymes which target the fibrin and collagen of the necrotic tissue. In comparative studies, none of the substances available on the market has shown to have a significant effect on the closure of the ulcer [21].

Autolytic debridement relies on the ulcer's own enzymes, in particular from necrotic cells and activated phagocytes. In this case, it is sufficient to keep the ulcer moist, where the moisture is stabilized using therapeutic support systems such as sterile moist compresses, hydrogels or superabsorbers. These support systems can be combined with local ulcer antiseptics such as hydrogels containing polyhexanide. Autolytic debridement is painless and safe, however, the time required for complete necrolysis is much longer than for mechanical procedures.

In the initial phase of the repair process, the debridement is necessarily more extensive than in later phases and may have a decisive advantage over leaving the repair process to its natural course. Devitalised tissue fragments are removed rapidly using a sharp instrument. Autolysis only needs to remove a few remaining fragments, allowing the second phase of ulcer repair to begin quickly.

It needs to be noted that when debridement takes place, it includes trauma to the wound, cooling of the ulcer, a change in the chemical environment and it may remove positive mediators of healing. Therefore, during phases in which the ulcer is closing satisfactorily, the so-called 'stable repair phase', every time the dressing is changed, a decision must be made as to whether debridement should be performed at all or whether it would make more sense to rest the ulcer.

21.4 Stable Necrosis

This alternative treatment concept for people with critical PAD means to stabilise a dry necrosis and to wait for the slow process of autolytic rejection. It is used in case an operative or interventional procedure to enhance perfusion is not suitable or may demand too much effort from a patient with important co-morbidities. An amputation in the inadequately perfused region may also be disadvantageous; as such intervention would extend the area of the ulcer and further impair the chance of wound closure. PAD limits the inflammation and the development of granulation tissue. In this non-reactive condition, the minimal remaining perfusion is sufficient. In this case, PNP is of benefit, since the whole process can take place either without pain or whilst keeping the use of analgesics to a minimum.

At first, necrosis develops with almost no reaction from the surrounding tissue. While the necrosis dries out and turns into a stable necrosis, a *demarcation zone* develops in the periphery including microabscesses. These microabscesses enable a spatially very limited autolytic rejection of the necrosis. At the same time, skin closure occurs on barely recognisable granulation tissue. The necrosis itself changes its consistency to a leather-like structure in the sense of mummification. It protects the surface of the ulcer and possibly fulfils other mechanical functions e.g. allowing the patient to transfer while using the necrotic limb for some steps. Finally, this is followed by autoamputation with often scarless skin closure (Fig. 21.7).

The therapeutic options are confined to supportive measures. Short periods of antibiotic therapy may be necessary. In addition, the original decision to leave the necrosis and forego revascularisation measures should be reviewed on a regular basis (Fig. 21.8). The demarcation zone must be cleared of detritus, so that any

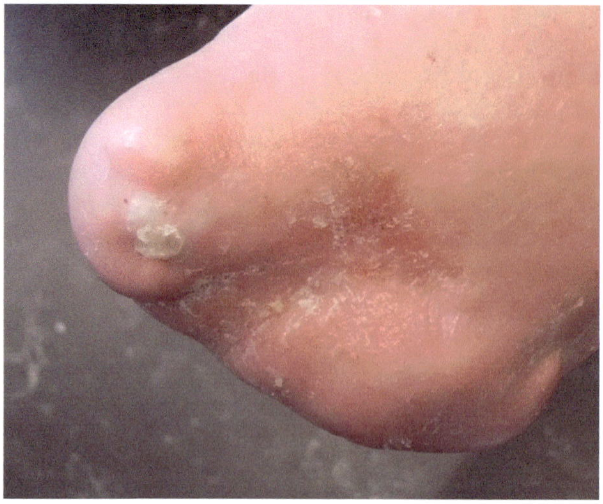

Fig. 21.7 Almost scarless skin closure after autoamputation of all toes

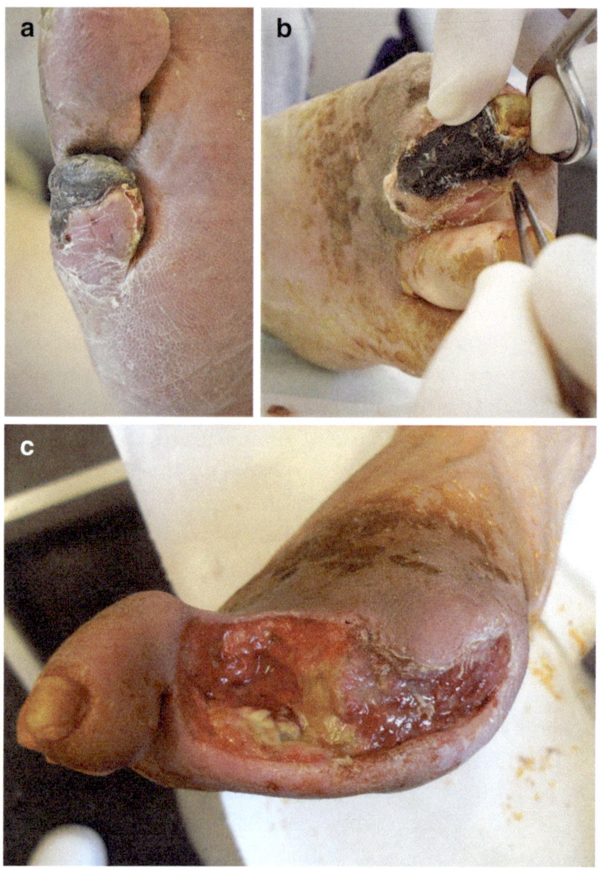

Fig. 21.8 Care of the border zone of a stable necrosis (**a**) early stage (**b**) advanced stage with predominantly autolysed border zone (**c**) after detachment of the toe

secretions can drain off. In the course of local treatment, there may be a detachment of the partially autoamputated necrosis (Fig. 21.8b, c). In this case, disinfectant dressing materials might be useful for longer than would otherwise be the case.

The primary goal of treatment, in this case, is not the closure of the ulcer. Most importantly the patients should not be restricted in their quality of life as a result of the ulcer, i.e. they should be able to walk or support themselves and not suffer pain. Life-threatening situations as a result of septicaemia or amputation while circulation is insufficient should be avoided.

The process is often protracted. Further difficulties ensue from the emotional burden of people caring for the patient, who may have difficulty in finding the appropriate reaction to the unusual appearance. In addition to providing detailed education for all those involved, an information sheet for relatives and caregivers can be very helpful.

The patient benefits, as the risks of a surgical major amputation can be avoided, and as autoamputation occurs at the precise borderline where perfusion is sufficient to ensure the survival of the tissue. The necrosis itself covers the ulcer and may fulfil other mechanical functions such as a brief bearing of the body's weight. For example, it might allow walking on a mechanically impaired but usable limb. In general, the process is not overly burdensome if pain and infections are kept to a minimum [22, 23] (Fig. 21.9).

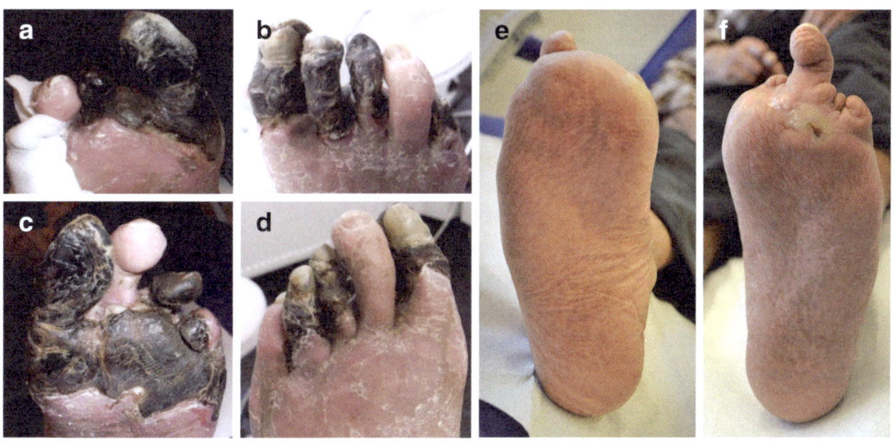

Fig. 21.9 Case report of stable necrosis: 70-year-old patient, haemodialysis for 15 years with renal insufficiency resulting from gout, interrupted for 10 years following a kidney transplant and long-term immunosuppressive therapy (Tacrolimus and corticosteroids), diabetes mellitus for 1 year, after PTA on both limbs with restored perfusion of the Arteriae tibialis anterior limited by several stenosis. A widespread inguinal haematoma followed the PTA, so that further revascularisation was not attempted, progress over 15 months. Mobile with walking frame, offloading with foam rubber insoles, 1 cm thickness in therapeutic shoe, use of dry antiseptics in the border zone of the necrosis and cotton wool to maintain warmth. Mobile and free from ulcers apart from superficial lesions 1 year after wound closure

21.5 Dressing Materials

The materials for dressings can be subdivided into primary dressings, which are in direct contact with the ulcer, secondary dressings, which regulate moisture, and external dressings, for support, warmth and protection from knocks and bumps. In other categorisations, these groups are described as 'ulcer fillers', 'ulcer coverings' and 'restraints'. Primary dressings may also be grouped into inactive (non-adherent gauze), hydroactive (moisture absorbent or moisture dispersing) and active dressings (having an influence on factors or enzymes).

21.5.1 Primary Dressings

Primary dressings are in contact with the ulcer. Their task is to create a microclimate that meets the needs of this phase of wound repair in terms of moisture and warmth. Some are said to reduce bacterial growth or attempt to influence mediators in order to intervene in the regulation of wound repair.

The order in which the materials are presented in this chapter reflects the phase of wound healing for which they are considered to be appropriate.

21.5.1.1 Amorphous Hydrogels

Hydrogels are three-dimensional polymer nets with a high water content which may be more or less solid. The amorphous wound gel preparations are only that firm as to not 'flow away' but do not resist pressure. They are offered in tubes or syringes, from which they can be squeezed out easily. They are used for rehydration. Keeping the ulcer moist, they help autolytic enzymes to exert their action.

Caution when using amorphous Hydrogels: In the case of a dry necrosis in an insufficiently vascularised limb, they should not be used.

21.5.1.2 Foams with Rough and Mixed Pore Sizes

These polymer foams (e.g. polyurethane foam) are good carriers for hydrogels and allow liquids to flow through their coarse mesh. They can be applied in the first and second phase of wound repair.

Caution when using these foams: (1) These foams may be very firm and must be cut in such a way that they lie on the surface of the ulcer with light pressure. The material should *not be pressed forcefully* into ulcer cavities or fistulae. (2) Since growing granulation tissue can invade these foams, they should not remain on the ulcer for more than *2–3 days*.

21.5.1.3 Alginates

Alginates (brown algae cell-walls, spirally twisted polysaccharides) turn into a gel in the ulcer and do not stick to its surface. They absorb fluids and transport them through their internal capillaries. They are applied in the first and second phase of wound repair. They can be soaked with antimicrobial additives such as silver compounds. Alginates are believed to have haemostatic properties resulting from the release of calcium ions (Ca^{++}).

Caution when using alginates: (1) Alginates should *not overlap the edge of the ulcer*, as they will transmit fluids through their capillaries to the surroundings and adhere to the skin. In a second moment, the overlapping capsule of alginate material may dry out and form a fixed bond with the edge of the ulcer creating a hard cover top preventing the drainage of secretions. (2) Due to the possibility of drying out, they should *not be applied to periosteum* or similar structures without first being moistened.

21.5.1.4 Fine Pore Foams

These foams have small and open pores which are partially sealed on the wound-facing surface. This prevents the growing granulation tissue from penetrating into their meshes. They are applied in the second and third phase of ulcer repair. There are foams containing silver, but in this phase of ulcer repair, disinfectants are not indicated and the combination is generally unnecessary. The integration of superabsorbers enables them to absorb a larger amount of liquids.

Caution when using fine pore foams: These foams are simple to use. However, under compression, the exudate can be pressed back into the ulcer. Foams with superabsorbers can be used for ulcers with heavy secretion.

21.5.1.5 Spacer Grids

Hydrophobic gauzes such as greased gauze merely prevent the surface of the ulcer from sticking to the dressing and therefore represent a basic form of primary dressing. They are used when the ulcer no longer needs moisture. When a marked reduction in exudation is required, the spacer grid can be combined with a highly absorbent dressing pad containing superabsorbers.

Caution when using spacer grids: Hydrophobic gauze is straightforward to use.

21.5.1.6 Solid Hydrogels

Solid hydrogels are three-dimensional polymer nets with less water content than the amorphous ones. They are available as pads, which as a result of the adhesive features of their material do not require additional adhesives and should not irritate the skin. They are occlusive and are used to prevent dehydration.

Caution when using solid Hydrogels: In the case of a dry necrosis in an insufficiently vascularised limb, they should not be used.

21.5.1.7 Hydrofibres

Hydrofibres consist of carboxymethylcellulose and are used in the second phase of wound closure. In contact with the ulcer secretion, they form a gel. They absorb liquids vertically and should not conduct them to the edge of the ulcer. They are used to rehydrate ulcers.

Caution when using Hydrofibres: They too should not be applied when dry necrosis is intended.

21.5.1.8 Hydrocolloids

Hydrocolloids were among the first of the so-called 'modern wound care' products, however, they have gone out of fashion. They are also used in the second phase. They close the wound and, in the occlusion, a malodorous pus-like fluid develops.

In the case of the diabetic foot, it is assumed that they are associated with infections of the ulcer.

21.5.2 Secondary Dressings

The secondary dressings cover the ulcer and the primary dressing. Their main role is to regulate the flow of fluids, either to absorb fluids or to keep them in the ulcer.

21.5.2.1 Compresses

A compress, possibly integrated into a plaster, is the simplest form of secondary dressing. It absorbs only very small quantities of fluids.

21.5.2.2 Simple Absorbent Dressing Pad

Simple absorbent dressing pads generally consist of cellulose. They can absorb limited quantities of fluids. Their main disadvantage is that they release the absorbed liquid under pressure (for example under a compression bandage).

21.5.2.3 Absorbent Dressing Pad with Superabsorbers

Absorbent dressing pads with superabsorbers absorb the fluid into a core of swelling material consisting of acrylates. These are highly hygroscopic substances which are capable of absorbing and retaining large quantities of fluids even under pressure, for example under a compression bandage.

21.5.3 External Dressing

The external dressing serves as mechanical protection, to keep the other ulcer dressings in place and to keep the extremity warm. In cases where the skin is irritated or where a known oversensitivity to adhesives is present ('plaster allergy'), alternatives such as tubular gauze, are used to keep the dressing in place. In other cases, adhesive dressings have the advantage that they can be applied quickly and do not slip off easily.

21.5.4 Adhesive Fleece

Adhesive fleece is amongst the most widely used products in outpatient departments dealing with diabetic feet. In general, they can only be stretched in one direction. In the other direction, they are tight.

21.5.5 Gauze Bandages and Tubular Bandages

Elastic gauze bandages are typically preferred over inelastic gauze bandages, as they are easier to apply and offer more support.

Tubular bandages are stretchable. Some return to their original shape, others do not. When compared to gauze bandages, they have the advantage of preventing any application errors that might lead to limb constriction. However, they should not be knotted at the end, as this may also lead to constriction and to pressure ulcers on the lower leg.

21.5.6 Surgical Cotton Wool

Surgical cotton wool consists of a synthetic material which does not irritate the skin and produces less microscopic materials than the natural product. It warms the covered area and can absorb small amounts of fluid if necessary. Cotton wool should not be used as the outer surface of the whole dressing and should not come into direct contact with the skin.

Cotton wool which has become moist with ulcer secretions and subsequently dries can become hard and apply harmful pressure. In addition, surgical cotton wool is relatively expensive. Therefore, it has been replaced in some areas by foam bandages. These are washable and thus contribute to cost reduction.

21.5.7 An Example of a 'Cotton Wool Shoe'

For patients with an angioneuropathic foot, a 'cotton wool shoe' can be used. The foot and the lower leg are covered with gauze or tubular bandages to a height which can be individually determined. Then the cotton-like padding bandage is applied to create an even layer covering the area and protecting the toes or heel from bumps. Three to five layers are placed on top of each other and these layers are placed on the toes and wrapped using the remaining material (Fig. 21.10). The material is wrapped around the heel in such a way that there is not too much material on the instep and still enough on the heel. The layers are wrapped around the heel in figure of 8 in the same way as with bandages used to stabilise the ankle (see also TCC Fig. 19.1d in Chap. 19). The stabilization is achieved by using a tubular bandage.

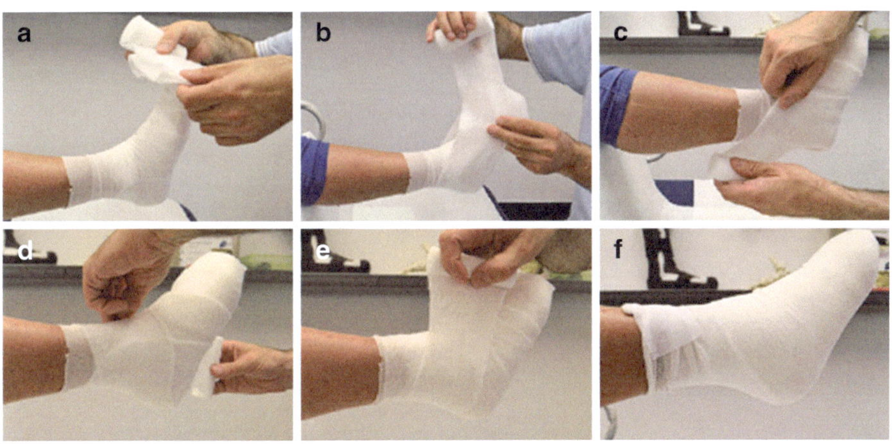

Fig. 21.10 Example of a 'cotton wool shoe' without particular protection for toes or heel: (**a**) three layers of cotton wool used as padded bandage to protect against bumps, (**b**) wrapping the bump protection, (**c, d**) form an 8 around the heel, (**e, f**) wrapping the leg upward until the desired height

Even though protection against impacts is ensured to a certain degree, the extent of pressure relief in the case of plantar ulcers is limited.

21.5.8 Choice of Material and Avoiding Mistakes

Many roads lead to Rome—and there is more than one way to cover an ulcer. 'Dressings have the magic power to induce the belief that they heal the ulcer while covering it.' Paul Brand, the pioneer of the treatment of neuropathic pressure ulcers in the western world is quoted as saying. The variety of alternatives in the dressings cupboard seems to have more to do with the character of the therapists than with the ulcers of their patients. Some prefer to have a wide choice of options available; others prefer a narrower range for a concise strategy. There is some evidence in favour of the use of MMP binding substances [1], which still needs to be confirmed.

The first decision concerns the question of whether the ulcer requires more moisture or if fluids should be drained off. This depends on formation of secretions and on what is currently best for the ulcer (Table 21.1). The specific decision for the material is based on ease of use (Intervals between dressing change, competence of the persons responsible for changing the dressings, sources of error and mechanical properties), price and personal experience.

It is particularly important to avoid any possible mistakes. Most of these errors involve a false estimation of the amount of fluid drained from the ulcer and the dressing's ability to handle it.

21.5.8.1 Aggressive Secretions Remain on the Ulcer and the Surrounding Area

The result is a self-sustaining inflammation. This is typical for the first phase of wound healing in highly inflamed wounds and is avoided by giving preference to dressings that drain fluids well.

21.5.8.2 Large Quantities of Secretion

Even if secretions have no aggressive characteristics, large quantities can lead to a maceration of the surrounding skin or to hypergranulation. This can be caused by high fluid production, for example in the case of oedema and dressings without sufficient drainage capacity. Dressings containing highly absorbent gels, so-called superabsorbers, are well suited to remove fluids from the ulcer can be applied in these cases.

Table 21.1 Criteria to determine the fluid requirements of an ulcer

More dry	More moist
Primary wound repair	Secondary wound repair
Acute minor wound (trivial wound)	Problem wound (due to site, depth, exposed structures, area)
Epithelisation phase	Infection and Granulation phase
Dry necrosis/PAD	

21.5.8.3 Excessive Fluids Under a Hard Cover When Using Alginates

Alginates can form a gel when in touch with ulcer secretions and dry out later. They can establish a firm connection with the surrounding skin and form a covering that looks like a scab. In contrast to a scab, the quantity of fluid under such an inconspicuous cover may increase and generate pressure. It then may lead to the formation of a fistula and damage of vital tissue.

21.5.8.4 Dehydration of Superficial Wounds After Opening Blisters

The result is the necrosis of layers of skin that are otherwise unaffected and the induction of extensive, deep ulcers. Simple greased gauzes on an open blister are therefore less effective, solid hydrogels or hydrocolloids are more suitable.

21.5.8.5 Moistening of Dry Necrosis in Critical PAD

It is particularly important that the necrotic material does not enter a process of bacterial decay and become the starting point of a bacterial invasion. It is equally important that a significant immune reaction is not required, as the available blood flow is insufficient to provide the necessary resources. For this reason, the activation of the process by moistening the ulcer in an attempt to stimulate an autolytic debridement is counterproductive.

21.5.9 Alternative Ulcer Therapy

Many substances, natural products or other materials are believed to have properties which promote wound repair. Some of them have a regional widespread use such as tea tree oil in Australia or olive oil in Mediterranean countries. None of them is an established standard treatment for the diabetic foot.

Available products are:

- Nutritional products (honey, sugar, olive oil…)
- Plant extracts (tea tree oil…)
- Hormone preparations from other fields of indication (insulin…)
- Vitamins or Provitamins (dexpanthenol, vitamin E…)
- Constituent parts of enzymes (zinc…)
- Other molecules of biological origin (haemoglobin…)

Some of these have been known for a long time, others are promoted as new and promising solutions. It is not possible to pass conclusive judgement at present as robust evidence for their use is not available. When using materials such as food that are not approved for the therapy of wounds, the possibility of legal consequences must be taken into account.

21.5.9.1 Disinfection of the Ulcers

In contrast to antibiotics, which are metabolised and specifically kill sensitive bacteria, disinfectants have a much less precise effect and inhibit or kill bacteria, fungi, viruses, protozoa and endogenous cells. For this reason, they cannot be administered systemically but only locally. The common term 'local disinfectant' is therefore redundant. For the disinfection of ulcers, substances are used which are supposed to be less harmful to the body's own cells. In choosing the right substance, the following possible unfavourable characteristics are relevant: inactivation of the disinfectant by proteins ('Protein error'), staining, prolonged application time needed, short shelf life, and pain. For this reason, only a few substances are in use. Examples are: Hypochlorous acid, Octenidine, Phenoxyethanol, Povidone iodine, Polyhexanide and compounds of silver. It is particularly important **not** to apply them routinely without considering the unwanted effects.

21.5.10 Physical Methods for Accelerating Wound Repair

There is very little which has not been attempted over the centuries to speed up the repair of wounds. Hardly any of the methods used have proven to be effective. The case of hyperbaric oxygen (HBO) therapy is controversial. In one well-conducted randomised double-blinded study this method was shown to cause faster wound closure in a mixed population of patients with adequate perfusion or non-reconstructable PAD [24]. Two subsequent studies have not shown statistically significant differences [25, 26].

On the other hand, Negative Pressure Wound Therapy (NPWT) is used widely, even by the authors, although there is no clear evidence of its effectiveness [27]. In this case, the ulcer is hermetically sealed with a foil dressing and the chamber thus created is subjected to a defined vacuum with the use of an electronically controlled pump. By using different dressings it can be ensured that the vacuum reaches all areas of the ulcer. These are mostly large-pored polyurethane foams or polyvinyl foams. Supporters of this therapy assume accelerated growth of granulation tissue [28, 29].

21.6 Methods of Plastic-Surgical Wound Closure

Diabetic foot ulcers might be hard to close by the endogenous repair process. In the case of large defects, plastic surgery methods can shorten the path and make wound closure conceivable in the first place. It depends in particular on the position and perfusion of the site, whether skin grafts, local flaps, pedicled flaps or free flaps are considered. These procedures are outlined on the following pages.

21.6.1 Skin Transplantation

In the case of skin transplantation, skin of the patient is removed from a distant and healthy area and transferred to the ulcer. The thickness and the way of further preparation of that skin are eponymous for the procedure. So a split-thickness skin graft can be distinguished from a full-thickness skin graft. Often it is not the entire wound surface that is covered, but the final wound closure is achieved as new skin grows from the transferred skin onto the surrounding granulation tissue.

Skin transplantation is an opportunity if ulcers are well perfused and covered with healthy granulation tissue.

21.6.1.1 Split Skin Graft

A split-thickness skin graft or split skin graft is taken with a dermatome. This is a tangential cutting blade that splits the superficial epidermis from the deeper dermis. The skin obtained is transferred and fixed at the recipient site. These methods are widely used as they achieve good rates of permanent wound closure and the donor site usually recovers rapidly. On the downside, the grafted area is not able to withstand pressure later on. Split skin grafts shrink by about 20%.

The split skin graft may be enlarged by various incisions in the graft. Precise cutting patterns leave the impression of a mesh which is responsible for the names 'meshed skin graft' or 'mesh graft'. It is the most widely used procedure for areas of skin which are not subject to pressure. Meshed skin graft shrinks by around 30%. It is particularly useful when only a small area of donor skin is available (Fig. 21.11).

21.6.1.2 Full-Thickness Skin Graft

Full-thickness skin grafts consist of the entire epidermis, the entire dermis and islands of subdermal fat tissue. They offer the best mechanical resistance and the best cosmetic result. Shrinkage is limited to about 10%. Full-thickness skin grafts are challenging since the tissue is thicker than split skin graft and the growth of new vessels to restore perfusion needs more time. In the transitional period, the graft may be rejected.

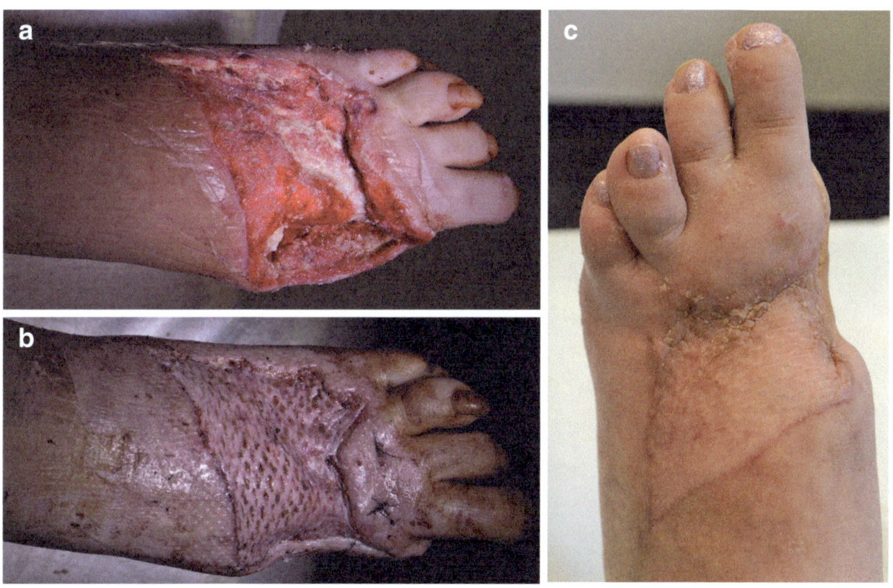

Fig. 21.11 (**a**–**c**) Deep ulcer on the dorsum of the foot after surgical debridement and preparation using negative pressure ulcer therapy. The ulcer is covered by split skin graft as mesh graft. Result after 9 months. The shrinking of the grafted skin might be relevant

Fig. 21.12 Reverdin graft (By kind permission of Dr. med. Peter Mauckner)

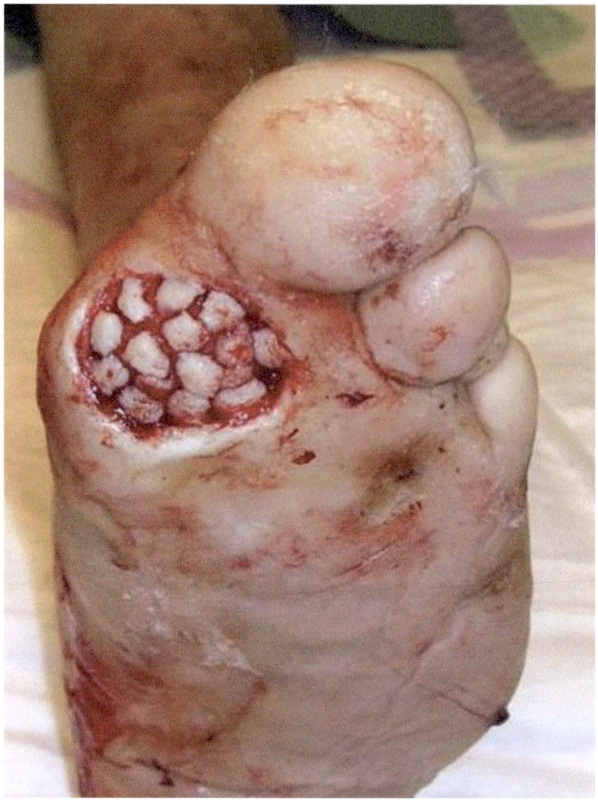

A popular method is so-called 'Reverdin graft' or 'pinch graft' as it is easy to perform. It consists of inserting little pieces of skin in a well-prepared ulcer and leaving the remaining parts of granulation tissue to be closed by growth from the graft and from the surrounding area. The small pieces of skin are lifted from a region which is not subject to pressure and separated tangentially using a scalpel. These patches are applied to the granulating ulcer and within days new capillaries attach to them providing nourishment. At the borders this is split skin, in the centre of the islands it is full-thickness skin (Fig. 21.12).

21.6.2 Local Flaps

Local flaps maintain their original perfusion through tissue beneath the flaps and from adjacent skin areas. Cuts are applied to the skin and the subdermal fat tissue to form a block in a predefined shape. One side of this block often remains connected to the original area to permit blood flow through the subdermal plexus, which helps to provide sufficient perfusion immediately after the operation. This block is then shifted to an adjacent position with as little tension as possible. It thus covers a larger area than before including the ulcer. These flaps are beneficial in weight-bearing areas of glabrous skin even if the intact skin has to be incised.

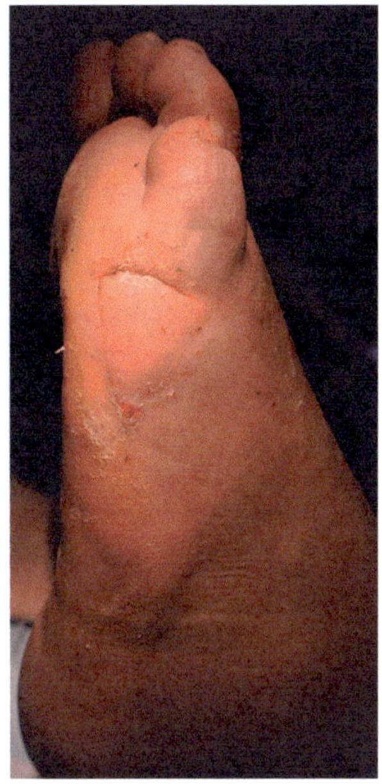

Fig. 21.13 Closing a lesion above the 5th MTH using a V-Y advancement flap

The incisions follow different patterns that often give the flap its name. An example might be the *Z-plasty*. This is a procedure involving the transposition of two interdigitating triangular flaps. The resulting suture has the shape of a Z.

21.6.2.1 V-Y-Advancement Flap

In order to perform these flaps, a triangular incision is made with its base close to the ulcer to be covered. This incision resembles the letter 'V' with the ulcer in the open part of the letter. The ulcer is removed and the base of the triangle is moved over the defect. The seam line then has the shape of the letter 'Y' (Fig. 21.13).

21.6.2.2 Double-V-Y-Advancement Flap

Larger defects may be covered using two *V-Y-advancement* flaps. The bases of the triangles are contiguous.

21.6.3 Pedicle Flaps

Pedicle flaps use an existing anatomical neighbourhood of arteries and veins, a so-called angiosome. The region which is supplied in this way is removed entirely and transferred to a neighbouring region. The stem serves the flap through its vessels. This has the significant advantage that the flap preserves its original source of blood supply. The circulatory situation is therefore less limiting than in the case of local advancement flaps. The designation of the flaps is taken from the area of origin. There are anatomically favourable standard areas for the removal of flaps and for covering defined neighbouring areas. For example, the 'sural flap' is generally preferred to cover defects on the heel. The donor site is closed using, for example, a split skin graft.

21.6.4 Free Flaps

If there is no possibility for any of the above-mentioned techniques the option of a free flap transfer should be considered. In the case of free flaps, the vessels in the stem are severed and microsurgically connected to suitable vessels at the transplantation site. This can be critical because a part of the blood flow is drained to the transplant, leading to a lack of perfusion to the remaining areas. This is described as a *steal phenomenon* and may even lead to tissue loss. If there are no appropriate vessels available to sustain a free flap, an additional blood supply to the region in question by a bypass may be considered. The vascular surgeon should first install a bypass to ensure sufficient flow. A free flap is connected in a second procedure later on. Distal to a bypass, the steal-phenomenon has advantages since it guarantees blood flow thus maintaining the bypass open.

The free transplant is not dependent on the specific conditions of the regions adjacent to the ulcer and can cover larger areas. There are numerous free flaps described. The selection is made taking into account various factors, which include the perfusion of the receiving region (Fig. 21.14).

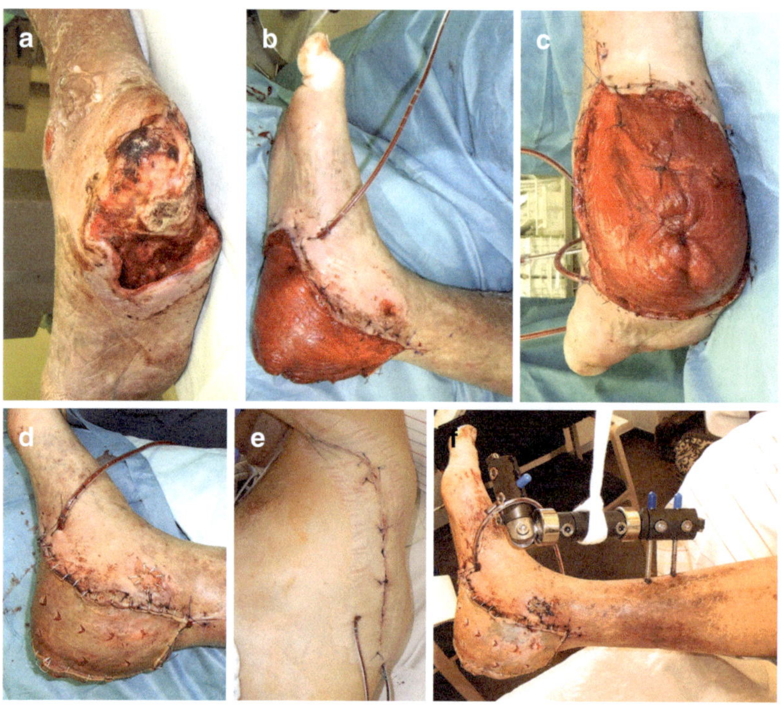

Fig. 21.14 (**a**) Extensive right heel lesion with osteomyelitis of the calcaneus, (**b**, **c**) covering with latissimus dorsi flap after partial removal of the calcaneus (**d**) covering the transplant with split skin, (**e**) donor site at the left thorax (**f**) securing the transplant by surgical offloading (**g**) postoperative doppler control of the perfusion of the transplant (**h**, **i**) postoperative condition after 4 weeks, (**j**, **k**) after 1 year and provision of orthopedic shoes

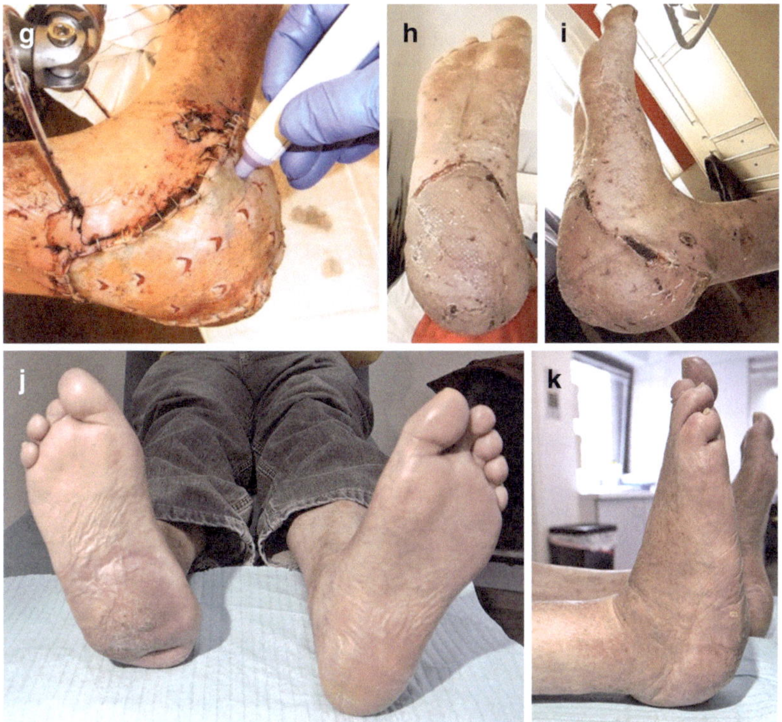

Fig. 21.14 (continued)

References

1. Edmonds M, Lazaro-Martinez JL, Alfayate-Garcia JM, Martini J, Petit JM, Rayman G, Lobmann R, et al. Sucrose octasulfate dressing versus control dressing in patients with neuroischaemic diabetic foot ulcers (Explorer): an international, multicentre, double-blind, randomised, controlled trial. Lancet Diabetes Endocrinol. 2017. https://doi.org/10.1016/S2213-8587(17)30438-2.
2. Game FL, Attinger C, Hartemann A, Hinchliffe RJ, Londahl M, Price PE, Jeffcoate WJ, Foot International Working Group on the Diabetic. IWGDF guidance on use of interventions to enhance the healing of chronic ulcers of the foot in diabetes. Diabetes Metab Res Rev. 2016;32(Suppl 1):75–83. https://doi.org/10.1002/dmrr.2700.
3. Bakker K, Apelqvist J, Schaper NC, Board International Working Group on Diabetic Foot Editorial. Practical guidelines on the management and prevention of the diabetic foot 2011. Diabetes Metab Res Rev. 2012;28(Suppl 1):225–31. https://doi.org/10.1002/dmrr.2253.
4. Medizin, Ärztliches Zentrum für Qualität in der. Nationale VersorgungsLeitlinie Typ-2-Diabetes Präventions- und Behandlungsstrategien für Fußkomplikationen. Programm für Nationale VersorgungsLeitlinien; 2006.
5. Ruttermann M, Maier-Hasselmann A, Nink-Grebe B, Burckhardt M. Local treatment of chronic wounds: in patients with peripheral vascular disease, chronic venous insufficiency, and diabetes. Dtsch Arztebl Int. 2013;110(3):25–31. https://doi.org/10.3238/arztebl.2013.0025.
6. Armstrong DG, Jude EB. The role of matrix metalloproteinases in wound healing. J Am Podiatr Med Assoc. 2002;92(1):12–8.

7. Lobmann R, Ambrosch A, Schultz G, Waldmann K, Schiweck S, Lehnert H. Expression of matrix-metalloproteinases and their inhibitors in the wounds of diabetic and non-diabetic patients. Diabetologia. 2002;45(7):1011–6. https://doi.org/10.1007/s00125-002-0868-8.
8. Lobmann R, Schultz G, Lehnert H. Proteases and the diabetic foot syndrome: mechanisms and therapeutic implications. Diabetes Care. 2005;28(2):461–71.
9. Winter GD. Effect of air exposure and occlusion on experimental human skin wounds. Nature. 1963;200:378–9.
10. Singer AJ, Clark RA. Cutaneous wound healing. N Engl J Med. 1999;341(10):738–46. https://doi.org/10.1056/nejm199909023411006.
11. Falanga V. Wound healing and its impairment in the diabetic foot. Lancet. 2005;366(9498):1736–43. https://doi.org/10.1016/s0140-6736(05)67700-8.
12. Coerper S. Indikation und Technik der limitierten, fußerhaltenden Knochenresektion beim Diabetischen Fußulcus. Zeitschrift f Wundheilung. 2003;5:169–74.
13. Dissemond J, Goos M. Optionen des Débridements in der Therapie chronischer Wunden. JDDG. 2004;9(2):743–51.
14. Steed DL, Donohoe D, Webster MW, Lindsley L. Effect of extensive debridement and treatment on the healing of diabetic foot ulcers. Diabetic Ulcer Study Group. J Am Coll Surg. 1996;183(1):61–4.
15. Steinsträßer L, Hasler R, Hirsch T, Langer S, Steinau HU. Therapieoptionen der Zukunft bei chronischen Wunden. Chirurg. 2008;79(6):555–9.
16. Baer WS. The classic: the treatment of chronic osteomyelitis with the maggot (larva of the blow fly). Clin Orthop Relat Res. 2011;469(4):920–44. https://doi.org/10.1007/s11999-010-1416-31931.
17. Armstrong DG, Salas P, Short B, Martin BR, Kimbriel HR, Nixon BP, Boulton AJ. Maggot therapy in "lower-extremity hospice" wound care: fewer amputations and more antibiotic-free days. J Am Podiatr Med Assoc. 2005;95(3):254–7.
18. Thomas S, Jones M, Shutler S, Jones S. Using larvae in modern wound management. J Wound Care. 1996;5(2):60–9.
19. Thomas S, Jones M, Wynn K, Fowler T. The current status of maggot therapy in wound healing. Br J Nurs. 2001;10(22 Suppl):S5–8, S10, S12.
20. Peters T, Rennekampf HO. Mechanisches débridement. Wund Manag. 2008;5:224–8.
21. König M, Vanscheidt W, Augustin M, Kapp H. Enzymatic versus autolytic debridement of chronic leg ulcers: a prospective randomised trial. J Wound Care. 2005;14(7):320–3.
22. Fikri R, Bicknell CD, Bloomfield LM, Lyons SP, Samarasinghe DG, Gibbs RG, Valabhji J. Awaiting autoamputation: a primary management strategy for toe gangrene in diabetic foot disease. Diabetes Care. 2011;34(8):e134. https://doi.org/10.2337/dc11-0848.
23. Levy L, Luft S. Healing in an uncontrolled diabetic following severe infection and spontaneous amputation of the fifth toe. J Am Podiatry Assoc. 1962;52:836–7.
24. Londahl M, Katzman P, Nilsson A, Hammarlund C. Hyperbaric oxygen therapy facilitates healing of chronic foot ulcers in patients with diabetes. Diabetes Care. 2010;33(5):998–1003.
25. Fedorko L, Bowen JM, Jones W, Oreopoulos G, Goeree R, Hopkins RB, O'Reilly DJ. Hyperbaric oxygen therapy does not reduce indications for amputation in patients with diabetes with nonhealing ulcers of the lower limb: a prospective, double-blind, randomized controlled clinical trial. Diabetes Care. 2016;39(3):392–9. https://doi.org/10.2337/dc15-2001.
26. Santema KTB, Stoekenbroek RM, Koelemay MJW, Reekers JA, van Dortmont LMC, Oomen A, Smeets L, et al. Hyperbaric oxygen therapy in the treatment of ischemic lower- extremity ulcers in patients with diabetes: results of the DAMO2CLES multicenter randomized clinical trial. Diabetes Care. 2018;41(1):112–9. https://doi.org/10.2337/dc17-0654.
27. Dumville JC, Hinchliffe RJ, Cullum N, Game F, Stubbs N, Sweeting M, Peinemann F. Negative pressure wound therapy for treating foot wounds in people with diabetes mellitus. Cochrane Database Syst Rev. 2013;10:Cd010318. https://doi.org/10.1002/14651858.CD010318.pub2.
28. Armstrong DG, Attinger CE, Boulton AJ, Frykberg RG, Kirsner RS, Lavery LA, Mills JL. Guidelines regarding negative wound therapy (NPWT) in the diabetic foot. Ostomy Wound Manage. 2004;50(4B Suppl):3S–27S.
29. Venturi ML, Attinger CE, Mesbahi AN, Hess CL, Graw KS. Mechanisms and clinical applications of the vacuum-assisted closure (VAC) Device: a review. Am J Clin Dermatol. 2005;6(3):185–94.

The Charcot Foot

22

The Charcot foot, also known as Charcot neuropathic osteoarthropathy (CN), diabetic neuropathic osteoarthropathy (DNOAP). It is an inflammatory syndrome, characterised by varying degrees of bone and joint disorganization secondary to underlying neuropathy, trauma, and perturbations of bone metabolism. The discussion of the underlying pathogenesis will not go into in great detail but only to the extent that is necessary for understanding the condition. Moreover, even 120 years after the death of Jean Martin Charcot some aspects of the pathogenesis are still controversial and have not progressed beyond the hypothetical.

22.1 Overview

'The diabetic Charcot foot syndrome is a serious and potentially limb-threatening lower-extremity complication of diabetes.' Thus begins the joint consensus document of the ADA and APMA on the Charcot foot [1]. In 1883 Jean Martin Charcot (1825–1893) described the destruction of the foot skeleton in patients with loss of pain sensation as a consequence of syphilis [2]. Even then discussion arose as to whether external factors such as continued weight-bearing on the affected extremity after trauma, or internal factors such as altered vascular regulation or impaired bone metabolism played a predominant role, a discussion which continues to this day [3, 4]. World-wide, diabetes mellitus is currently the most common disease underlying neuropathic osteoarthropathy. Numerous distal neuropathies (alcohol or drug-induced, leprosy) and disorders of the spinal cord and the nerve roots (e.g. syringomyelia) can also be associated with Charcot foot.

There is meanwhile a consensus that there is no single factor that leads to the development of a Charcot foot but that various risk factors or preceding events increase the propensity for its development.

D. Hochlenert et al., *Diabetic Foot Syndrome*,
https://doi.org/10.1007/978-3-319-92055-9_22

What can be said with certainty today is that

1. **Neuropathy is a consistent feature of affected extremities, with diminished pain response to otherwise painful injury.** Only continued weight-bearing on the relatively painless injured foot leads to the extensive pictures which Charcot described in syphilitic polyneuropathy and which can occur in all other clinical forms of neuropathy (e.g. diabetic neuropathy, hereditary neuropathy, alcohol-induced neuropathy, neuropathy in leprosy) [5].
2. **Blood supply is sufficient to mount an inflammatory response.** Development of an active Charcot foot in the presence of severe disruption of peripheral blood flow is probably rare. In fact, the period following normalisation of blood flow as a result of bypass surgery or angioplasty is even considered a particular risk for the development of Charcot foot [6]. So, the presence of peripheral arterial occlusive disease does not fundamentally rule out the possibility of Charcot foot [7].

There are, in addition, a number of hypotheses which attempt to provide a pathophysiological explanation for the clinical observations about a Charcot foot:

1. Charcot himself suspected a neuropathy-related defect of bone metabolism as the underlying feature of the condition [2]. Pre-existing *osteopenia* may play a causal role in people with type 1 diabetes [8].
2. The role of *obesity* as a risk factor for the development of Charcot foot is controversial [9].
3. For a long time, the presence of a peripheral autonomic neuropathy with dysregulation of capillary blood flow (*luxury perfusion*) was also considered an important pathological mechanism for the development of acute Charcot foot [10, 11]. A more recent investigation found severe impairment of C-fibre function in patients with diabetic neuropathy irrespective of whether they developed neuropathic osteopathy or not. However, in the patients who developed a Charcot foot the maximum microvascular hyperaemic (MMH) response was surprisingly considerably better preserved than in those who did not [12]. Finally, in a publication from the year 2011 the authors interpret their observations as showing that the hyperaemia present in acute Charcot foot is merely the expression of the local inflammatory processes and not of a peripheral sympathetic neuropathy [13].
4. Today it is generally assumed that the condition is precipitated by (often unnoticed) trauma and is maintained in predisposed individuals by the development of an uncontrolled inflammatory reaction. However, fever, leucocytosis or CRP elevation are often far less marked than the clinical picture of inflammation with swelling, erythema and increased temperature [14] would suggest. The described inflammatory process is triggered by the release of proinflammatory cytokines (TNF-α, Interleukin-1β), which in turn leads to increased expression of the receptor activator of NF-κB ligand (*RANKL*) by various local cell types. RANKL triggers the synthesis of NF-κB. Under physiological conditions, this stimulates both the maturation of osteoclasts (cells which break down bone substance) from

precursor cells and the production of the antagonist osteoprotegerin from osteoblasts (cells which build bone substance). The continued production of pro-inflammatory cytokines, RANKL, NF-κB and osteoclasts as a result of continued trauma of the damaged extremity leads to the osteolytic processes typical of the Charcot foot [15].

5. It is also postulated that *surgical trauma* can trigger the processes underlying a Charcot foot [16]. A British registry study found that in 12% of the patients diagnosed with an active Charcot foot a surgical procedure of some kind had been performed on the affected foot in the 6 months prior to diagnosis [17]. The explanation may include postoperative bone infection or insufficient aftercare with continued weight-bearing. It is important to note that on account of the loss of protective pain sensation people with neuropathy need different protection after surgical procedures.

The initial presentation of the Charcot foot is usually mild in nature (Phase 1 and 2) but can rapidly become more pronounced as a result of repeated unnoticed trauma of the affected extremity (Phase 3). On account of the relative insensitivity which is a universal feature in these patients, information from the patient concerning a history of preceding trauma is often not reliable [18]. The classical clinical finding in this phase consists of a markedly swollen, hot and often reddened foot with only mild or moderate pain or discomfort [19] (Fig. 22.1). Measurement of the *temperature* of the affected foot often shows a difference of several degrees compared with the contralateral foot [20]. In addition to the clinical assessment, comparative measurement of the skin temperature is a suitable method both for diagnosis [21] and for monitoring of the acute Charcot foot [22]. The *difference in temperature* is established using a surface thermometer and is pathological from a one degree higher temperature on the affected side (Fig. 22.2). For the measurement it is important to carefully scan the skin over the suspicious region. The temperature increase may only be present in a small area and can be a key pointer for the evaluation of radiological findings.

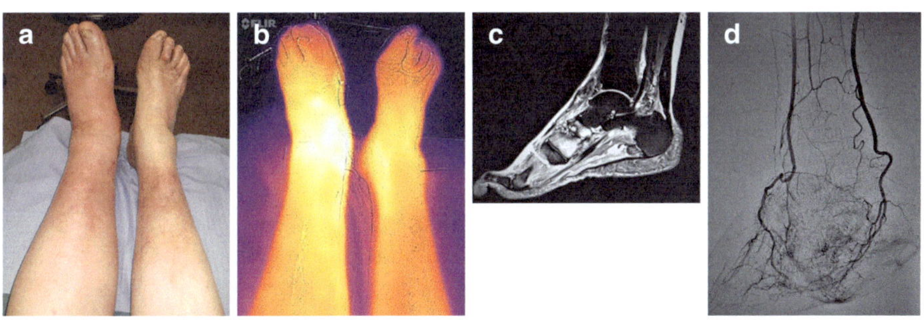

Fig. 22.1 (**a**) Clinical picture of an acute Charcot foot; (**b**) Infrared picture taken with FLIR ONE™ and an android™ smartphone; (**c**) MRI T2 with the fat suppression technique STIR; (**d**) DSA showing hypervascularisation

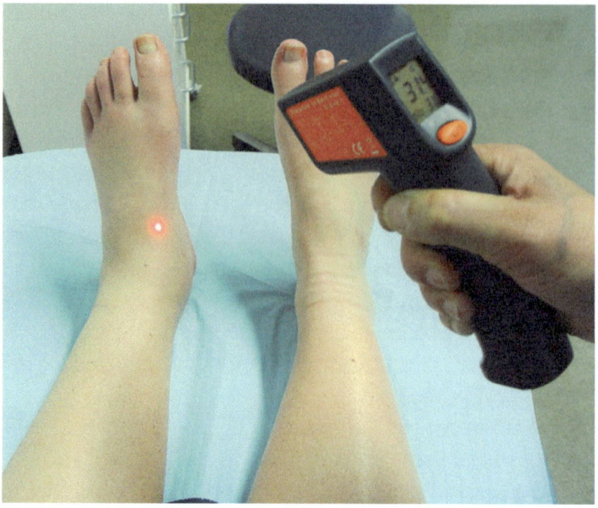

Fig. 22.2 Pinpoint temperature measurement with a surface (infrared) thermometer

Conventional X-ray is recommended as the primary imaging procedure for diagnosis and evaluation of the Charcot foot [1]. The method is low-cost and universally available, but in early stages of the Charcot foot (Phase 1–3) the findings may be normal [22]. Because identifying the disease at these initial stages is crucial for the prognosis of the Charcot foot, classifications based only on X-ray findings [23] are no longer considered state of the art [24]. In these early stages magnetic resonance imaging (*MRI*) [25] or nuclear medicine procedures [26] are therefore preferred for confirmation or exclusion of the diagnosis.

Bone marrow oedema as a consequence of a post-traumatic overloading injury or stress damage is the first finding in the chronology of the condition which is identifiable in an imaging procedure. It forms the basis of the grading system developed by *Kiuru* et al. for classification of the MRI findings [27]:

- Grade I: Endosteal marrow oedema (X-ray negative)
- Grade II: Periosteal and endosteal oedema (X-ray negative)
- Grade III: Muscle oedema, periosteal oedema and endosteal marrow oedema (X-ray negative)
- Grade IV: Fracture line (X-ray negative/positive)
- Grade V: Callus in cortical bone (X-ray positive)

Without treatment, the pathological bone and joint changes present in the acute stage can lead to the development of fractures (Phase 4), dislocations (Phase 5) and, depending on the location of the findings, more or less pronounced deformities (Phase 6) of the affected foot [28] (see phases in the Sect. 22.2).

The classification system of *Sanders & Frykberg* has become established for describing these different location patterns [29]. However, this only permits a

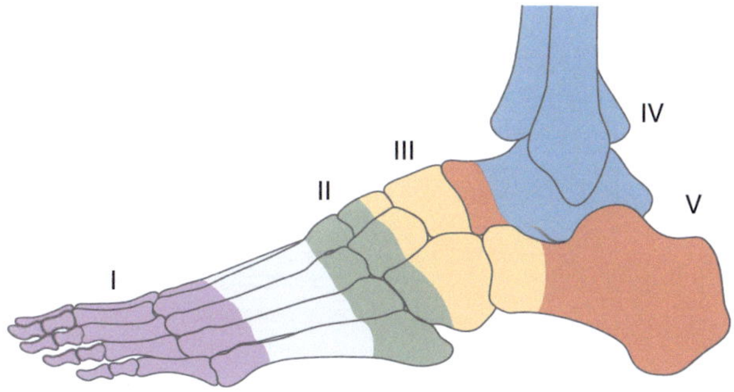

Fig. 22.3 Classification by location (Sanders I–V) modified after Baumgartner [30]

radiological classification, involvement of several joint complexes is possible, and a stringent treatment recommendation cannot be derived from this classification.

Sanders I—Metatarsophalangeal joints (15%)
Sanders II—Lisfranc complex (40%)
Sanders III—Chopart joint (30%)
Sanders IV—Ankle joint (10%)
Sanders V—Calcaneus (5%) (Fig. 22.3)

Practical consequences: It is generally agreed that termination of the continued weight-bearing leads to reestablishment of intact structures. Early diagnosis and consistent offloading are currently regarded as the cornerstones of treatment. Delayed diagnosis leads to a worse prognosis with an increasing complication rate [31].

NB: Simply telling a person with neuropathy to avoid weight-bearing after an injury (sprain etc.) is an omission on the part of the physician. Knowing about the neuropathy, everything must be done to ensure that any stress on the foot, which the patient will not notice and can therefore scarcely avoid, does not cause damage.

22.2 Natural History

Figure 22.4 shows the pathology and diagnostic work-up of Charcot foot according to the different phases.

- From Phase 3 onwards (Inflammatory response) a "Charcot foot" can be defined.
- The initial trauma can go unnoticed by the patient, for example when getting off a bicycle.
- Up to Phase 4 (non-displaced fracture) complete healing of the condition is possible, after that only partial healing with a persistent defect is possible.
- Although phase 5 can be present without an antecedent typical fracture, at the very least an avulsion fracture is usually present.

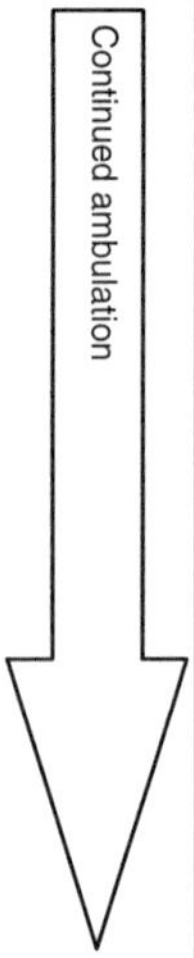

Phase	Pathology	Clinical picture	Medical Imaging
1	Initial trauma	E.g. sprain, soft tissue swelling	
2	Latency	Continuing damage with no identifiable or characteristic signs	MRI: possible minimal bone marrow oedema as incidental finding
3	Inflammatory response	Raised skin temperature, swelling, erythema and possibly pain	MRI: bone marrow oedema Scintigraphy: bone remodelling
4	Fractures	As above, possibly hypermobility or crepitation of the bone ends	X-ray: fractures, sequelae of ruptured ligaments such as widening of the space between M1 and M2 due to rupture of the Lisfranc ligament
5	Dislocation	As above	X-ray: dysfunctional position of the fragments
6	Deformity	Outwardly visible architectural changes	X-ray/CT: fractures and altered position of bones
7	Deviation	Displacement of the functional weight-bearing axis	
8	Functional loss of the extremity	Deviation making walking impossible	
Apart from the Charcot lesion itself ulcers or swelling can developat new and unphysiological bony prominences			
A	No ulcer		
B	Ulcer	Ulceration without connection to the fractured region	Defect
C	Fistula	Ulceration with connection to the fractured region and additional destruction	Possibly fistula, gas formation

Fig. 22.4 Phases of the natural history of Charcot foot

22.3 Charcot Foot with Corresponding Ulcer

When there is a coexisting ulcer the differential diagnosis between Charcot arthropathy and osteomyelitis is often very difficult. Here magnetic resonance imaging (MRI) plays an important role [32]. In future, *DWI (diffusion weighted imaging)* techniques may also be of assistance [33] (Fig. 22.5).

The **infected Charcot foot** as independent entity is associated with a high rate of major amputation and requires specialised treatment in dedicated centres. This treatment follows the criteria of septic surgery. In the case of early, thorough removal of the infected tissue (bone, tendons, joints) it is, however, often possible to preserve a residual foot capable of weight-bearing (Fig. 22.6).

22.4 Immobilisation

Immobilisation of the joints whose bony parts are affected is the cornerstone of treatment.

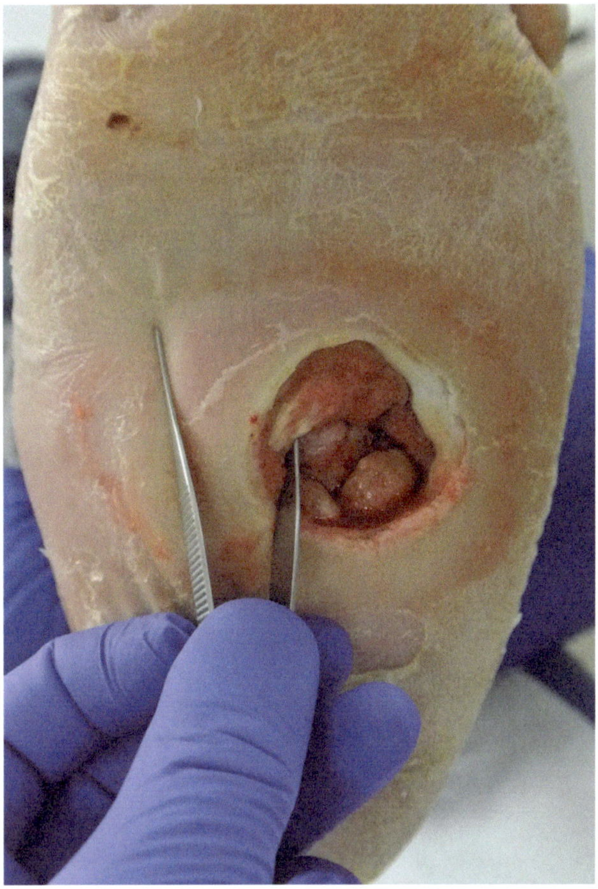

Fig. 22.5 Charcot foot with plantar ulcer, fistula and bone involvement

22.4.1 Suspected Charcot Foot: A Medical Emergency!

Since full recovery (restitutio ad integrum) is no longer possible once Phase 5 (dislocation) has been reached and this stage can occur at any time and suddenly with unprotected ambulation, **steps to provide appropriate immobilisation must be taken immediately, without delay, with any suspicion of Charcot foot**. This is the case if the foot shows a unilateral painless inflammatory reaction with markedly elevated skin temperature and swelling but with little systemic reaction. Confirmation of the diagnosis may have to be postponed until later and consists of conventional X-ray and, if there is no evidence of a fracture/dislocation, MRI with a fat-suppressing technique. Initiation of adequate immobilisation cannot wait for confirmation of the diagnosis [34]!

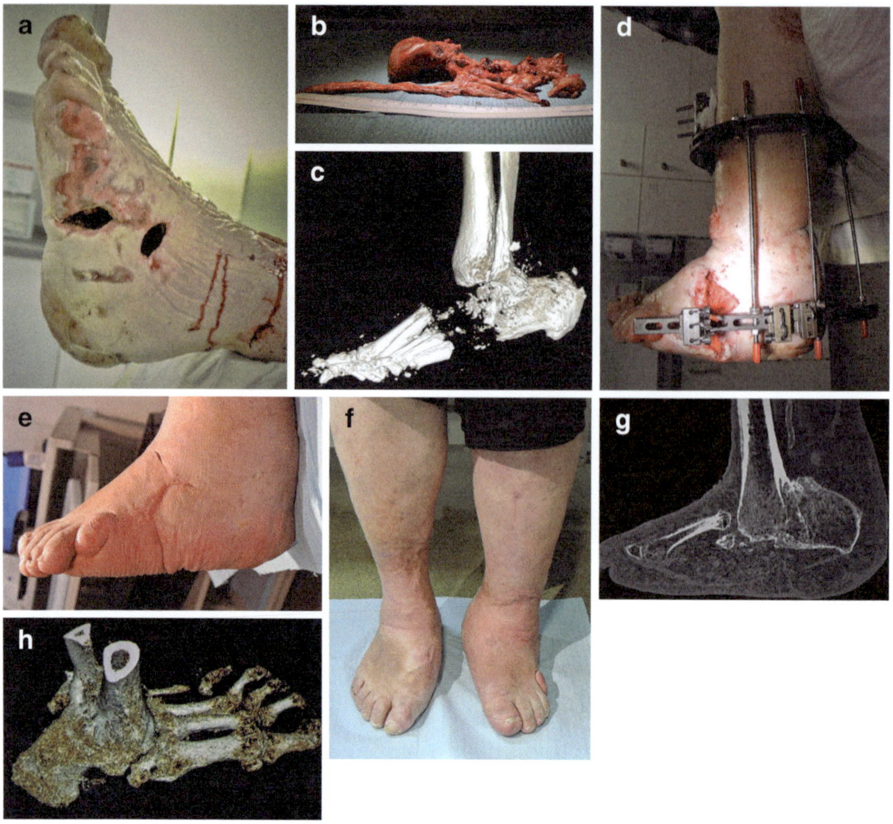

Fig. 22.6 (**a**–**h**) Infected Charcot foot, initial debridement with resection of infected bony structures, calcaneotibial fusion with hybrid ring external fixator. Outcome after 9 months

22.4.2 Immobilisation Versus Non-Weight-Bearing

The most important measure is immobilisation of the joints which exercise leverage on the diseased structures. The standard procedure is the use of a total contact cast (TCC) or a removable bivalve cast [35]. This provides three-dimensional immobilisation which prevents all movement including movement in the ankle joint and between the forefoot and the toes. The load is transferred to the entire plantar surface and partially to the shin and calf.

Non-weight-bearing by reducing the number of steps is desired initially but not later on. During the phase of bone regeneration mechanical loading of the bone is essential for normal remodelling. However, in the case of locations on the hindfoot (calcaneus or talus) a longer duration of reduced weight-bearing is probably appropriate. This can be achieved with a bivalve cast which supports the tibial condyles.

22.4.3 Duration of Immobilisation

How long the immobilisation should be continued has not been finally established [36]. If some weeks have passed since the clinical signs, particularly the swelling and raised skin temperature, have subsided and this is maintained, a careful transition to a custom-made shoe can be considered. To avoid unnecessarily prolonged waiting-time until mobilisation can start, the time needed to build all the necessary shoes should be borne in mind. An interim MRI can be useful but signs such as bone marrow oedema recede very slowly. It is a matter of controversy whether the stable phase corresponds to the complete disappearance of the bone marrow oedema on the MRI or whether a permanent disappearance of clinical signs is sufficient.

22.4.4 Venous Thromboembolism Prophylaxis?

It is not clear whether a neuropathic patient who walks on the fractured leg and activates the muscle pump benefits from venous thromboembolism prophylaxis with heparin or whether this actually causes more harm than good. In a study of 184 people who received 879 non-removable TCCs and no heparinisation, during 18 months of observation in 26 patients a deep vein thrombosis (DVT) was ruled out with DVT-scan. The others showed no clinical evidence of DVT. Thus, in no case was the diagnosis of a DVT made [37]. In conclusion, in this large group, there was no problem that could have been addressed prophylactically with heparinisation.

22.5 Surgical Treatment

The national and international guidelines published to date do not make any explicit recommendations regarding structured surgical treatment.

A systematic review of published studies on surgical algorithms for the treatment of Charcot neuroarthropathy covering 95 uncontrolled retrospective cohort analyses on exostosectomy, Achilles tendon lengthening and fusion found that all reports constituted only Level IV or V evidence [38].

Treatment currently follows the principles of 'best clinical practice'. There is a definite need for controlled studies. A first step towards structuring surgical management of Charcot foot can be found in a German-Austrian consensus document [39].

22.5.1 Removing Bony Prominences

Dislocated bony structures of the tarsus in an otherwise stable plantigrade foot can lead to increased plantar pressures with the risk of development of new or recurrent lesions. If these cannot be accommodated by appropriate footwear,

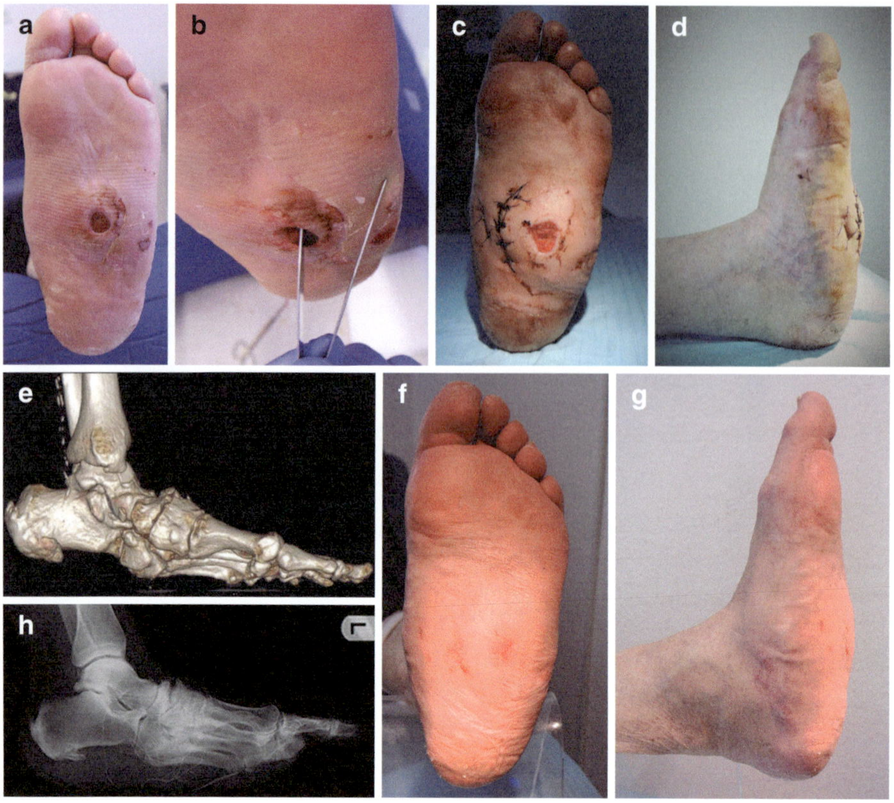

Fig. 22.7 (**a**–**h**) Example of resection of a bony prominence

resection of such a 'pseudoexostosis' is a surgical option to reduce increased plantar pressure (Fig. 22.7). Minimally invasive surgical therapy is also suitable in this indication (Fig. 22.8).

22.5.2 Reconstruction

In the case of acute dislocation or marked instability, conservative therapy such as repositioning and retention in a TCC is not usually successful. Therefore, early consideration should be given to the use of surgery once the initial swelling has subsided. In this phase stabilisation in an anatomically correct position is easier to achieve than when the foot has 'healed' in a deformed position (Fig. 22.9).

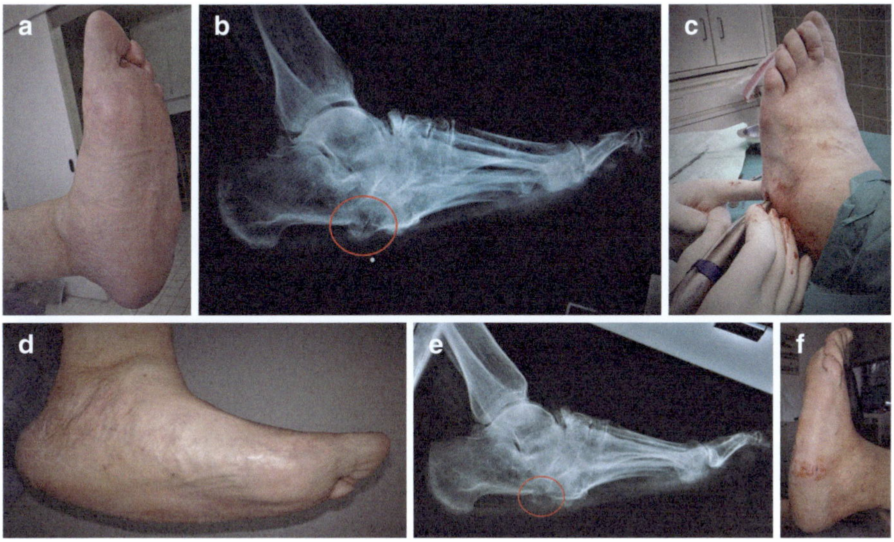

Fig. 22.8 Example of minimally invasive ablation of a bony prominence in the area of the calcaneocuboid joint in a patient who has suffered recurrent plantar lesions in the repeatedly adapted orthopaedic bespoken shoe: (**a**, **b**) preoperative (**c**) intraoperative (**d**, **e**) postoperative (**f**) 7th postoperative day

Reconstruction is usually performed if injury-free weight-bearing of the foot with appropriate bespoke footwear is not possible. Existing ulcers are not a fundamental contraindication for surgical management. Surgery should provide correction in all spatial dimensions whereby, in contrast to other orthopaedic surgical procedures, a subtractive rather than an additive strategy is pursued, i.e. bone is sacrificed rather than built up.

22.5.3 Achilles Tendon Lengthening

An *equinus deformity* is frequently present and may be corrected by Achilles tendon lengthening (Fig. 22.10) [40]. Percutaneous procedures can be used in this case. Complete severing of the Achilles tendon is not recommended on account of the risk of a calcaneal gait and subsequent plantar heel ulceration [41].

If the *equinus deformity is combined with a pes cavus*, dislocation in the region of the lateral column can occur, sometimes even with exposed joint structures. This kind of deformity cannot be managed with conventional offloading techniques and a surgical strategy is indicated (Fig. 22.11).

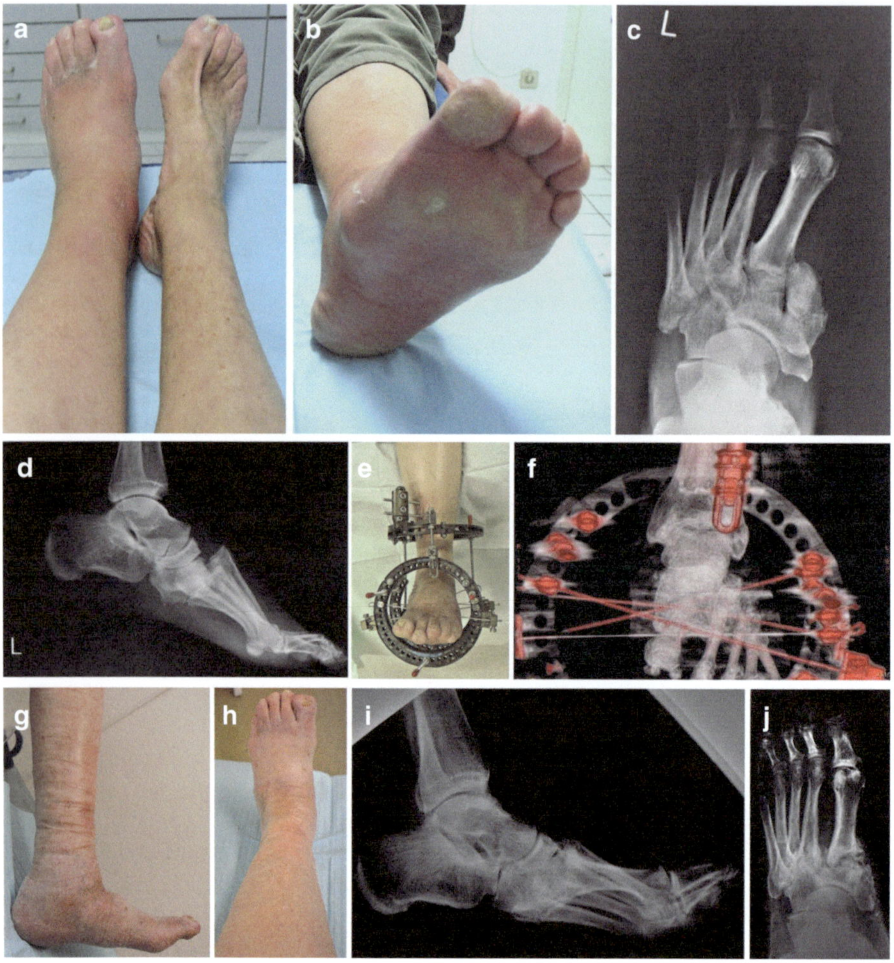

Fig. 22.9 (**a–d**) Acute dislocation of the Lisfranc complex 5 days after a fall and continued weight-bearing, (**e**, **f**) after surgical correction of the medial column and resection of the medial (first) cuneiform bone, retention in a hybrid ring fixator (**g–j**) outcome after 6 months in the phase of shoe treatment, clinically and radiologically, respectively

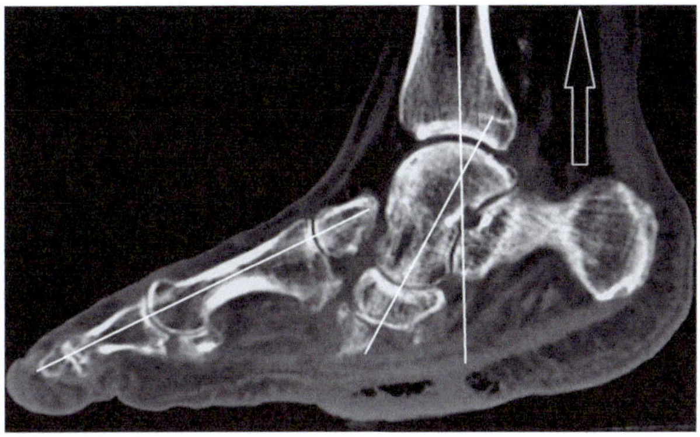

Fig. 22.10 Sagittal CT-scan: the equinus deformity was 'compensated' by dislocation in the region of the Lisfranc complex during painless ambulation, resulting in a typical rocker bottom deformity

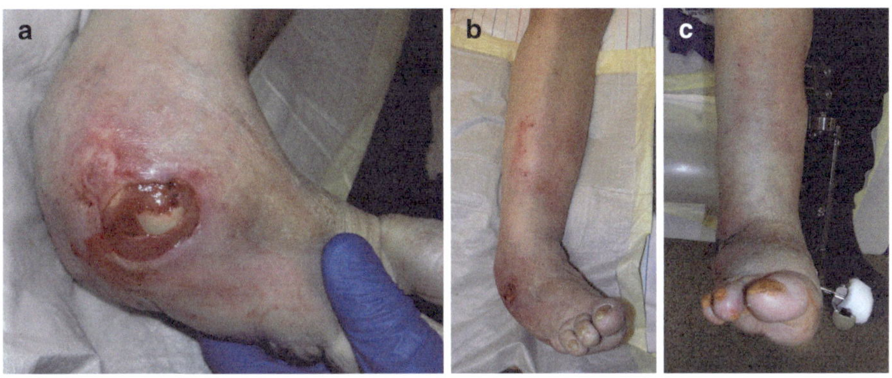

Fig. 22.11 (**a**–**c**) Subtalar dislocation with a skin defect over the talus with exposed talar bone, reduction and stabilisation with external fixation and Z-plasty of the Achilles tendon

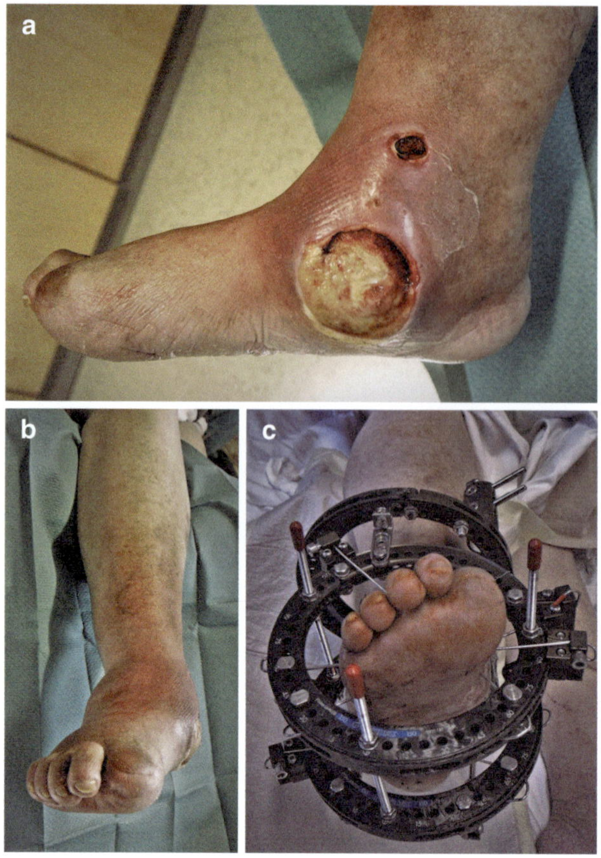

Fig. 22.12 (**a**–**c**) Medially perforated talonavicular joint, fixated with hybrid ring fixator following reduction and Z-plasty of the Achilles tendon

In the case of *pes planovalgus and shortening of the calf muscle complex* there is often dislocation in the talonavicular joint and corresponding bony perforation. This situation is not suitable for weight-bearing in accommodating footwear either and surgery is indicated (Fig. 22.12).

22.6 Summary

- **Immobilisation is the cornerstone of treatment of the Charcot foot. It can be supplemented by surgical procedures.**
- **Suspected Charcot foot is a medical emergency. Early interruption of the destructive process through prompt initiation of appropriate treatment can prevent functional impairment or even functional loss of the leg. Even if the diagnosis cannot initially be confirmed this should on no account delay the start of treatment.**

22.7 Recommended Literature

Robert G. Frykberg (Ed.).: The Diabetic Charcot Foot: Principles and Management.

Comprehensive text with individual chapters by many American and European authors, addressing topics from pathogenesis, to natural history to conservative and surgical management of all relevant aspects of the diabetic Charcot foot. First international book publication dealing exclusively with this topic. 1st edition 2009, 294 pages, ISBN-13: 978-1-57400-130-3

References

1. Rogers LC, Frykberg RG, Armstrong DG, Boulton AJ, Edmonds M, Van GH, Hartemann A, et al. The Charcot foot in diabetes. Diabetes Care. 2011;34(9):2123–9. https://doi.org/10.2337/dc11-0844.
2. Hoche G, Sanders LJ. On some arthropathies apparently related to a lesion of the brain or spinal cord, by Dr J.-M. Charcot. January 1868. J Am Podiatr Med Assoc. 1992;82(8):403–11.
3. Chantelau E, Onvlee GJ. Charcot foot in diabetes: farewell to the neurotrophic theory. Horm Metab Res. 2006;38(6):361–7. https://doi.org/10.1055/s-2006-944525.
4. Sanders LJ. The Charcot foot: historical perspective 1827-2003. Diabetes Metab Res Rev. 2004;20(Suppl 1):S4–8. https://doi.org/10.1002/dmrr.451.
5. Wienemann T, Chantelau EA, Richter A. Pressure pain perception at the injured foot: the impact of diabetic neuropathy. J Musculoskelet Neuronal Interact. 2012;12(4):254–61.
6. Edelman SV, Kosofsky EM, Paul RA, Kozak GP. Neuro-osteoarthropathy (Charcot's joint) in diabetes mellitus following revascularization surgery. Three case reports and a review of the literature. Arch Intern Med. 1987;147(8):1504–8.
7. Palena LM, Brocco E, Ninkovic S, Volpe A, Manzi M. Ischemic Charcot foot: different disease with different treatment? J Cardiovasc Surg. 2013;54(5):561–6.
8. Petrova NL, Foster AV, Edmonds ME. Difference in presentation of charcot osteoarthropathy in type 1 compared with type 2 diabetes. Diabetes Care. 2004;27(5):1235–6.
9. Stuck RM, Sohn MW, Budiman-Mak E, Lee TA, Weiss KB. Charcot arthropathy risk elevation in the obese diabetic population. Am J Med. 2008;121(11):1008–14. https://doi.org/10.1016/j.amjmed.2008.06.038.
10. Duncan CP, Shim SS. J. Edouard Samson Address: the autonomic nerve supply of bone. An experimental study of the intraosseous adrenergic nervi vasorum in the rabbit. J Bone Joint Surg Br. 1977;59(3):323–30.
11. Edmonds ME, Roberts VC, Watkins PJ. Blood flow in the diabetic neuropathic foot. Diabetologia. 1982;22(1):9–15.
12. Baker N, Green A, Krishnan S, Rayman G. Microvascular and C-fiber function in diabetic charcot neuroarthropathy and diabetic peripheral neuropathy. Diabetes Care. 2007;30(12):3077–9. https://doi.org/10.2337/dc07-1063.
13. Christensen TM, Simonsen L, Holstein PE, Svendsen OL, Bulow J. Sympathetic neuropathy in diabetes mellitus patients does not elicit Charcot osteoarthropathy. J Diabetes Complicat. 2011;25(5):320–4. https://doi.org/10.1016/j.jdiacomp.2011.06.006.
14. Petrova NL, Moniz C, Elias DA, Buxton-Thomas M, Bates M, Edmonds ME. Is there a systemic inflammatory response in the acute charcot foot? Diabetes Care. 2007;30(4):997–8. https://doi.org/10.2337/dc06-2168.
15. Jeffcoate WJ, Game F, Cavanagh PR. The role of proinflammatory cytokines in the cause of neuropathic osteoarthropathy (acute Charcot foot) in diabetes. Lancet. 2005;366(9502):2058–61. https://doi.org/10.1016/s0140-6736(05)67029-8.

16. Aragon-Sanchez J, Lazaro-Martinez JL, Hernandez-Herrero MJ. Triggering mechanisms of neuroarthropathy following conservative surgery for osteomyelitis. Diabet Med. 2010;27(7):844–7. https://doi.org/10.1111/j.1464-5491.2010.03019.x.
17. Game FL, Catlow R, Jones GR, Edmonds ME, Jude EB, Rayman G, Jeffcoate WJ. Audit of acute Charcot's disease in the UK: the CDUK study. Diabetologia. 2012;55(1):32–5. https://doi.org/10.1007/s00125-011-2354-7.
18. Armstrong DG, Todd WF, Lavery LA, Harkless LB, Bushman TR. The natural history of acute Charcot's arthropathy in a diabetic foot specialty clinic. Diabet Med. 1997b;14(5):357–63. https://doi.org/10.1002/(SICI)1096-9136(199705)14:5<357::AID-DIA341>3.0.CO;2-8.
19. Caputo GM, Ulbrecht J, Cavanagh PR, Juliano P. The Charcot foot in diabetes: six key points. Am Fam Physician. 1998;57(11):2705–10.
20. McGill M, Molyneaux L, Bolton T, Ioannou K, Uren R, Yue DK. Response of Charcot's arthropathy to contact casting: assessment by quantitative techniques. Diabetologia. 2000;43(4):481–4. https://doi.org/10.1007/s001250051332.
21. Armstrong DG, Lavery LA, Liswood PJ, Todd WF, Tredwell JA. Infrared dermal thermometry for the high-risk diabetic foot. Phys Ther. 1997a;77(2):169–75; discussion 176–167.
22. Armstrong DG, Lavery LA. Monitoring healing of acute Charcot's arthropathy with infrared dermal thermometry. J Rehabil Res Dev. 1997;34(3):317–21.
23. Eichenholtz SN. Charcot joints. Springfield, IL: Charles C Thomas; 1966.
24. Chantelau EA, Grutzner G. Is the Eichenholtz classification still valid for the diabetic Charcot foot? Swiss Med Wkly. 2014;144:w13948. https://doi.org/10.4414/smw.2014.13948.
25. Morrison WB, Ledermann HP, Schweitzer ME. MR imaging of the diabetic foot. Magn Reson Imaging Clin N Am. 2001;9(3):603–13, xi.
26. Palestro CJ, Mehta HH, Patel M, Freeman SJ, Harrington WN, Tomas MB, Marwin SE. Marrow versus infection in the Charcot joint: indium-111 leukocyte and technetium-99m sulfur colloid scintigraphy. J Nucl Med. 1998;39(2):346–50.
27. Kiuru MJ, Pihlajamaki HK, Ahovuo JA. Bone stress injuries. Acta Radiol. 2004;45(3):317–26.
28. Sinha S, Munichoodappa CS, Kozak GP. Neuro-arthropathy (Charcot joints) in diabetes mellitus (clinical study of 101 cases). Medicine (Baltimore). 1972;51(3):191–210.
29. Frykberg RG, Zgonis T, Armstrong DG, Driver VR, Giurini JM, Kravitz SR, Landsman AS, et al. Diabetic foot disorders. A clinical practice guideline (2006 revision). J Foot Ankle Surg. 2006;45(5 Suppl):S1–66. https://doi.org/10.1016/s1067-2516(07)60001-5.
30. Baumgartner R, Möller M, Stinus H. Orthopädieschuhtechnik. 2. Aufl.: C. Maurer Druck und Verlag GmbH & Co. KG; 2013.
31. Pakarinen TK, Laine HJ, Maenpaa H, Mattila P, Lahtela J. Long-term outcome and quality of life in patients with Charcot foot. Foot Ankle Surg. 2009;15(4):187–91. https://doi.org/10.1016/j.fas.2009.02.005.
32. Berendt AR, Lipsky B. Is this bone infected or not? Differentiating neuro-osteoarthropathy from osteomyelitis in the diabetic foot. Curr Diab Rep. 2004;4(6):424–9.
33. Herneth AM, Friedrich K, Weidekamm C, Schibany N, Krestan C, Czerny C, Kainberger F. Diffusion weighted imaging of bone marrow pathologies. Eur J Radiol. 2005;55(1):74–83. https://doi.org/10.1016/j.ejrad.2005.03.031.
34. Tan AL, Greenstein A, Jarrett SJ, McGonagle D. Acute neuropathic joint disease: a medical emergency? Diabetes Care. 2005;28(12):2962–4.
35. Petrova NL, Edmonds ME. Charcot neuro-osteoarthropathy-current standards. Diabetes Metab Res Rev. 2008;24(Suppl 1):S58–61. https://doi.org/10.1002/dmrr.846.
36. Christensen TM, Gade-Rasmussen B, Pedersen LW, Hommel E, Holstein PE, Svendsen OL. Duration of off-loading and recurrence rate in Charcot osteo-arthropathy treated with less restrictive regimen with removable walker. J Diabetes Complicat. 2012;26(5):430–4. https://doi.org/10.1016/j.jdiacomp.2012.05.006.
37. Stafford M, Bates M, Jemmott T, Tang W, Lucas J, Walton D, Mottolini N et al. Total contact casting is a safe treatment modality for acute charcot osteoarthropathy and neuropathic ulceration and is not associated with increased incidence of deep vein thrombosis. In Diabetic Foot Study Group, 14th Scientific Meeting 2017, Porto; 2017.

38. Lowery NJ, Woods JB, Armstrong DG, Wukich DK. Surgical management of Charcot neuroarthropathy of the foot and ankle: a systematic review. Foot Ankle Int. 2012;33(2):113–21. https://doi.org/10.3113/FAI.2012.0113.
39. Koller A, Springfeld R, Engels G, Fiedler R, Orthner E, Schrinner S, Sikorski A. German-Austrian consensus on operative treatment of Charcot neuroarthropathy: a perspective by the Charcot task force of the German Association for Foot Surgery. Diabet Foot Ankle. 2011;2. https://doi.org/10.3402/dfa.v2i0.10207.
40. Mueller MJ, Sinacore DR, Hastings MK, Strube MJ, Johnson JE. Effect of Achilles tendon lengthening on neuropathic plantar ulcers. A randomized clinical trial. J Bone Joint Surg Am. 2003;85-A(8):1436–45.
41. Colen LB, Kim CJ, Grant WP, Yeh JT, Hind B. Achilles tendon lengthening: friend or foe in the diabetic foot? Plast Reconstr Surg. 2013;131(1):37e–43e. https://doi.org/10.1097/PRS.0b013e3182729e0b.

23 Organisation of an Outpatient Clinic

In this chapter, the authors summarise their thoughts and experiences concerning an ongoing challenge in every outpatient clinic: How can we be better organised? The aim is to provide a resource of suggestions that need to be adapted to local requirements if found useful. This topic will never be fully resolved with a result that satisfies everyone. However, it is a topic of great importance, as so much depends on good organisation: work satisfaction of the staff, patients' waiting time and therefore satisfaction, and the economic success necessary to finance an outpatient foot clinic. The willingness to adapt as soon as there are opportunities for improvement seems to be the best guarantee in a difficult economic environment.

23.1 Overview

Care for people with DFS is provided in the patient's home, in outpatient clinics, community general practitioners' surgeries and sometimes in inpatient facilities. It is not necessarily the case that one institution covers all the necessary services but by linking to other healthcare providers, all needs should be met. 'Do what you do best and link to the rest' [1]. The German working group for the diabetic foot requires a minimum of commitment in coordination with the most important partners by means of a written cooperation agreement for certification. **Efficient organisation of the processes in an outpatient foot clinic is demanding because planning ahead may be difficult due to unpredictable events. Inadequate reimbursement in many countries means that staffing levels are below what would be considered ideal.**

The division of labour in some countries is planned in such a way that each patient visiting the clinic usually sees a doctor. This varies, however, from country to country depending on professional skills and legal aspects. In the *occupational profile* in the field of podiatry, for example, there are major differences ranging from

D. Hochlenert et al., *Diabetic Foot Syndrome*,
https://doi.org/10.1007/978-3-319-92055-9_23

toenail cutting to podiatrists prescribing drugs or devices and performing surgery. International standardisation would be much appreciated. In people with DFS it is to be remembered that the foot problem is a consequence of diabetes and many other comorbidities. Taking this into account, a sensible allocation of duties between doctors and other professionals is desirable. If the decision-maker is the doctor it is imperative that they expose themselves to as many cases as possible to increase their knowledge. Their position should not only be based on hierarchy but on better education and more experience.

The typical workflow steps are as follows:

- reception and administration
- undress the patient's feet
- control the efficiency of any offloading
- removal of dressings so that the wound can be accessed
- debridement
- documentation
- treatment and evaluation by the healthcare professional
- support and guidance for patients and relatives
- apply dressing to any ulcers
- dress the patient and check the offloading
- administrative duties such as prescriptions and new appointments
- cleaning and preparation of the room for the next patient

The way the work is organised depends on the number of rooms, the number of staff members and the possibility to group patients in a meaningful way. Possible groupings might be: people with active DFS, people in remission, emergencies and people carrying special bacteria. As far as costs are concerned, personnel costs are the most expensive part and usually amount to 3–5 times the cost of rooms. Therefore, a careful allocation of resources aims to organise a perfect working environment for employees and no limitation on budgets for instruments, materials or rooms. For example, in the case of caring for 10 people it might be more efficient to treat them over 2–3 h in three rooms with two professionals rather than in one room with one professional over a whole day. Optimising the working environment is important for economic success.

Efficiency increases dramatically with the number of rooms available. It shouldn't be the speed of the patient undressing and dressing that determines the pace of work. Maximum efficiency is achieved if at least two rooms are available for one employee and if more personnel is available, at least three rooms are accessible.

The elements of an efficient workflow are as follows:

- Always having one person in charge to oversee who is waiting, who is expected and what is happening in each room. This person must be organised but does not necessarily have to have much experience in treating the disease. This coordinator might help other staff members, but for brief periods only.

- Deciding carefully which team member will be in charge of dealing with severe cases as these may be very time-consuming. It might be more efficient if this work is not undertaken by the most experienced staff members.
- Not allowing a situation to develop where staff members are unable to perform because other members or rooms are not available.

One of the most difficult challenges is to keep the consequences of unexpected scenarios to the minimum through careful planning. Typical scenarios might be emergency cases or patients who come to check-up appointments and have developed major diseases. Other inefficiencies might arise if patients don't attend appointments or patients that have been thought to be time-consuming require less time than predicted. Therefore it should be laid down:

- Which administrative tasks can be done during periods when not attending to patients?
- Which steps might be safely postponed in times of high workload?
- At which moment during times of high workload staff members ask others for assistance so as not to make it a personal conflict.

The team has to adapt the pace rapidly if the situation arises. The staff member in charge of overseeing the situation has to recognise when the waiting time for a patient has reached a predefined limit and advise the need for an accelerated tempo.

The time required for a single patient might be similar to the time required at a previous contact. It might be useful to note this at a specific place in the documentation.

23.2 Equipment with Furniture

A treatment room is usually furnished with the following:

- a treatment chair or plinth
- a chair for the therapist
- a shelf for the patient's clothes
- a washbasin with all the accessories required for a legal hand washing area
- sufficient illumination

Additional other equipment:

- a computer with a keyboard that can be disinfected
- a dressing trolley (that can be moved outside if the patient is a carrier of multi-resistant bacteria)
- movable tray for sterile instruments and other material
- camera and monitor for documentation and to show the patient what is under the foot
- desk or standing desk

23.3 Equipment with Instruments

In the order of frequency of usage these are:

- Instruments typically needed for each patient
  - forceps
  - scissors
  - scalpel
- Instruments of frequent use usually stored near the treatment area
  - ring curette
  - sharp spoons/curettes
- Instruments of rare use that can be stored centrally
  - cutting pliers in different shapes to cut nails and edges
  - Luer forceps (small and large)
  - probes to explore fistulas
  - suture set (needle holder, curved clamp, scissors, surgical forceps)
- Blood glucose monitors and equipment for the treatment of hypoglycaemia and cardiovascular emergencies are stored close to patient care. This is also where legal regulations and the individual probability in this institution come into play.

Dressing material. This is a very individual decision. The following is a possible selection of commonly used products

- foam with small pores
- foam with large pores
- pads used for infected wounds
- spacer grids
- compresses, sterile and non-sterile
- cotton wool
- gauze
- tubular bandage
- adhesive fleece
- adsorbent compresses
- compresses with superabsorbers
- self-adhering felt

Offloading equipment

- Bandage shoes in different size
- Therapeutic offloading shoes in different sizes
- Walkers in different sizes
- Cast materials

23.4 Documentation and Storage of Pictures

Documentation of ulcers should contain at least: diagnosis of causes (conditions and triggers), measured dimension, description of the wound bed, margin and surrounding area, debridement, dressing, motivation for a changing [2].

'A picture is worth a thousand words'—documenting a wound that is probably true (Fig. 23.1). In most cases, however, one picture is not enough. In special situations, such as the start of treatment, a fixed series of images should be taken. In other situations, two images are usually required: one to depict the wound in detail and one to document the wound including the surrounding area. The photographic documentation does not replace the written documentation. It must also be recorded in writing what the wound looked like, what was done and the concept to pursue.

It is best to document immediately and also to file the photo documentation correctly right away. Unfortunately, this is often not well supported by the software used in medical facilities and additional software may be needed.

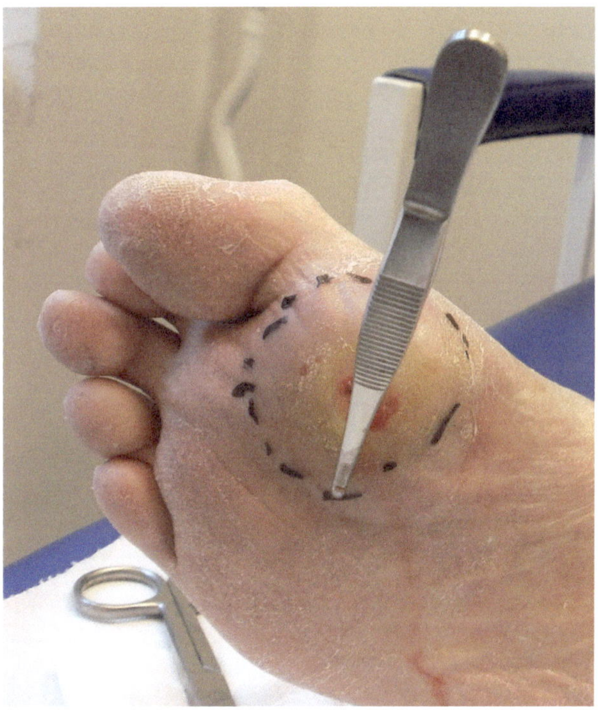

Fig. 23.1 Photo documentation: undermining wound margins

23.5 Patients in Remission

The high incidence of reactivation determines the need to offer support to the patient in remission. Shoes and overall foot care should be controlled on a regular basis. To maximise the benefit for the patient it is necessary to control not only the shoes the patient is wearing at the time of the visit, but all shoes in use (Fig. 23.2). Doctors must be understanding of patients not wearing prescribed footwear at all times. If inadequate shoes are worn at the consultation it shows a level of trust by the patient. How to deal with it? The concept of selective authenticity (see below) is helpful in this case, sometimes supplemented by some humour and plenty of empathy.

23.6 Emergencies

Each patient with a foot problem (ulcer or unilateral swollen, hot foot) that has not been seen in the foot clinic or has worsened is an emergency. If such a patient is already present in the clinic they cannot be sent away with an appointment but must be seen. In the case of a telephone call, the patient must be seen within one working day. Comments that minimise the problem, whether by patients, relatives or unspecialised medical professionals, mustn't lead to postponed appointments. If the clinic isn't able to provide a timely appointment, a realistic alternative has to be found.

Contact with these patients may represent time-consuming effort. Proper planning minimises the disruption of scheduled appointments. The following organisational points may assist:

- Precise instructions for the patient when making the appointment as to what to bring in. These include the last medication and all available medical reports.
- Hand out a questionnaire for the patient's history which may be filled out in the waiting area together with any other documents the patient has to complete.

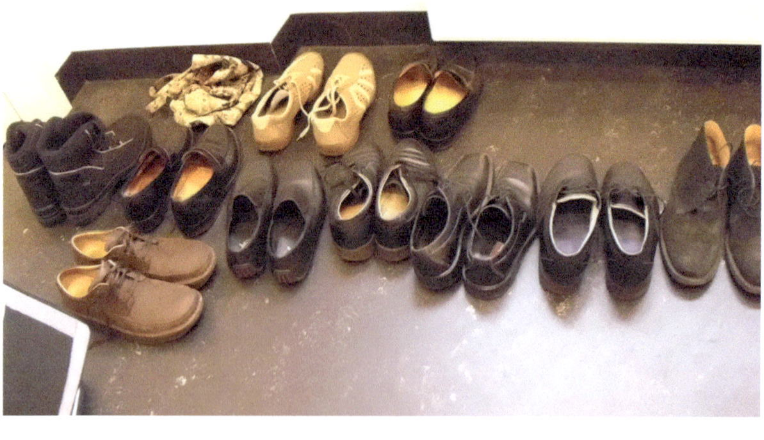

Fig. 23.2 Shoes in use in the inactive phase are controlled during the remission visit

- Defer the detailed history and discussion of the diabetes therapy until the 2nd appointment, when the patient is more receptive, if this is reasonable. The first contact is highly stressful for the patient as many new facts have to be handled. An overload of the patient with too much information should be avoided at this stage.
- Prepare information in written form. This is necessary to document that all legal requirements to inform the patient have been properly met. These sheets cannot be simply handed out but have to be discussed with the patient and possibly also with the relatives.
- All documentation has to be accessible to the patient and all caregivers involved.

23.7 Overloaded Therapists

Unrealistic goals or the lack of any goal is the basis for the condition marked by the fashionable term '*burnout*'. A typical and unrealistic expectation of healthcare professionals is that they are able to help everyone. To avoid frustration it is useful to know the performance of the whole team, which realistic goals exist and especially when they are achieved. Occasions to celebrate might be the end of a difficult time or a particularly good result in benchmarking. If there are no goals, a sense of achievement is never reached and a feeling of 'it is never enough' may prevail.

There are also concepts to deal with aggressive patients such as *selective authenticity* (Ruth Cohn). In simple terms, this concept means that everything that is said has to be true but not everything that is true has to be said. An appropriate response is not based on the mood of the member of staff but on the needs of the patient. It is important to be authentic, but it is also important to realise the situation as a whole and select how to be authentic. A decision must be made to be either direct or sympathetic, i.e. if an aggressive patient is basically in despair and doesn't know how to go on. As a result, it may also be adequate to express feelings for example by being shocked about a repeated ulcer reactivation in stylish shoes in a direct manner using strong language to reach the patient. A trigger for being aggressive may also be hypoglycaemia and in that case, it would be a tragic error to follow the first impulse of perhaps 'Throw him out'. To do so, **a moment of reflection is needed as well as a cool head as part of expected professional behaviour**. It might be useful to offer a question that works like a buffer: 'What do you mean exactly?' or 'Has there been something else you've noticed?' By doing so it is possible to gain time and be able to understand the background of the situation. Communication skills like these are taught in special seminars.

23.8 Error and Complaint Management

'Your worst customer is your best friend' [1]—There are a few regular faultfinders, who always find something to complain about. Their complaints are useful for the facility when analysed with a cool head and enable the team to perform in a more professional manner in the future. Therefore, it is useful that these critics can be seen and evaluated without causing stress for the whole team. The team should be sufficiently confident to look beyond any perceived injustices and personal hostilities to choose one of the fields to improve and tackle the task.

Other situations which are useful as a starting point for learning processes are *near misses*. They show what could have happened. They also have to be seen and judged by the whole team. They are observed by team members and should be discussed in an open-minded fashion without stress.

Suggestions for improvement can be elaborated in team meetings and the results become part of the handbook of the facility. Efficient team meetings have a structure:

- Topics are fixed in advance and known to all
- Problems are identified but not necessarily solved
- All participants have to do with the topics discussed and all necessary team members are present.
- A time limit must be set for problemsolving. If time overruns it may be necessary to postpone this discussion. The decision as to who is working on a proposal for the next meeting will be made at this time.
- Each meeting has a protocol. Topics are clear before the next meeting and have become part of the handbook or they are still open and a basis of the next meeting.

23.9 Recommended Literature

Jeff Jarvis: What Would Google Do? Reverse-Engineering the Fastest-Growing Company in the History of the World

Many considerate observations regarding the relationship between companies and their clients in the age of internet and social networks—inspiring and humorous 416 pages.

References

1. Jarvis J. What would google do? Reverse-engineering the fastest-growing company in the history of the world. New York: HarperCollins Publishers; 2009.
2. Ruttermann M, Maier-Hasselmann A, Nink-Grebe B, Burckhardt M. Local treatment of chronic wounds: in patients with peripheral vascular disease, chronic venous insufficiency, and diabetes. Deutsches Arzteblatt international. 2013;110(3):25–31. https://doi.org/10.3238/arztebl.2013.0025.

Organisation of Shared Care 24

This chapter is dedicated to the cooperation of independent healthcare providers. They combine knowledge and skills to achieve solutions for all aspects of care for people with DFS, knowledge and skills each member alone would not be able to achieve. In this chapter we've combined the experience of the authors in their own environments and in the networks they support. The result should be considered a resource of ideas and possibly even some solutions.

24.1 Why a Network?

A network for the treatment of people with DFS integrates all specialists in a region. This group has the overall responsibility for the result of the treatment of people in the area. The network therefore has to try to involve all necessary partners of sufficient quality. The network as a whole is only however as good as the weakest link.

A network must act in two ways. Firstly, it allows the treatment of single patients in the best possible way, as each component of the network does only what they do best and leaves other aspects of care to other members. Secondly, it optimizes the delivery of care in the region. In some networks, the organisation of care is the exclusive goal of the network.

24.1.1 Shared Care for Individual Patients

The pursuit of improving quality is the driving force to build systems that allow shared care between different healthcare specialists. This not only satisfies the needs of patients, but caregivers, insurance companies (where relevant) and politicians. Standardisation of clinical roles, responsibilities, training and competency allows each healthcare professional to efficiently perform their designated task, which improves both quality of care and economic efficiency.

D. Hochlenert et al., *Diabetic Foot Syndrome*,
https://doi.org/10.1007/978-3-319-92055-9_24

24.1.1.1 Improved Competence

A network can provide professional **education** and training, for example, standardisation of roles such as 'podiatrist', 'podiatry assistant', 'cast technician', or 'orthotist'. **Transparency** of descriptions of roles and responsibilities and of their outcomes contributes to improving competence.

24.1.1.2 Coordinated Cooperation

The basis of coordinated cooperation requires a shared view of what has to be achieved. A network can develop guidelines, organise the distribution of tasks, describe interfaces, and develop this into a treatment pathway. It can also structure the availability of information, for example, the production of medical reports or sharing audit outcomes.

24.1.2 Delivering Care to a Region or Country

A network may be the solution to problems in the delivery of care to a region or country. In developing a network, not only are the needs of the patient improved by better coordination of care through better trained professional, but it can also be a contact point for politicians or other partners in the wider social environment (e.g. insurance companies, patient organisations, adult education services, scientific societies, and professional associations).

Improving care should start as early as possible in the chronological development of the disease:

Early **consultation with the general practitioner or other healthcare professional** can be improved by information and awareness campaigns, lectures in meetings with patient organisations, poster advertising, radio and television broadcasts, print media, diabetes-websites, local 'diabetes days'. In the UK the charity Diabetes UK has rolled out several successful campaigns for patients. One in particular, 'Putting Feet First', amongst other initiatives, has issued information directly to patients about what to expect in their annual check of diabetes, including an annual foot examination and what they should look for on a daily basis [1].

Easy and early **access to specialised care** with the help of:

- Meetings for professionals
- Trainings and workshops for general practitioners, pharmacists and their teams, professionals engaged in wound treatment, podiatrists and shoemakers.
- An Emergency Phone Number
- An internet site
- A P.R. campaign (for example—'Putting feet first' as above.)

Reduction of supposed unnecessary amputations by:

- **External second opinion** before major amputations (for example by discussion with the full multi-disciplinary team)

24.2 Elements of a Network

The following medical disciplines and providers are needed to care for people with DFS: diabetologists, foot and ankle surgeons/orthopaedics, vascular surgeons, angiologists/interventional radiologists, plastic/reconstructive surgery, dermatology, interdisciplinary inpatient departments, domestic care services, shoemakers, other casting/offloading specialists and podiatrists (Fig. 24.1). Each element is equally important as the network is only as strong as its weakest link. If there is one that is more important it would be the primary care provider (e.g. General practitioner, community nurse or community podiatrist). These professionals have to identify the patient most in need of care amongst many other patients. Primary care practitioners may not part of the network in its narrowest sense and don't have to comply with specialist quality criteria, but they are the most important referrers. Therefore, the network depends on primary care professionals and their liaison with the specialist network; common successes must be shared.

The key position in a network is the service that coordinates specialised treatment. Usually, these are the outpatient services of the 'Diabetic foot clinics' (Fig. 24.2). In German networks, this outpatient services position is called an 'outpatient coordinator'. Usually, these are diabetologists taking responsibility for specialised

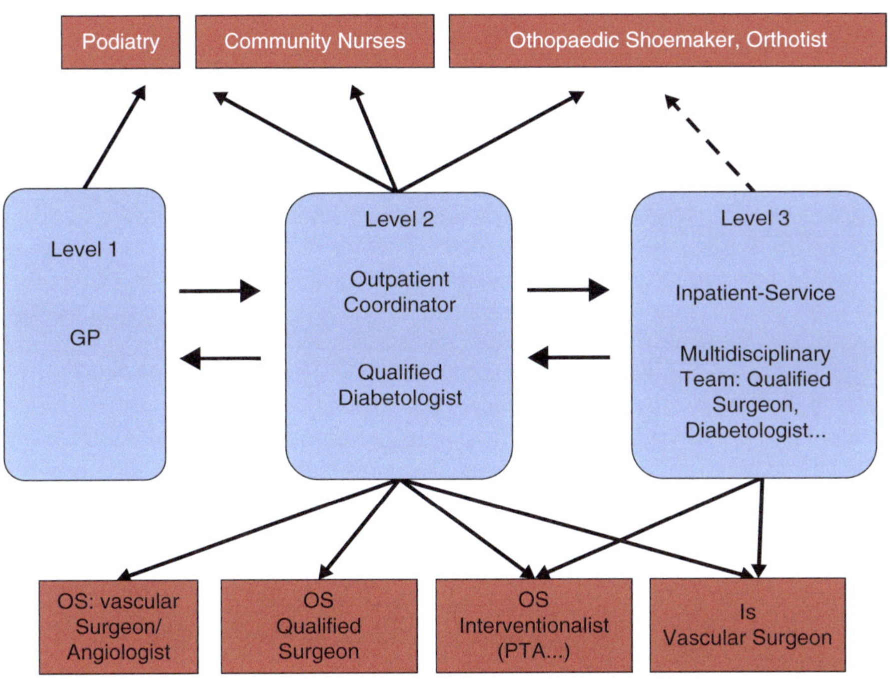

Fig. 24.1 Scheme of collaboration in the DFS network Northern Rhineland in outpatient-services (OS) and inpatient-services (IS)

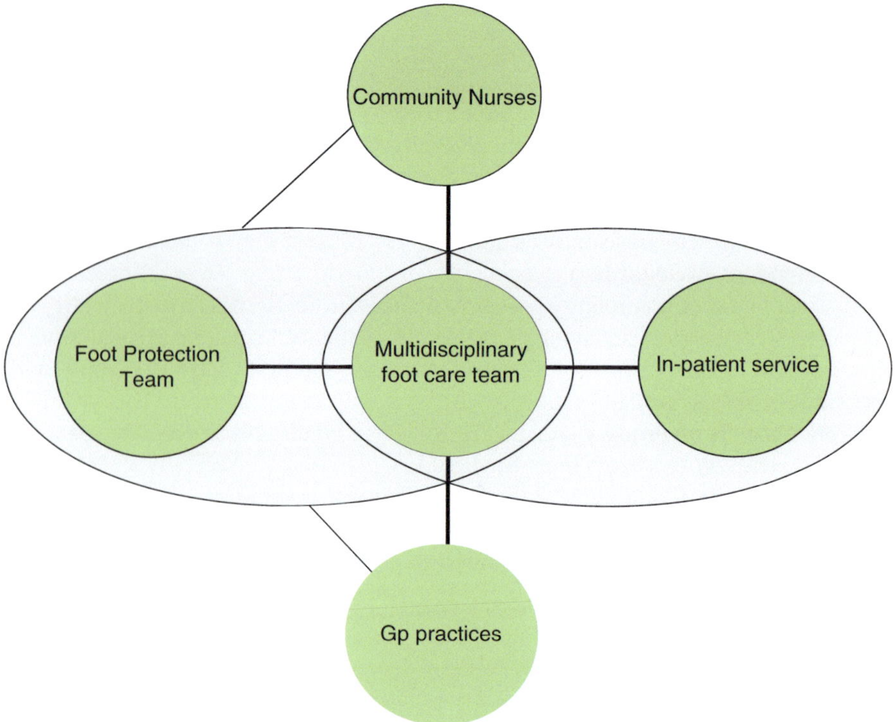

Fig. 24.2 Scheme of the network care in Suffolk

medical and management concerns. As these areas do not form part of their professional training, they are trained during intensive courses.

Each service should be defined by its duties, interfaces and quality requirements. This is the basis that allows good outcomes to be achieved. As a forum to exchange information and allow decision-making a quality-circle might be useful (Fig. 24.3). These circles are used for continuous education, cases are discussed and external speakers invited to attend. In some circles, results are exchanged based on the data provided. Each participant knows the number of patients and the results of all members. The validity of the data is tested using a random sample of 10 patients that is controlled during an external audit once a year. To achieve this each participant audits one other member in a random sequence once a year.

In South West England impressive improvements have been noted in major amputation rates with a system of 'peer reviews'. A peer review is a system whereby a team of individuals from one multidisciplinary team reviews the services, guidelines, procedures, pathways, facilities, and outcomes of another in a non-judgmental fashion, using the feedback to create a report to improve services throughout the region [2].

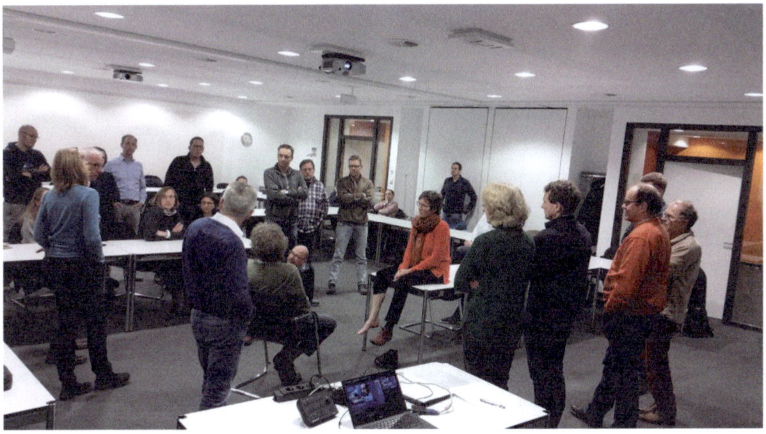

Fig. 24.3 Quality-circle in Cologne discussing issues on the criteria for a biomechanical examination of a diabetic foot

24.2.1 Examples of Elements to Enable Shared Care

24.2.1.1 Hand Held Records Folder

A hand-held record folder might be used to exchange medical records. This folder has to be carried by the patient to each visit of each of the providers and copies of all findings are collected in the folder. Hence all data is available for everyone to whom the patient hands the record folder. No access to computers, internet or specific programs is needed. However, the folder can be lost and requires completion by all healthcare professionals, which may in some cases require duplication of record keeping.

24.2.1.2 Digital Technology

The German 'mobile WoundASS' is an experienced nurse equipped with telecommunication tools who visits the affected person at home. The role is not to simply change dressings but the 'WoundASS' acts as a substitute for an outpatient clinic. The major advantage is avoidance of transportation to the clinic. Specialised medical treatment, to a large extent, may be given in the patient's home. Legal aspects, structural requirements and medical skills are taught during a special training course.

A similar system in Derbyshire in the UK, uses a digital technology to provide podiatry based care in community clinics closer to the patients home, improving waiting times in local clinics and patient experience [3].

24.2.1.3 External Second Opinion

One area of Germany has instituted external second opinion before amputation. The hospitals involved have agreed to request a second opinion before each major amputation. The contract stipulates rights and obligations and defines accepted indications for major amputations: untreatable pain, untreatable sepsis and massive impairment of quality of life by a leg unusable for locomotion. Following 2 years of evaluation of activity, in 10 out of 22 cases a major amputation was considered not necessary after this measure [4]. The procedure is further promoted in personal communications and specialised media. The aim is to achieve an overall recognition of this procedure as a basis for coverage of costs of a major amputation.

24.2.2 Examples of Elements to Improve Structure

24.2.2.1 Audit and Feedback

Auditing is a well-known instrument for quality improvement. It is carried out once a year by a colleague in a round-robin procedure or by a central institution or by 'peers'. Since 2005, Belgian multidisciplinary diabetic foot clinics are recognised by health authorities. Amongst other tools, they have implemented a system of audits [5]. Other examples of this method have been German and British initiatives. The review work of peers helping to provide resources for better organisational structures was also central to the initiatives in the South West England [2].

24.2.2.2 Feedback on Results

Feedback should attempt to match results of outcome with the risk profile of the patients treated by the facility. Results depend on the complexity of cases and averaging case mix can be misleading. The main topics of concern are:

- Data collection (only a selected population or all patients?)
- Quality of the data (are control mechanisms implemented and how well do they work?)
- What are the benchmark items and how are they calculated?
- Communication of the results (written report or open discussion?)

24.2.2.3 Professional Education

The professional training of doctors and staff is a cornerstone for improving the care of people with DFS. For example, DFSG's "step-by-step" programme in cooperation with diabetes organisations throughout the world has brought about a huge improvement [6]. Professional education might be:

- Courses for Medical Education: National and international courses for physicians have been implemented by societies and by private organisations.
- Courses training cast techniques.
- Courses training dressing techniques and how to apply felt to redistribute load.
- Courses on behaviour issues and communication.

24.2.2.4 Emergency Telephone Numbers

Emergency telephone numbers (the 'Hot Foot Phone'). Callers can be directed to general information or specific services, ensuring that a patient promptly receives the correct treatment by an appropriate specialist.

24.2.2.5 Internet

Internet sites (e.g. www.Amputation-verhindern.de, www.diabetes.org.uk/guide-to-diabetes/complications/feet/taking-care-of-your-feet) On the site patients may find information about the care and treatment of diabetic feet. Meetings and events are also communicated here.

24.2.2.6 P.R. Campaign

Information and awareness campaigns (Fig. 24.4). The campaign was aimed at caregivers as well as a wider public, patients and their relatives. The methods included press releases, activities with both local health authorities and adult education centres as well as others.

Similar events run by Diabetes UK have raised awareness of amputation rates in patients with diabetes [7].

24.3 Results

Networks have increased the numbers of treated patients as sign of general acceptance and improved results [8] (Fig. 24.5).

A network is a regional structure of specialised, shared care. It communicates with patients, general practitioners, insurance companies and large parts of society. Thus, the network participates in the improvement of the quality of care of individual patients and of the delivery of care in the region.

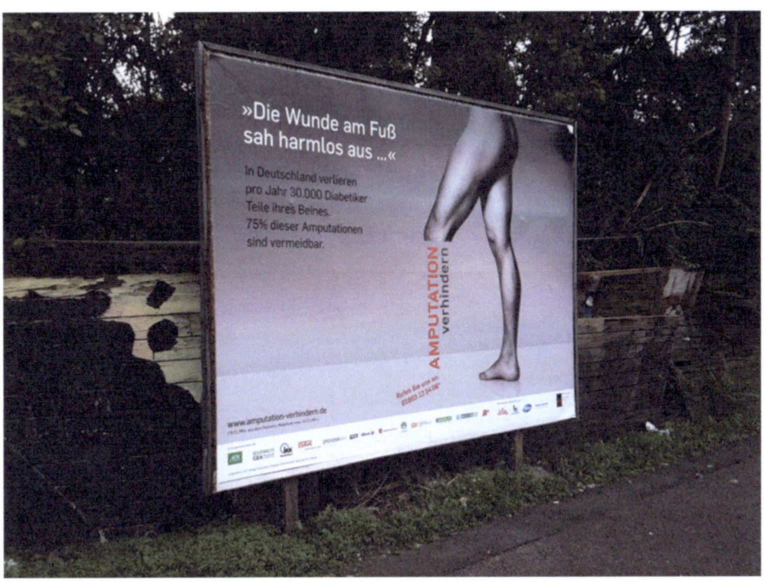

Fig. 24.4 Poster advertising during the awareness campaign 2010 in Cologne gave DFS a greater public awareness and spread the emergency telephone number

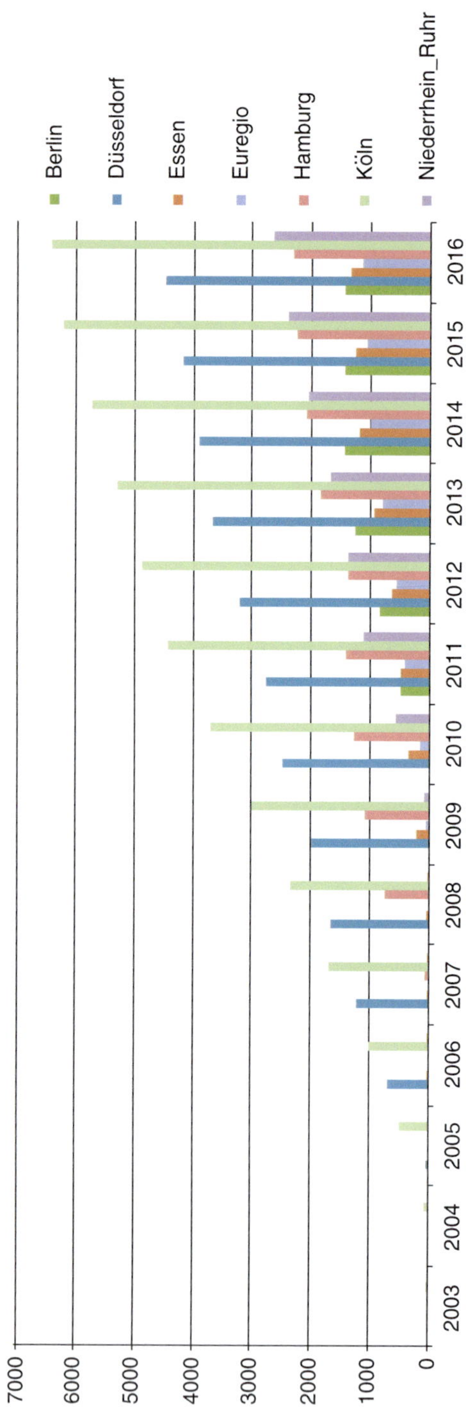

Fig. 24.5 Number of patients treated each year in the German networks

References

1. Diabetes UK. Putting Feet First. 2018. https://www.diabetes.org.uk/get_involved/campaigning/putting-feet-first. Accessed 1 Apr 2018.
2. Paisey RB, Abbott A, Levenson R, Harrington A, Browne D, Moore J, Bamford M, Roe M, South-West Cardiovascular Strategic Clinical Network peer diabetic foot service review team. Diabetes-related major lower limb amputation incidence is strongly related to diabetic foot service provision and improves with enhancement of services: peer review of the South-West of England. Diabet Med. 2018;35(1):53–62. https://doi.org/10.1111/dme.13512.
3. NHS. New digital camera technology for diabetic foot patients to be expanded across Derbyshire. 2018. Accessed 18 Mar 2018.
4. Hochlenert D, Engels G, Hinzmann S, Ardjomand P, Riedel M, Schneider S. Externe Zweitmeinung zur Verhinderung von Majoramputationen bei Menschen mit Diabetischem Fußsyndrom. Diabetologie und Stoffwechsel. 2013;8:P229.
5. Morbach S, Kersken J, Lobmann R, Nobels F, Doggen K, Van Acker K. The German and Belgian accreditation models for diabetic foot services. Diabetes Metab Res Rev. 2016;32(Suppl 1):318–25. https://doi.org/10.1002/dmrr.2752.
6. Abbas ZG, Lutale JK, Bakker K, Baker N, Archibald LK. The 'step by step' diabetic foot project in Tanzania: a model for improving patient outcomes in less-developed countries. Int Wound J. 2011;8(2):169–75. https://doi.org/10.1111/j.1742-481X.2010.00764.x.
7. The_Diabetes_Times. Shoe shop raises amputation awareness. 2016. http://diabetestimes.co.uk/shoe-shop-raises-amputation-awareness/. Accessed 1 Apr 2018.
8. Hochlenert D. Qualitätsbericht der Netzwerke Diabetischer Fuß Nordrhein, Hamburg und Berlin. 2017. http://www.fussnetz-koeln.de/Start/Dokus/Qualitaetsbericht_2017.pdf

Grading and Classification 25

The essential classifications of the diabetic foot syndrome are presented below in the wording of the respective original publication. Supplementary remarks are only made where it was considered absolutely necessary for to understand and correctly apply the respective classification.

25.1 The Dysvascular Foot: A System for Diagnosis and Treatment [1]

Foot lesions are divided in six grades. The determination of grade is based on the depth of the skin lesion and the presence or absence of infection and gangrene.

Grade Zero

There are no open lesions in the skin although there may be evidence of healed lesions. There may be bony deformity, such as clawtoes, depressed metatarsal heads, Charcot joint changes, and partial amputations such as toe, toe and ray, transmetatarsal, Lisfranc and Chopart, calcanectomies, partial or complete, and Syme's amputations.

Grade One

There is a superficial ulcer without penetration to deeper layers. Again, bony deformity may be present and bony prominence frequently underlies the ulcer.

Grade Two

The ulcer is deeper and reaches tendon, bone, or joint capsule. Bony prominence of some degree is usually present.

Grade Three

Deeper tissues are involved and there is abscess, osteomyelitis, or tendinitis, usually with extension along the midfoot compartments or tendon sheats. Such eternal signs of infection as heat, redness, and swelling may be less than would have been expected when the degree of infection is exposed at surgery.

D. Hochlenert et al., *Diabetic Foot Syndrome*,
https://doi.org/10.1007/978-3-319-92055-9_25

Grade Four

There is gangrene of some portion of the toe, toes, and/or forefoot. The gangrene may be wet or dry, infected or noninfected, but in general, surgical ablation of a portion of the toe or foot is indicated.

Grade Five

Gangrene involves the whole foot or enough of the foot that no local procedures are possible and amputation must be carried out, at least, at the below the knee level.

25.2 The University of Texas Diabetic Foot Classification System [2]

		Grade			
		0	I	II	III
Stage	A	Pre or postulcerative lesion completely epthelialised	Superficial Wound not involving tendon, capsule, or bone	Wound penetrating to tendon or capsule	Wound penetrating to bone or joint
	B	Infection	Infection	Infection	Infection
	C	Ischemia	Ischemia	Ischemia	Ischemia
	D	Infection and Ischemia	Infection and Ischemia	Infection and Ischemia	Infection and Ischemia

25.3 PEDIS: A Diabetic Foot Ulcer Classification System for Research Purposes [3]

25.3.1 Perfusion

Grade 1 No symptoms or signs of PAD in the affected foot, in combination with

- palpable dorsal pedal and posterior tibial artery or
- ankle-brachial index 0.9–1.10 or
- toe-brachial index >0.6 or
- transcutaneous oxygen pressure ($tcpO_2$) >60 mm Hg.

Grade 2 Symptoms or signs of PAD, but not of critical limb ischemia (CLI):

- Presence of intermittent claudication (in case of claudication, additional non-invasive assessment should be performed), as defined in the document of the International Consensus on the Diabetic Foot or
- Ankle-brachial index <0.9, but with ankle pressure >50 mm Hg or
- Toe-brachial index<0.6, but systolic toe blood pressure >30 mm Hg or
- $TcpO_2$ 30–60 mm Hg or
- Other abnormalities on non-invasive testing, compatible with PAD (but not with CLI).

Note: if tests other than ankle or toe pressure or $tcpO_2$ are performed, they should be specified in each study.
Grade 3 Critical limb ischemia, as defined by

- systolic ankle blood pressure <50 mm Hg or
- systolic toe blood pressure <30 mm Hg or
- $tcpO_2$ <30 mm Hg.

25.3.2 Extent/Size

Wound size (measured in square centimetres) should be determined after debridement, if possible. The outer border of the ulcer should be measured from the intact skin surrounding the ulcer.

25.3.3 Depth/Tissue Loss

Grade 1 Superficial full-thickness ulcer, not penetrating any structure deeper than the dermis.
Grade 2 Deep ulcer, penetrating below the dermis to subcutaneous structures, involving fascia, muscle or tendon.
Grade 3 All subsequent layers of the foot involved, including bone and/or joint (exposed bone, probing to bone).

25.3.4 Infection

Grade 1 No symptoms or signs of infection.
Grade 2 Infection involving the skin and the subcutaneous tissue only (without involvement of deeper tissues and without systemic signs, as described below). At least two of the following items are present:

- Local swelling or induration
- Erythema >0.5 to 2 cm around the ulcer
- Local tenderness or pain
- Local warmth
- Purulent discharge (thick, opaque to white or sanguineous secretion).

Other causes of an inflammatory response of the skin should be excluded (e.g. trauma, gout, acute Charcot neuro-arthropathy, fracture, thrombosis, venous stasis).

Grade 3 Erythema >2 cm plus one of the items described above (swelling, tenderness, warmth, discharge) or infection involving structures deeper than skin and subcutaneous tissues such as abscess, osteomyelitis, septic arthritis, fasciitis. No systemic inflammatory response signs, as described below.

Grade 4 Any foot infection with the following signs of a systemic inflammatory response syndrome This response is manifested by two or more of the following conditions:

- Temperature >38 or <36 °C
- Heart rate >90 beats/min
- Respiratory rate >20 breaths/min
- $PaCO_2$ <32-mm Hg
- White blood cell count >12.000 or <4.000/cu mm
- 10% immature (band) forms.

25.3.5 Sensation

Grade 1 No loss of protective sensation on the affected foot detected, defined as the presence of sensory modalities described below.
Grade 2 Loss of protective sensation on the affected foot is defined as the absence of perception of the one of the following tests in the affected foot:

- Absent pressure sensation, determined with a 10-g monofilament, on two out of three sites on the plantar side of the foot, as described in the International Consensus on the Diabetic Foot.
- Absent vibration sensation, (determined with a 128-Hz tuning fork) or vibration threshold >25 V (using semi-quantitative techniques), both tested on the hallux.

25.4 The Society for Vascular Surgery Lower Extremity Threatened Limb Classification System: Risk Stratification Based on Wound, Ischemia, and Foot Infection (WIFi) [4]

1. **W**ound
2. **I**schemia
3. foot **I**nfection

W I fI score

1. **W: Wound/clinical category**

SVS grades for rest pain and wounds/tissue loss (ulcers and gangrene): 0 (ischemic rest pain, ischemia grade 3; no ulcer) 1 (mild) 2 (moderate) 3 (severe)

Grade	Ulcer	Gangrene
0 Clinical description: ischemic rest pain (requires typical symptoms + ischemia grade 3); no wound	No ulcer	No gangrene
1 Clinical description: minor tissue loss. Salvageable with simple digital amputation (1 or 2 digits) or skin coverage	Small, shallow ulcer(s) on distal leg or foot; no exposed bone, unless limited to distal phalanx	No gangrene
2 Clinical description: major tissue loss salvageable with multiple (≥3) digital amputations or standard TMA (trans metatarsal) ± skin coverage	Deeper ulcer with exposed bone, joint or tendon; generally not involving the heel; shallow heel ulcer, without calcaneal involvement	Gangrenous changes limited to digits
3 Clinical description: extensive tissue loss salvageable only with a complex foot reconstruction or nontraditional TMA (Chopart or Lisfranc); flap coverage or complex wound management needed for large soft tissue defect	Extensive, deep ulcer involving forefoot and/or midfoot; deep, full thickness heel ulcer ± calcaneal involvement	Extensive gangrene involving forefoot and /or midfoot; full thickness heel necrosis ± calcaneal involvement

2. **I: Ischemia**

Hemodynamics/perfusion: Measure TP or $TcPO_2$ if ABI incompressible (>1.3): SVS grades 0 (none), 1 (mild), 2 (moderate), and 3 (severe).

Grade	ABI	Ankle systolic pressure	TP, $TcPO_2$
0	≥0.80	>100 mm Hg	≥60 mm Hg
1	0.6–0.79	70–100 mm Hg	40–59 mm Hg
2	0.4–0.59	50–70 mm Hg	30–39 mm Hg
3	≤0.39	<50 mm Hg	<30 mm Hg

ABI ankle-brachial index, *PVR* pulse volume recording, *SPP* skin perfusion pressure, *TP* toe pressure, *$TcPO_2$* transcutaneous oximetry
Patients with diabetes should have TP measurements. If arterial calcification precludes reliable ABI or TP measurements, ischemia should be documented by $TcPO_2$, SPP, or PVR. If TP and ABI measurements result in different grades, TP will be the primary determinant of ischemia grade. Flat or minimally pulsatile forefoot PVR = grade 3

3. **fI: foot Infection:**

SVS grades 0 (none), 1 (mild), 2 (moderate), and 3 (severe: limb and/or life-threatening)

SVS adaptation of Infectious Diseases Society of America (IDSA) and International Working Group on the Diabetic Foot (IWGDF) perfusion, extent/size, depth/tissue loss, infection, sensation (PEDIS) classifications of diabetic foot infection

Clinical manifestation of infection	SVS	IDSA/PEDIS infection severity
No symptoms or signs of infection	**0**	Uninfected
Infection present, as defined by the presence of at least 2 of the following items: • Local swelling or induration • Erythema >0.5 to ≤2 cm around the ulcer • Local tenderness or pain • Local warmth • Purulent discharge (thick, opaque to white, or sanguineous secretion)	**1**	Mild
Local infection (as described above) with erythema >2 cm, or involving structures deeper than skin and subcutaneous tissues (e.g., abscess, osteomyelitis, septic arthritis, fasciitis), and no systemic inflammatory response signs (as described below)	**2**	Moderate
Local infection (as described above) with the signs of SIRS, as manifested by two or more of the following: • Temperature >38° or <36 °C • Heart rate >90 beats/min • Respiratory rate >20 breaths/min or $PaCO_2$ <32 mm Hg • White blood cell count >12,000 or <4000 cu/mm or 10% immature (band) forms	**3**	Severe

$PACO_2$ partial pressure of arterial carbon dioxide, *SIRS* systemic inflammatory response syndrome
Ischemia may complicate and increase the severity of any infection. Systemic infection may sometimes manifest with other clinical findings, such as hypotension, hypotension, confusion, vomiting, or evidence of metabolic disturbances, such as acidosis, severe hyperglycemia, new-onset azotemia.

Note: The complete system should be used to describe the initial situation of all patients with ischaemic rest pain or wounds in the context of chronic peripheral circulatory disorder if treatment outcomes are reported, regardless of the therapy performed. The system should not be used in patients with acute ischemia, inflammatory vascular disease or traumatic vascular injuries. Treatment outcomes of patients with and without diabetes mellitus should be analysed separately. The presence of neuropathy in patients with diabetes should be noted in long-term examinations of wound healing, ulcer recurrences and amputations as far as possible, as this affects the probability of recurrence.

Further details on the exact application of the different systems can be found in the respective original publication.

References

1. Wagner FW Jr. The dysvascular foot: a system for diagnosis and treatment. Foot Ankle. 1981;2(2):64–122.
2. Armstrong DG. The University of Texas Diabetic Foot Classification System. Ostomy Wound Manage. 1996;42(8):60–1.
3. Schaper NC. Diabetic foot ulcer classification system for research purposes: a progress report on criteria for including patients in research studies. Diabetes Metab Res Rev. 2004;20(Suppl 1):S90–5. https://doi.org/10.1002/dmrr.464.
4. Mills JL Sr, Conte MS, Armstrong DG, Pomposelli FB, Schanzer A, Sidawy AN, Andros G. The society for vascular surgery lower extremity threatened limb classification system: risk stratification based on wound, ischemia, and foot infection (WIfI). J Vasc Surg. 2014;59(1):220–34.e1–2. https://doi.org/10.1016/j.jvs.2013.08.003.

Index

D. Hochlenert et al., *Diabetic Foot Syndrome*,
https://doi.org/10.1007/978-3-319-92055-9

MIX
Papier aus verantwortungsvollen Quellen
Paper from responsible sources
FSC® C105338

If you have any concerns about our products,
you can contact us on
ProductSafety@springernature.com

In case Publisher is established outside the EU,
the EU authorized representative is:
Springer Nature Customer Service Center GmbH
Europaplatz 3, 69115 Heidelberg, Germany

Printed by Libri Plureos GmbH
in Hamburg, Germany